W0228074

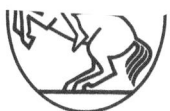

# Advances in Neurotraumatology

*Published under the Auspices of the Neurotraumatology Committee of the World Federation of Neurosurgical Societies*

*Editor-in-Chief: R. P. Vigouroux*

*Volume 1*

# Extracerebral Collections

*Managing Editor: R. L. McLaurin*

*Springer-Verlag Wien New York*

Professor ROBERT P. VIGOUROUX
Clinique Neuro-chirurgicale, C.H.U. Timone, Marseille, France

Professor ROBERT L. McLAURIN, M.D.
Neurological Surgery, University of Cincinnati, Ohio, U.S.A.

With 72 Figures

ISSN 0178-3696
ISBN-13:978-3-211-81876-3     e-ISBN-13:978-3-7091-8805-7
DOI: 10.1007/978-3-7091-8805-7

# Foreword

This series of yearly books on Advances in Neurotraumatology is being published under the auspices of the Scientific Committee of Neuro-traumatology of the World Federation of Neurological Surgeons. For some years neurotraumatology was perhaps too much looked upon as a secondary part of neurosurgery. But the constant increase of cases has provoked a renewal of interest all over the world, involving not only neurosurgeons but also any surgeon who has to take care of such patients. Each volume, in order to cover the whole of neurosurgery, will be concerned with a special topic, the various chapters of which being envisaged in detail, and followed by a practical "How to do it". Every volume will also contain chapters outside the envisaged topic regarding some up-to-date problems. The authors, chosen from various countries for their special competence, will try to offer an efficient contribution to the knowledge of neuro-traumatology, and also to present a bedside series of handy books helping those who tend these cases. The first volume will deal with "Extracerebral Collections", the second "Dorsal and Lumbar Spine and Spinal Cord Injuries", the third "Cerebral Contusions, Lacerations and Hematomas", and the next ones will continue to successively approach all the other neurotraumatological topics.

ROBERT P. VIGOUROUX

# Contents

# List of Contributors

Becker, Donald P., M.D., Division of Neurosurgery, Department of Surgery, University of California Los Angeles School of Medicine, Los Angeles, California, U.S.A.

Brihaye, Professor Jean, Clinique de Neurochirurgie, Hôpital Universitaire St. Pierre, Institut Bordet, 1, rue Héger Bordet, B-1000 Bruxelles, Belgium.

Choux, Dr. Maurice, Département de Neurochirurgie pédiatrique, Hôpital des Enfants, C.H.U. Timone, Boulevard Jean Moulin, F-13385 Marseille Cedex 4, France.

Guillermain, P., M.D., Clinique Neuro-chirurgicale, C.H.U. Timone, 264, Rue Saint-Pierre, F-13385 Marseille Cedex 5, France.

Marshall, Lawrence F., M.D., Division of Neurological Surgery H-893, University of California Medical Center, 225 Dickinson Street, San Diego, CA 92103, U.S.A.

Matsumoto, Professor Satoshi, M.D., Department of Neurosurgery, Kobe University School of Medicine, 7-5-1 Kusunoki-cho, Chuo-Ku, Kobe 650, Japan.

Miller, Professor J. Douglas, M.D., Department of Surgical Neurology, Western General Hospital, Crewe Road, Edinburgh EH4 2XU, U.K.

Tamaki, N., M.D., Department of Neurosurgery, Kobe University School of Medicine, 7-5-1 Kusunoki-cho, Chuo-Ku, Kobe 650, Japan.

# Traumatic Extradural Hematomas

P. GUILLERMAIN*

Neurochirurgien des Hôpitaux, Clinique Neuro-chirurgicale (Professeur
Robert P. Vigouroux), C.H.U. Timone, Marseille (France)

With 16 Figures

## Contents

An extra-dural hematoma (EDH) is an epidural collection of blood situated between the dura and the bone. When it happens it is a neurotraumatological emergency but it is also the rarest complication of cranial traumas. The EDH is well known and has been described long ago (J. L. Petit 1750: Queloz[171]). It has led to several publications since the first typical clinical description of an EDH originating from the rupture of the middle meningeal artery was attributed to Jacobson (1885) by other authors (Gallagher[55], McKissock[133], Weaver[215], Zuccarello[229]). These publications have been included in a review in 1974 by Zander and Campiche[223] who underlined the frequency of atypical forms and the importance of an early diagnosis by angiography in order to operate as soon as possible, before an irreversible point, the EDH appearing to be an absolute operative indication.

Other studies have been published since, which tend to show the interest linked to that type of lesion, including global statistics[30, 83, 105, 114, 117, 140, 166, 228], physio-pathological studies based on experiments[41, 79, 80, 230] or emphasizing a particular topographical[3, 13, 17, 59, 148, 192, 226, 227] or clinical aspect where chronic[15, 25, 111, 169, 229] or delayed forms[22, 51, 64, 149, 173] prevail. A renewed interest can be linked to the use of the CT scan as a means of diagnosis and in the monitoring of brain-traumatized patients. The hematoma can be detected in conscious patients, and its evolution can be watched and in some cases, the operative indications can be discussed[43, 54, 67, 94, 159, 215]. The previous studies from our department[20, 24, 68, 75, 128, 207, 208, 210] and our present series (648 cases of EDH) confirm the general impression obtained from the literature that the pattern of the EDH of the young adult, in its classical form, either clinical (troubles of consciousness after a free interval) or evolutional (acute) or topographical (temporo-parietal), is far from being the norm: the free interval can be lacking or very long, the evolution subacute or chronic, the troubles of consciousness can be missing, and the lesion can be found anywhere or occur at any age, including the elderly and the infant.

## A. Anatomy

The epidural space is only virtual because of adherences (fibrous and vascular tracts) between the dura (inner periosteum) and the bone. In the infant and the child, these adherences are very tight, particularly near the sutures, and the vascular exchanges very numerous between the dura and the bone. In the older child and the adult, the adherences are generally less visible and the vascular exchanges less important, but several arterial meningeal ramifications move from one point to another. In the elderly, on the contrary, the adherences are nearly total because of fibrous tracts which are so thick that they make the detachment of the bone-flap difficult.

There is a detachable temporo-parietal and anterior occipital area which was depicted by Gerard Marchand in 1890[223] but some areas are more easily detachable than others (frontal region, spheno-temporal region, detachable occipital zone of kromleim). The temporo-parietal region is particularly liable to trauma and 65 to 75% of fractures prevail in this area, which explains the great number of EDHs in this zone, especially as the meningeal vascularization is richer here than elsewhere.

The origin of the bleeding can vary but in most cases the hematoma has an arterial origin due to the lesion of meningeal blood vessels. It occurs less often from the anterior or posterior meningeal artery than the middle meningeal artery which vascularizes most of the convexity. In the child, these arteries run between the two sheets of the dura and until he is five, they have no direct relationship with the bone, but later they constitute part of the inner table so they can be injured by a blow and particularly if there is a fracture. The tiny perforating ramifications going from these vessels to the diploe, the vascular tracts of meningeal adherences can be equally torn or pulled away by a trauma and they can provoke a bleeding. Bleedings of venous origin are less frequent: meningeal veins, granulations of pacchioni, or the venous sinus which can be linked to a fracture. The dura itself is vascularized between its sheets so, that even without damage to a large meningeal vessel, its laceration can lead to a bleeding and that a fracture bleeds because of the lesion of diploic vessels. All these conditions contribute to hematoma development in this area.

## B. Physio-Pathology

We must make a difference between the phenomena linked to cranial trauma and those following the development of the EDH.

### I. The Cranial Trauma

A cranial trauma is responsible for the immediate signs. At the moment of the trauma, the kinetic energy can be more or less absorbed by the skull above if the bone is fractured. The shock-wave can be fully transmitted or not to the underlying structures. In the axial direction, the lesion can be either direct or provoked by a contracoup. In the lateral direction, the shock wave can be transmitted to the base and particularly to the foramen magnum. So the brain undergoes movements due to the phenomena of acceleration-deceleration described by Gurdjian and Webster[77], which are responsible for superficial or peripheral lesions, where as deformations (translation, rotation, and mainly distortion) described by Ommaya et al.[154] are responsible for deep lesions. Whether they are localized or diffuse, macro or microscopic, superficial or deep, organic or functional, these lesions, when they exist, develop by themselves and worsen the EDH because of the secondary reactions they involve, reactions which lead to oedema. Thus we may explain the initial symptomatology, the clinical future and the prognosis of the EDH with intracranial associated lesions.

## II. The EDH

At the moment of the shock, first there is a crushing of the skull which forms a concavity open to the outside (inbending) around which the bone has a reaction of a sinusoidal type with a convexity to the outside (outbending); the fracture tends to be around the shock area[77]. Because of the different resilience of the bone and of the dura, at the moment of the shock, when the depression—cone takes form, the dura moves with the bone table but sometimes leaves it when release takes place. So, there may be an epidural detachment which precedes and "promotes" the bleeding detachment whether there is a fracture or not. This phenomenon already described by Erichsen (1779), Bell (1816) (Gallagher[55]), and later by Duret (1919)[40] has been corroborated through experiments by Ford and MacLaurin[50].

If there is vascular damage, the bleeding collects and if the source of the bleeding does not cease, the hematoma spreads, detaching the dura more and more. The adherence of the sutures does not limit the collection: Choux et al.[24] have injected hot gelatin into the epidural area and have shown that the meningeal adherence to the coronal suture alone was able to limit the spreading hematoma for a while. Once present, the blood collection works like an expansive process and results in a more or less serious symptomatology depending on its localization. The localized oedema can be visualized by the CT scan as hypodense areas surrounding the hematoma[81, 118]. As soon as the hematoma reaches a crucial volume it brings about lesions by mass-effects leading to the compression of the III (ipsilateral mydriasis) and later of the lateral part of the peduncle (contralateral hemiplegia) because of the hernia of the uncus and of the parahyppocampal gyrus with a blocking of the cistern ambians and of the aqueduct and meanwhile the state of consciousness is affected. In the last period, there are blows to the contralateral peduncle which knocks on the tentorium cerebelli. There are also lesions of the contralateral III (bilateral mydriasis) with bilateral paralysis and decerebration. A vicious circle appears which stops only if the hematoma is removed, because some lesions directly linked to the hematoma: cortical compression, diencephalomesencephalic blows, and other indirect ones due to vascular compression (communicant and posterior cerebral arteries) responsible in the CT scan for images of softening sometimes visualized, occur at the same time and worsen each other. All these factors can lead to an oedema which itself worsens both direct and indirect lesions.

The main feature of the EDH is the appearance, after a free interval, of troubles of consciousness and signs of localization. However, the evolution of the hematoma with course of time is not easily specified because there is some discrepancy between experimental and clinical facts. Indeed, Ford and MacLaurin[50] have shown that in the dog, the hematoma reaches its maximum size a little time after the start of the bleeding and this seems to be corroborated by Lofgren[132], Ecrison's studies and the Oslo School[41, 79, 80, 230] who showed that the hematoma reaches 80% of its volume in a very short time (1/10th of the bleeding time) but this one is longer (half an hour). Now, from a clinical point of view, the hematoma evolution can be acute, subacute or chronic depending on how long the free interval will last. Then it is admitted that the free interval does not necessarily correspond to the time of anatomical appearance and to the development of the hematoma, but rather to that space of time during which the compensating mechanisms of the cerebral lesion have been exhausted[50, 51, 167]. Furthermore, if the EDH always follows a vascular lesion, all meningeal vascular lesions are not complicated by an EDH[56, 182, 185]. Further, if the bleeding starts with the trauma, how could we explain in some cases the visualization by arteriography[64] or in the CT scan[22, 51, 112, 149, 169, 177] of a hematoma several hours or days after a previously "normal" investigation, when the vascular lesion was found in most cases during operation. Some protective mechanisms do exist and they do not work adequately when the epidural bleeding takes place[51, 169, 182, 185].

So, the clinical features of the EDH, its immediate or delayed appearance, the existence or not of a free interval, its acute, subacute or chronic evolution, depends on the more or less important parts played by vascular protective mechanisms at the moment of the bleeding and also depends on how much the brain can compensate a compression. Several factors must be considered:

1. The patient: varying individual tolerance[50] according to the age, the cerebral circulatory condition, anatomical variations.

2. The hematoma: its size, its localization in a functional or not cerebral zone, or in a region in which the dura can be more or less detachable.

3. The origin of the bleeding: arterial or sinus originating bleedings implying a considerable flow, evolve faster and are more important than venous or diploic originating bleedings, which are responsible in most cases for a slowly evolving hematoma.

4. The protective mechanisms: *Some* of them provide the hematoma decompression: escape of blood outside through a fracture and particularly in children[18, 24, 91, 97]. *Others* provide a provisional hemostasis: spasmodically injured vessel, formation of a False aneurysm and of an arteriovenous fistula between the meningeal and diploic vessels[41]. According to Habash *et al.*[79] and Zwetnow *et al.*[230], the hematoma volume and the duration of

bleeding depend either on the distance between the fistula and the origin of the bleeding or on the dimensions of the fistula[80]. A low blood pressure can interfere and if it does, the reestablishment of a correct blood pressure and blood volume for a previously hypotense patient could be responsible for the delayed appearance of an EDH[22, 64]. The same process with the existence of brain lesions or a connected edema which, because of a mass-effect, may play a compressive part by a "tampon"-effect, all this leading to an eventual hematoma delayed during the curing of these connected lesions or during a treatment based on a hyperosmolar agent or on hyperventilation[22, 51, 72, 112].

## C. General Data

*I. Frequency:* ordinarly, the EDH worsens 1 to 4% of cranial traumas, the frequency varying according to the series: 1 to 2%[6, 101, 117, 121, 136], 2 to 3%[86, 120, 180], 3 to 4%[92, 119, 133], though others state a larger frequency: 10 to 16%[14, 103, 165, 228]. These figures increase in autopsy cases: 21 to 26%[23, 124, 204] which emphasizes the gravity of these hematomas.

In the child the same frequency is to be found, from 1.8% (Campbell[18]) to 3.7% (Svendsen[194]), 3.7% in our series (172 cases), greater by Pang[159] (5%).

In the elderly (over 65) we have noted 1 to 3% in one of our previous studies[212].

Since the introduction of CT, the EDH frequency has increased: 3% Koo[110], 5.5% Gardeur[57], 6.8% Zimmerman[224], 8% Lanksgh[118], 10% Clifton[26]. So, the frequency of our cases has gone from 4% before the CT scan (507 cases) up to 9% since its nearly systematic use (141 cases).

*II. Sex, age: 1. Sex:* Males are predominant in 71% (our series) to 98% (McKissock[133]) of cases, the average is of 80% (Jamieson[101]), 4 men : 1 woman. In children, the proportion is of 3 to 1 (Queloz[171]) but up to the age of 2, the occurrence is equal for boys and girls. In contrast, in the elderly, it is 2 to 1.

*2. Age:* usually, the EDH affects young adults. It is particularly frequent between 20 and 40 years (Gallagher[55]) or between 30 and 40 years (Heyser[86]). The average age of McKissock's patients is 24[133]. In our series, 51% of the adults are under 30, as in Kvarnes' series[117]. Under 15, the EDH represents 22% (McKissock[133]) to 31% (Gerlach[61]) of the observed EDH, 26.5% in our series, but over 65, they are not rare (5% of our cases).

*III. Aetiology:* the EDH are rare in war time: from 2,000 scars, Schorstein[187] only noticed 3 EDH.

In peace time (Fig. 1) traffic accidents provide the highest and the most seriously injured patients; crashes are to be found in more than half of the cases. Falls represent the 2nd most, common etiology, they are frequent in the old or children. Direct trauma are fairly numerous. We should note that for the EDH, the trauma is more often less important than for other cranial

| | Pouyanne[168] 1965 | Gallagher[55] 1968 | Kvarnes[117] 1978 | Cordobes[30] 1981 | Grevsten[67] 1982 | Our series 1983 |
|---|---|---|---|---|---|---|
| Traffic accidents | 66% | 30% | 35% | 67% | 52% | 60% |
| Falls | 26% | 46% | 54% | 15% | 24% | 31% |
| Direct trauma | 4% | 20% | 11% | 18% | 11% | 8% |

Fig. 1. Nature of trauma

| | Pouyanne[168] 1965 243 cases | Jamieson[101] 1968 167 cases | Cordobes[30] 1981 82 cases | Our series 1983 648 cases | Others |
|---|---|---|---|---|---|
| Lateral | 89% | 70% | 81% | 70% | 80 à 95%[55,114,117] |
| Frontal | 7% | 11% | 13% | 20% | 5 à 25%[91,125,180,193,207] |
| Vertex | 1% | 2% | | 2% | 1 à 3%[93,133,227] |
| Basal | | 6% | 5% | 4% | |
| Occipital | 1% | 7% | 1% | 2% | 3 à 14%[9,46,131,216] |
| Posterior fossa | 2% | 7% | | 2% | 3 à 12%[5,90,117,202] |

Fig. 2. Lesional topography

trauma complications because it is the local impact which is involved in its genesis and not the movements of the brain at the moment of the trauma.

Because of the nature of trauma, a polyneurotrauma is noticed in 20 to 30% of the cases, involving, according to the connected lesions, with the dreadful problem of the most urgent emergency measures.

## D. Anatomico-Pathology

### I. The Hematoma

*1. Localization:* As Zander and Campiche[223] have noticed, the location of the hematoma is not always described in the same way by authors. Some only quote large regions (frontal, parietal, temporal...), while others take transition areas into account (fronto-temporal, parieto-temporal...) and finally, some localizations (vertex, base) are not always made distinct. In Fig. 2 we have quoted the repartition of hematoma in some series which are different because of their dates and the number of cases.

*a) Temporo-parietal* or *lateral EDH:* we have gathered temporal and parietal hematomas and their anterior and posterior extensions. This is the most usually frequent localization in more than 70% of the cases. This proportion, noted by most authors, is linked to the presence of the middle meningeal artery and of its branches, and it is also linked to the frequency of traumas in this area.

*b) Atypical localizations:*

*Frontal:* they are hematomas specific to the anterior fossa and they do not spread over the little wing of the sphenoid[207]. 2 times out of 3, they are present in children and the young patients but we have never seen it in an infant. Basal forms are exceptional: we have found 9 cases/128, Andreoli[3] 2/23.

*Occipital:* they are located opposite the occipital lobe and limited by the longitudinal superior and transverse sinuses[208]. They appear to be rare in children: 1 case/18 in our series, 2 cases/62 EDH Mazza[149].

*Subtemporal:* they are seldom distinguished from the temporal EDH of the convexity. We have noticed 4% (29 cases), Jamieson[101] 6%. In these cases, the hematoma is located under the temporal lobe and does not spread over the convexity.

*Vertex:* they are located in the apex, pressing on the superior longitudinal sinus.

*Posterior fossa:* they are the most frequent hematomas in this region[49, 221], and their incidence varies from 1 to 12%.

The evaluation of the spreading of the hematoma can differ according to the authors, since localized collections are reported with such different frequencies: 19% (Gallagher[55]) and 90% (Pouyanne[168]). Owing to the use of the CT scan which provides a precise topographical diagnosis, in our series, localized collections appear to be more frequent (62%) than those spreading over 1 or 2 sutures (38%), more often in children (56%) than in adults (50%). This tends to be linked to the fact that adherences are tighter between the dura and the bone near the sutures for young children. Moreover, a more systematic use of the CT scan has enabled us to detect more numerous hematomas in the posterior fossa (the frequency has gone from 2 up to 4%) and in localizations that only lead to very few complications: the frontal EDH frequency has increased (16 to 21%), so has the temporo-basilar EDH (3 to 8%).

Bilateral forms are rare[178, 184], when they are put down in the series: 4 cases/167[55], 5 cases/167[101], 2 cases/243[168], 3 cases/125[133], 7 cases/192[6] and 5 cases/648 in ours.

Two ideas must be taken into account in the EDH topography:

1. On the one hand, while lateral hematomas are more often linked to acute clinical forms, in chronic forms atypical localizations prevail: in more than 50% of the cases collected by Young[222], in 73% of our series, chronic EDH were located outside the parieto-temporal region.

2. On the other hand, the dura is detachable at every point near the convexity and the base, and the hematoma can be located anywhere. But if we only consider the temporal region, it is only involved in 50% of our studies and of Cordobes's[30], 57% of Weinman's[216], 58% of Kvarnes's[117], 41% of Gros's[69], 61% of Pouyanne's[168] and this seems to be fundamental for 40 to 60% of EDH "escaped" a temporal exploratory burr hole.

*2. Aspect:* If it may be fluid at the beginning of the bleeding, the hematoma quickly turns into clots sticking to the dura, and looks like "currant jelly" in early cases and a brown thicker "flat-cake" in late cases. Many chronic EDH possess capsules that histologically resemble the chronic subdural fibro vascular membrane[123, 146] and they are sometimes calcified[105, 123, 160], as happened in 3 of our cases. A capsule with a brown fluid center have been reported and the "capsuling" starts between 21 days and 3 months[29, 36, 62, 81, 97, 99, 138, 213] but it is variable. Iwakuma[97] only noticed it 2 times in 21 chronic cases and Punt[170] did not see it in a case evolving for 33 years.

*3. Origin of the bleeding:* The prevailing importance of an arterial lesion in the EDH formation is shown by all statistics. Indeed, in more than half of the cases, the hematoma has an arterial origin (middle meningeal artery or anterior or posterior branch). In 40% of the cases, the origin is either venous or osseous and in 10% of the cases, a diffuse bleeding of the dura is noticed. However, in about 25 to 35% of the cases, the bleeding origin is unknown either because it is not specified in the surgical protocol or because it is not discovered. In this high percentage the hematoma has probably no arterial or sinus origin because its removal or the numerous contacts of the sucker would have probably shown one of these bleedings. We have noted that whilst most lateral hematomas have an arterial origin, frontal hematomas can have an arterial or venous origin, whereas the hematomas of the vertex are linked to the injury of the superior longitudinal sinus in all cases. The basilar temporal hematomas can have an arterial origin as well as a venous one (sinus of brechet).

## II. Bone Lesions

Fractures, classical signs of the EDH are found in 85 to 90% of the cases[223]. Several authors have noticed this frequency but in a variable proportion according to the radiological, surgical, autopsy or CT scan considerations: 86% for Arseni[6] or Kvarnes[117], 76% in our series on radiological outlines alone, 91% on radiological, surgical, or autopsy findings (Gallagher[55]) or in the CT scan (Zimmerman[224]), but during the autopsy of 211 EDH, Freytag[53] observed a bone lesion 205 times. Usually the type of the lesion is a fracture but we must point out that in 9% of our cases we did not find a real correlation between the fracture and the location of the hematoma, particularly in occipital localizations. We also noticed that in 11 cases/495 bone lesions, the fracture was contralateral to the lesion a discrepancy underlined by other authors (Josephson[106], McLaurin[134]). Moreover, we have pointed out the relative incidence of EDH which were underlying a depressed skull fracture (66 cases/495), this type does not usually involve an EDH (6% of the depressed skull fractures we observed). The osseous lesions seem to be less frequent in frontal EDH where they are to be found in about 50 to 60% of the cases, though it is nearly constant in the vertex and occipital hematomas.

According to general statistics, 10 to 15% of the EDH are said not to go along with bone lesions radiologically (24% in our series). Mealey[141] reports 17% in an article devoted to that sort of hematoma and Young[222] 40% in chronic forms. In children, the fracture is more often absent: 28% in our series 21 to 30% of the cases[18, 24, 65, 133]. This can be explained by the greater elasticity of a child's skull.

## III. Associated Lesions

We have only considered the lesions which worsen the patients' prognosis (Fig. 3). They were noted in about ⅓ of the cases before the use of the CT scan but their frequency has increased since and are similar to the autopsy data: 47%[55, 101]. Those lesions are more often either brain contusion-dilacerations or acute subdural hematomas, than intracerebral hematomas and their existence increases the gravity of EDH prognosis. According to us and to other authors[18, 20, 24, 68, 101], the frequency of associated lesions in children seems to be less (18% of them) than in the

a) Frequency
Before CT scan: Bourhis[14] 37%, Mendelow[142] 34%, Kvarnes[117] 32%, Our series 30%, Jonker[105] 24%, Cordobes[30] 22%, Teasdale[199] 27%, Pouyanne[168] 21%, McKissock[133] 11%
With CT scan: Cordobes[30] 48%, Our series 45%, Ericson[43] 42%

b) Topographic parting

|  | Pouyanne[168] | Jamieson[101] | Our series |
|---|---|---|---|
| Lateral | 20% | 46% | 35% |
| Frontal | 22% | 47% | 29% |
| Vertex |  | 33% | 25% |
| Occipital | 0% | 40% | 44% |
| Basal |  | 67% | 31% |
| Posterior fossa | 40% | 58% | 37% |

Fig. 3. EDH with associated lesions

adult where it is noticed in 40% of our cases, and their distribution according to the hematoma localization is noted in Fig. 3. We have observed the frequency of contracoup lesions associated with lateral and occipital EDH and underlying the hematoma in a frontal localization.

### E. Clinical Study

The clinical study of the EDH is ruled by the existence of troubles of consciousness whose evoluting modalities must be dealt with when chosing the course to follow and it is also ruled by localization signs. This pattern is not always constant and it is not specific for EDH. Indeed from a clinical point of view, nothing can enable us to differentiate EDH from other complications of cranial traumas.

### I. Troubles of Consciousness

They are quite variable from author to author, according to the classification and the terminology used (coma or obnubilation are not always stipulated). Moreover, some series include all EDH, others separate pure EDH from EDH with associated lesions; this explains some discrepancies.

*1. Immediate signs* (Fig. 4): They depend on the brain injury and do not correspond to the hematoma development.

A loss of consciousness is noted in 70 to 85% of the cases. It seems to be more frequent in adults (80%) than in children (57% of the cases) and it is particularly rare in infants, according to our findings.

Usually, the trauma does not lead to anything noteworthy at once. Indeed, in more than half the cases, the state of consciousness is normal or becomes normal again after a brief loss of consciousness. However, immediate trouble of consciousness is not rare and it can conceal the evolution of the hematoma. On the whole, in our series, it was more often a coma (32%) than an obnubilation (25%).

In our findings in children, the trauma has appeared to be minor in the beginning (in 62% of our cases) but an immediate coma was noted in 20%. In contrast, in adults, in ⅓ of the cases, there was an immediate coma, in ⅓ of the cases an obnubilation and in the last ⅓ there was a lucid state.

For comparison, immediate signs occurred in other cranial trauma complications at a rate noted in Fig. 4 b for cases in our department[32, 76, 211].

*2. Secondary troubles of consciousness:* the notion of a free interval is important when dealing with EDH because it constitutes part of the classical pattern. However, it is variably interpreted by different authors. Some of them speak of a lucid interval, patent or latent, true or false whether there is obnubilation or not; others speak of a free interval from all neurological signs. That is why we find such variable frequencies (Fig. 5).

a) Frequency

| | Pouyanne[168] | Gallagher[55] | Jamieson[101] | Kretschmer[114] | Cordobes[30] | Our series |
|---|---|---|---|---|---|---|
| Unconscious | 30% | 39% | 43% | 35% | 12% | 57% |
| Conscious | 70% | 61% | 57% | 65% | 88% | 43% |

b) Comparative pattern

| | Contusion dilacerations[211] | Subdural hematomas[32] | Intracerebral hematomas[76] |
|---|---|---|---|
| Unconscious | 74% | 86% | 74% |
| Conscious | 26% | 14% | 26% |

Fig. 4. Immediate signs

a) Frequency (O: EDH only)
(A: EDH with associated lesions)

| | Pouyanne[168] | Jamieson[101] | Gallagher[55] | Kvarnes[117] | Cordobes[30] | Our series |
|---|---|---|---|---|---|---|
| Lucid interval | 61% O: 63% A: 55% | 12% O: 6% A: 19% | 61% | 11% | 43% | 35% O: 42% A: 24% |

Free-lucid interval Pecker[162] 82%, Loew[131] 72%, Heyser[86] 75%, Huber[92] 70%, Grevsten[67] 66%, da Pian[35] 51%, Kretschmer[114] 46%, McKissock[133] 27%

b) Comparative pattern

| | Contusion dilacerations[211] | Subdural hematomas[32] | Intracerebral hematomas[76] |
|---|---|---|---|
| | 22% | 7% | 21% |

Fig. 5. Secondary disturbed consciousness

14 P. Guillermain:

Because of our belief in the predominence of the conscious state, we would rather use the term of lucid interval as it is noted in some series (Fig. 5). It seems to us to be more frequent in children (51%) than in adults (29%) and, unlike Jamieson[101] but like Ericson[43], it is more frequent when the hematoma is alone than when it is with associated lesions.

The classical 3-times pattern: loss of consciousness, lucid interval, secondary coma, is rare. It occurred in 8% of our cases, 2% of Jamieson's[101], but seems to be more frequent for Kretschner (20%)[114].

The free interval can either last some hours (in ¾ of the cases in acute forms) or some days or months in subacute and chronic forms.

The free or lucid interval can be missing in numerous EDH, either because it is concealed by primary trouble of consciousness or because consciousness remains normal. Anyway, its absence can, in any case, rule out the possibility of an EDH and its presence can neither prove it because other neurotraumatical complications can evolve with a lucid interval (Fig. 5 b).

*II. Neurological Signs*

*1. Classical signs: a) localization signs* (Fig. 6).

*Motor deficit:* It does exist in all series in the form of hemiplegia more often than a hemiparesis or a monoparesis that would be contralateral to the lesion. We know how difficult it is to find it in a decerebrate or comatose patient and that is why the deficit quite often appears after the amelioration of the state of consciousness.

*Mydriasis:* it is a classical sign which is to be found in 30 to 60% of the cases. It is usually one-sided with regard to the hematoma. When mydriasis goes along with the deficit, it leads to an alternate pseudo-syndrome.

*Other signs* can be noted, because of the lesion of cranial nerves or because of the lesional topography: aphasia, frontal or cerebellar syndrome, hemianopsia[139], exophthalmos[70, 179] . . .

Localization signs are noted in 55 to 67% of the cases, 60% in our series. In our experience, later appearing signs seem to be more frequent (68%) than those existing from the moment of the trauma or its immediate consequences (32%). They are more frequent in children (75%) than in adults (60%) and signs are more likely to be found associated with other lesions (71%) than in the presence of a hematoma alone (62%).

The way signs help localization is important but the hemiplegia can be found ipsilaterally to the lesion (9% of our cases, 5% of McKissock's[133]), and the mydriasis can be found contralateral (15% of our cases, 14% of McKissock's[133], 11% of Kvarnes's cases[117]).

As the CT scan more often detects asymptomatic lesions, the frequency of localization signs has risen, in our series, from 66% before its use to 49% since.

| | McKissock[133] | Jamieson[101] | Gallagher[55] | Grevsten[67] | Cordobes[30] | Our series |
|---|---|---|---|---|---|---|
| a) Frequency | | | | | | |
| Hemiplegia | 68% | 33% | 67% | 30% | 26% | 34% |
| Mydriasis | 60% | 33% | 63% | 43% | 49% | 34% |

| | Contusion dilacerations[211] | | Subdural hematomas[32] | | Intracerebral hematomas[76] | |
|---|---|---|---|---|---|---|
| b) Comparative pattern | | | | | | |
| Hemiplegia | 41% | | 44% | | 53% | |
| Mydriasis | 36% | | 40% | | 13% | |

Fig. 6. Neurologic signs

*b) Other signs.*

Bradycardia, which is a classical sign of brain compression seems rare in our experience, and that of Pouyanne[168] or Larghero[119]. It was noted in 15% of our cases, unlike Gallagher[55] who noticed it more often (50% of his cases). Like Jamieson[101] or Grevsten[67], we have found it more often in frontal than in the posterior fossa hematomas.

Anemia did not arouse our interest, except in the infant where the NF is low in ⅓ of the cases[24].

Finally, we would like to point out first the value of cranial impact when there is no radiological lesion and, secondly, late vomiting especially in children.

*2. Diffuse signs:* We do not insist on this part. Indeed we have noted, like others, in comatose patients, a diffuse pyramidal syndrome, neurovegetative, breathing or thermic disorders and decerebration, all signs whose importance is essential in a prognosis. Generalized comitial seizures are not rare (3 to 5%), like a meningeal syndrome noted in 15 to 20% of the cases.

### III. Evolutive Forms

From a trauma, the evolving pattern of the EDH is not unequivocal, and we tend to insist on the way the evolution takes place and its rapidity.

*1. Evoluting pattern* (Fig. 7): 3 forms seem to become apparent:

*a) Immediatly grave forms:* we are speaking of patients who immediatly after the trauma are in a coma. This condition only changes a little, keeps stationary or worsens little by little. We find them in 15 to 40% of cases in which the lucid interval is concealed by a coma. In more than half the cases there are immediate localization signs. They are grave forms since we note more than 50% result in death and they are more likely to be found when the hematoma is associated rather than pure and they are more frequent in the adult (31% of the cases) than in the child (17%), in our experience. One must remember that an immediate coma does not preclude vital further investigations.

*b) Aggravated forms:* Here, troubles of consciousness are evolutive and a real aggravation can be noted. It happens either because the trauma has been followed by an agitated obnubilation; a state which will worsen and will not enable us to speak of a lucid interval. These deteriorations, whatever step they make the patients reach, are progressive in 2 cases/3, but they may also be extremely quick in 1 case/3 and they always lead to a coma. Or it happens if trouble of consciousness appears after a lucid interval. This can progressively lead to a coma but in about 40% of the cases the process is sudden. This form has a variable frequency of 30 to 60% of the cases. While the state of consciousness is deteriorating we note the existence of

a) Frequency (O: HED only) (A: HED with associated lesions)

| | Pouyanne[168] 243 cases | Gallagher[55] 167 cases | Jamieson[101] 167 cases | Kvarnes[117] 132 cases | Cordobes[30] 82 cases | Our series 648 cases |
|---|---|---|---|---|---|---|
| Grave forms | 15% O: 10% A: 31% (death: 57%) | 21% | 23% O: 19% A: 27% | 40% | 24% (death: 50%) | 27% O: 19% A: 42% (death: 58%) |
| Aggravated forms | 62% O: 64% A: 55% (death: 47%) | 61% | 33% O: 26% A: 41% | 29% | 50% (death: 15%) | 48% O: 51% A: 42% (death: 32%) |
| Benign forms | 23% O: 26% A: 16% (death: 2%) | 18% | 44% O: 55% A: 32% | 31% | 26% (death: 5%) | 25% O: 30% A: 16% (death: 1%) |
| (Always conscious) | | | (25%) | (8%) | (10%) | (8%) |

b) Comparative pattern

| | Contusion dilacerations[211] | Subdural hematomas[32] | Intracerebral hematomas[76] |
|---|---|---|---|
| Grave forms | 49% | 57% | 28% |
| Aggravated forms | 33% | 25% | 28% |
| Benign forms | 18% | 18% | 44% |

Fig. 7. Evolutive forms

localization signs more often appearing during the clinical aggravation. It is the most frequent form, whether the hematoma is alone or associated and we have noted it in 58% of children, 44% of adult cases in our series.

*c) Forms without major trouble of consciousness:* They concern either patients who have rapidly improved a primarily trouble of consciousness or patients who have at the onset of trauma presented with obnubilation lasting without great variation, or patients who never presented with trouble of consciousness. This form is characterized by its benignity and in more than 60% of the cases, the patients present no evident neurological signs. This form is to be found in 20 to 40% of the cases, more often when the hematoma is alone than with associated lesions, and we have noted it as often in children (26%) as in adults (25%).

So the EDH evolution pattern does not seem to be characteristic since we find either immediatly grave forms, or forms with a lucid interval, or forms without major trouble of consciousness. All authors have pointed out that comaless forms were not rare in 20[114] to 40% [117] of the cases (31% in our series), and that a good deal of patients (in 8 to 25% of the cases) remain conscious during the evolution except with sometimes a temporary loss of consciousness loss[89, 95, 99, 134, 196, 200]. But the fact is that since the CT scan is largely used for cranial traumas, surgical lesions have been detected at a stage when the symptomatology was missing or reduced and wherever the lesion was located[51, 167, 199].

So, in our series, before using the CT scan we have noted 23% of benign forms and 6% of evolution with a normal conscious state. Since the use of CT those frequencies are 33% and 11% respectively.

*2. Forms depending on the rapidity of evolution* (Fig. 8).

*a) Acute forms:* they are the most frequent: 60 to 80% of the EDH are detected and operated in the first 24 hours, sometimes more (85%) in some series[45, 114, 168]. Most EDH with associated lesions and more than half of EDH alone are to be found in this category. However, we must point out that when 6-hour evolving hyperacute forms are individualized, typical acute forms (from the 6th to the 24th hour) are linked to only 20% of the EDH (our series, and those of Pouyanne[168] and Bourhis[14]) and the gravity of these hyperacute forms has been underlined[14, 106, 134, 142]. The rapidity of the EDH evolution depends on the origin of the bleeding: most acute or hyperacute forms are linked to a arterial originating bleeding.

*b) Subacute forms:* They are little described in the literature[95, 165, 184, 196] because they depend on the moment EDH are said to be chronic. If, like Fenelon[45], we regard as subacute the EDH evolving between the 24th hour and the 7th day, this form frequency can vary from 9[45, 168] to 39% [101] of the cases.

*c) Chronic forms:* Chronicity being in theory linked to the subdural hematomas, chronic EDH have resulted in several publications. Even if they were known a long time ago[66,97,99,151,181,190,200,222] they have been studied more recently[15,16,25,62,89,111,169,229]. The moment hematomas are said to be chronic can change according to the authors: 3 days (Loew[131], Sparacio[190],

| | Pouyanne[168] 233 cases | Jamieson[101] 163 cases | Our series 648 cases | Kvarnes[117] 133 cases |
|---|---|---|---|---|
| O—24 H | 85% O: 83% A: 92% (death: 37%) | 56% O: 47% A: 66% (death: 22%) | 69% O: 63% A: 81% (death: 43%) | 71% (death: 29%) |
| 24 H—7 D | 9% O: 11% A: 5% (death: 14%) | 39% O: 47% A: 30% (death: 5%) | 21% O: 25% A: 14% (death: 7%) | 14% (> 5 D) (death: 0%) |
| 7 D and more | 6% O: 6% A: 3% (death: 0%) | 5% O: 6% A: 4% (death: 0%) | 10% O: 12% A: 5% (death: 0%) | 15% (< 5 D) (death: 10%) |

Fig. 8. Rate of development of signs (O: EDH only) (A: EDH with associated lesions)

Clavel[25]), 7 days (Pouyanne[168], Jonker[105], us), 10 days (Hooper[91]), or 13 days (Iwakuma[97], Zuccarello[229]). Some hematomas have evolved for years: 6 (Grant[66]), 33 (Punt[170]). So they are noted with different frequencies: 2% (Clavel[25]), 4% (Zuccarello[229]), 12% (Jonker[105]), 10% in our series (62 cases). In practice, these hematomas behave like tumors, they evolve without important trouble of consciousness in most cases and generally it is because of their persistence or the appearance of headaches, of vomiting, of a deficit even of an papilloedema that further investigations are done. Favouring factors to the hematoma chronicity are chiefly linked to its topography and to the bleeding origin. They are most often bleedings from a venous origin[25,99,151,229], the hematoma being more often located in so-called atypical regions[29,71,191,222], probably because the dura is more sticky there than in the temporo-parietal area, as we already pointed it out. We must make a difference between those chronic hematomas and the delayed EDH which are visualized some hours or days later after a previous normal examination, angiography or CT scan[22,51,64,112,149,169,177]. These late forms are linked to the suppression of protective mechanisms which made the hemostasis possible, mechanisms we studied in the physiopathologically section of this article.

## IV. Topographic Forms

We are going to recall the EDH clinical aspects according to their localization when not associated with intracranial lesions which exercise influence on symptomatology. However, they are seldom described in the literature in their pure form and that is why we will use our personal studies.

*1. Lateral EDH:* They are the most frequent. A fracture is noted in about 85% of the cases for this region is particularly liable to trauma. In our series we had 446 lateral EDH, and among them 288 pure ones. Grave and acute forms are the most frequent (75% of our cases), the bleeding having an arterial origin. In 60% of the cases, there are localization signs and we had about 1 death/5 (23%). Chronic forms have been rare in our series (6% of the cases).

*2. Frontal EDH:* Long ago individualized[71, 125, 193, 207], they have been recently studied by Andreoli[3] in their pure form. Our series consists of 91 pure/128 frontal EDH. The fracture there is rarer than elsewhere (52% of Andreoli's cases[3], 55% of ours). Clinically speaking it is the "hematoma of the extremes"[162, 193]. Indeed, the pattern is either immediately grave or gets more and more grave (70% of Andreoli's cases, 43% of ours) with 1 time/2, localization signs, or the hematoma progresses with minor trouble of consciousness and no localization signs (in 57% of our cases). In 1 time/2 it is only obnubilation with an ICH syndrome which will evolve for several days, 1 time/2 consciousness has remained normal throughout the evolution, the EDH being detected at random during surgery on the anterior fossa. 32% of our cases are chronic forms. Ipsilateral exophthalmos is noticed by Gruskiewicz[70] or Romano[179] but we think it is rare (one case). Frontal EDH prognosis is said to be relatively good (13% fatality in our series).

*3. Temporo-basilar EDH:* These hematomas' clinical aspects have been pointed out by Guillaume and Pecker[74] and like them, we think their pattern is characteristic in pure forms. While 3 have led to an acute form, in 17 cases the evolution has been several days lasting obnubilation with a minor ICH syndrome and psychic troubles. But we have only found early mydriasis because of injury of III in 5 cases. This is a benign localization, death only having occurred in acute forms.

*4. Vertex EDH:* They have been distinguished from parasagittal EDH (Hooper[91]) by Alexander[1] and Columella[27]. In 1965, Pouyanne[168] found 16 cases in the literature, Columella[28] 32 in 1968. Published series are short[1,19, 28, 34, 98, 191], except Borzone[13]: 12 cases or Zuccarello[227]: 14 cases. In ours they are 12 and among them 9 are pure. These hematomas are characterized by the always present fracture crossing the LSS (bleeding origin in most cases). Their clinical form can vary: more often acute according to Zuccarello[227] and in our cases chronic according to

Columella[28], or both for Borzone[13]. The typical description is paraplegia. Early papillary edema because of venous congestion is rare (1 to 2 cases). These are serious hematomas: 50% fatality (Zuccarello[227]), 4/9 in our series.

*5. Posterior fossa EDH:* they have been studied for a long time: Reigh[174] finds 80 of them published in 1962, Calbucci[17], Besson[10] each 108 and 100 cases in 1977 and 1978. The importance of this localization is pointed out in studies formerly published on this topic[5, 59, 116, 126, 148, 192]; there are 15 cases in our series, 10 of them pure. This localization is frequent in children[10, 17, 192], 5 cases in our series. In most cases there is an occipital fracture crossing the lateral sinus often responsible for the bleeding. Acute forms with or without a lucid interval quickly lead to a serious coma with signs of brain stem dysfunction, acute hydrocephaly and early respiratory troubles. Chronic forms are not rare (4% of the cases)[10] simulating a tumor of this region[12, 29, 99, 192]. The death rate is similar to the acute forms being 4 deaths/10 in our series. A good deal of posterior fossa EDH probably escape notice for hyperacute forms lead to quick death before hospitalization. Nevertheless, the possible existence of an EDH in this region justifies its systematic exploration with the CT scan[202].

*6. Occipital EDH:* very few cases have been studied in this localization[9, 168, 178, 208]. We have noted 18 of them, 10 pure and their clinical aspect remind us of frontal hematomas, 6 had acute, 4 subacute or chronic evolutions, but the prognosis is less favourable (4 deaths/10 cases).

As regards to EDH, typical and atypical forms are classically opposed[69, 82, 156, 195]. In fact, on analysis of observations, there does not seem to be a specific type of EDH. Indeed it can have different forms according to the patient's age, the existence or not of associated lesions and the lesional topography. Nevertheless, from a clinical point of view, nothing enables us to be sure of the diagnosis facing other cranial trauma complications (particularly brain contusion-dilacerations and acute subdural hematomas), these can evolve similarly because we can observe immediately grave forms, others with a lucid interval and others without any trouble of consciousness. This stresses the importance of complementary investigations, above all because localization signs can be missing.

## F. Complementary Investigations

They have not equally worthy of interest because in emergency cases the paraclinical check-up is necessarily limited to indispensable examinations so that a diagnosis may be made.

### I. Standard Investigations

*1. The radiography* remains a routine examination in the standard check-up of a cranial trauma. It can detect a fracture and an eventual shifting of the calcified pineal gland. If everybody agrees with the importance of a detected fracture, no absence of a fracture during radiography (10 to 15% of the cases) can exclude a possible EDH, above all because these missing fractures during radiography can be found during surgery (more often in children than in adults).

*2. Electroencephalography:* It is of little interest particularly in an emergency, most examinations being conducted after surgery. However, in subacute and chronic asymptomatic forms, the presence of an asymetry, of slow localized waves, or of a focal depressed activity sometimes occurred after a true electric free interval must lead to investigations, particularly in the frontal and subtemporal localizations.

*3. Ophthalmological investigations:* It is of no use in an emergency but, however, in some chronic forms, the persistence of a papillary stasis has led to investigations.

## II. Diagnostic Methods

they have been improving but they are more or less used because of one or another contribution.

*1. Diagnostic burr hole:* It is still relevant in angiography and the CT scan time for its indication depends on the impossibility to achieve one of the two examinations in an emergency on patients whose state is deteriorating fast, or in cases when these examinations cannot be carried out.

*2. Cerebral angiography:* The importance of this examination in the detection of intracranial hematomas is no longer to be underlined as several publications show [11, 93, 113, 122, 135, 186, 214, 218] and studying EDH [31, 37, 46, 63, 108, 109, 126, 216, 225].

*a) EDH only:* Its shape is well known: the cranio-cortical detachment is characteristic and gives evidence of an extracerebral collection which causes an avascular biconvex space between the brain convexity and inner table of the calvaria. It seems to be obvious on a *towne* projection for lateral hematomas (Fig. 9), in profile for vertex and posterior fossa hematomas (Fig. 10), in anterior and posterior oblique projections for frontal and occipital hematomas (Fig. 11), and finally on *hirtz* incidence for subtemporal hematomas.

Vessel shiftings and vascular emptiness depend on the lesional topography and size.

The extradural characteristic of the bleeding can sometimes be certain when there is a detachment of the middle meningeal artery [88], or if there is a traumatic lesion of this artery [92, 129]. False aneurysm [4, 58, 87, 115, 157], extravasation of contrast material (Fig. 12) as several authors, after Lindgren [130] have noted [85, 145, 163, 183], arterio-venous shunts between meningeal and diploic vessels [42, 48, 96, 100, 188, 219]. Habash *et al.* [79] have recently insisted upon the importance of those shunts whose dimensions and distance between the

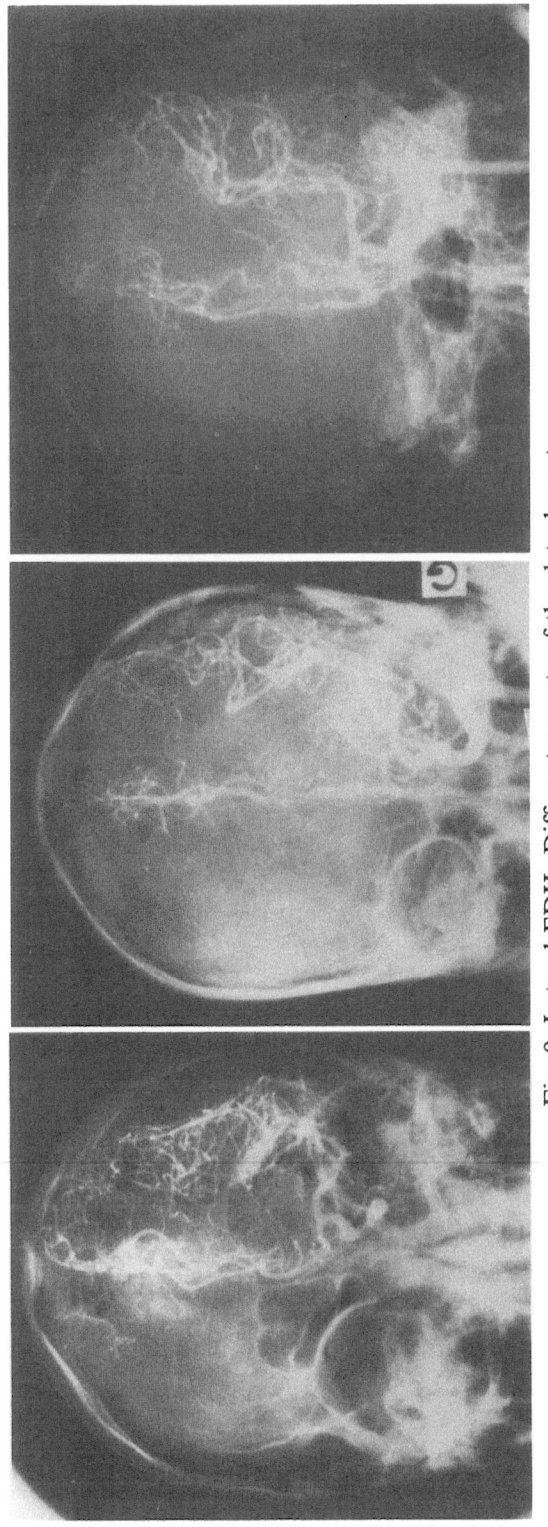

Fig. 9. Lateral EDH: Different aspects of the detachment

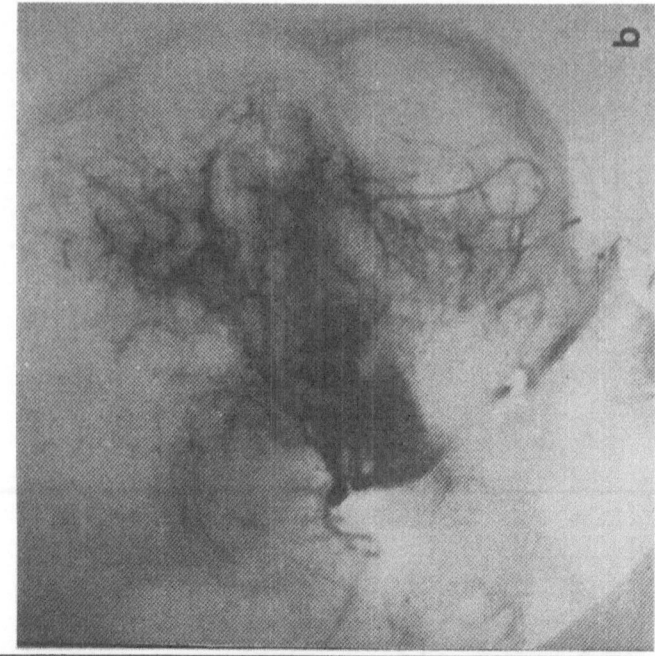

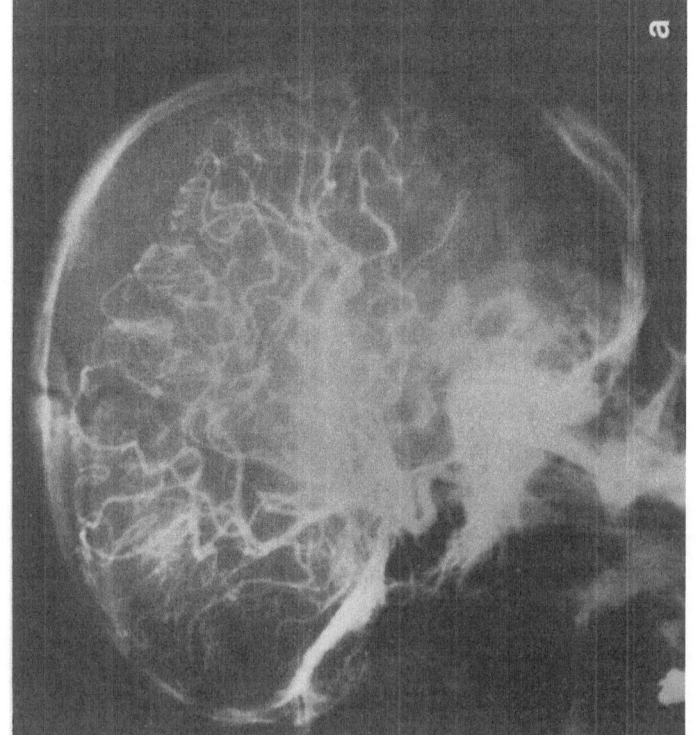

Fig. 10. Vertex (a) and posterior fossa (b) hematomas

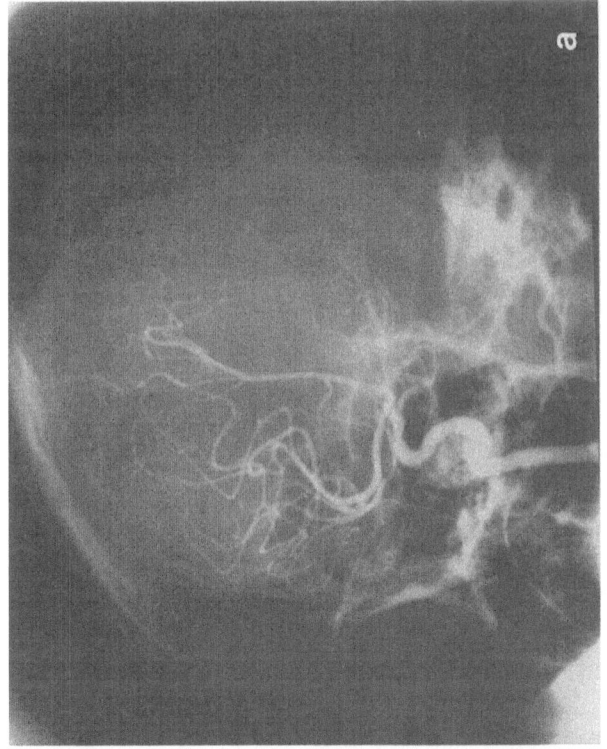

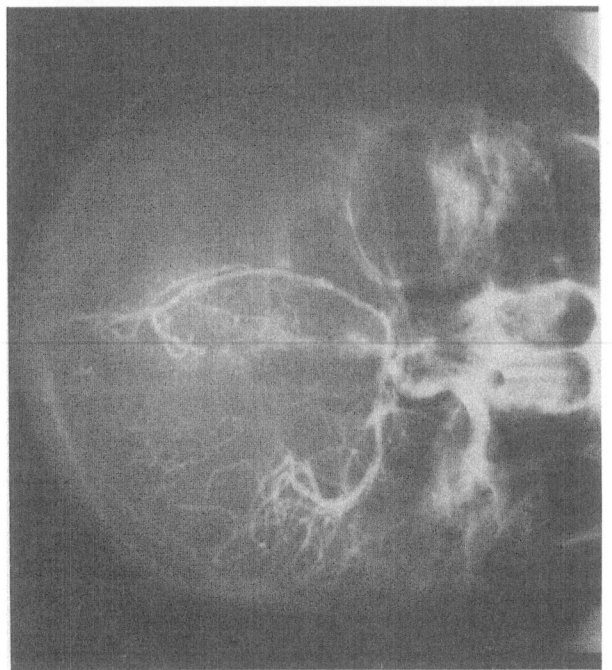

Fig. 11. Frontal (a) and posterior (b) hematomas: anterior and posterior oblique projection showing detachment

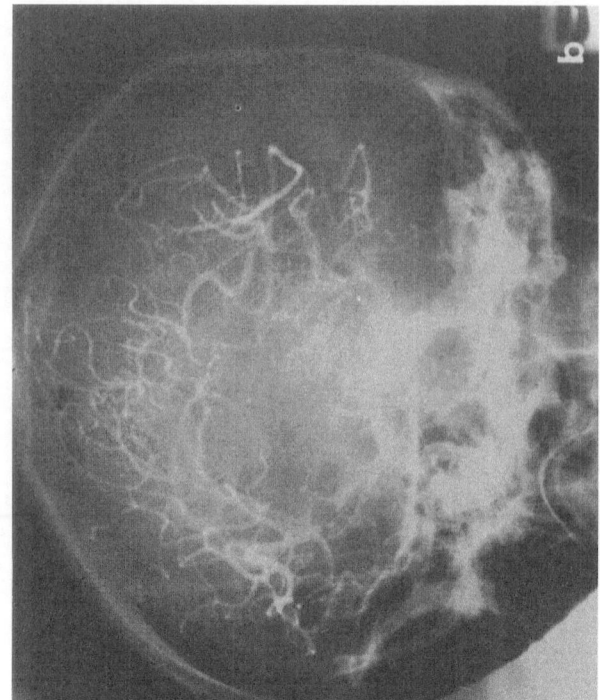

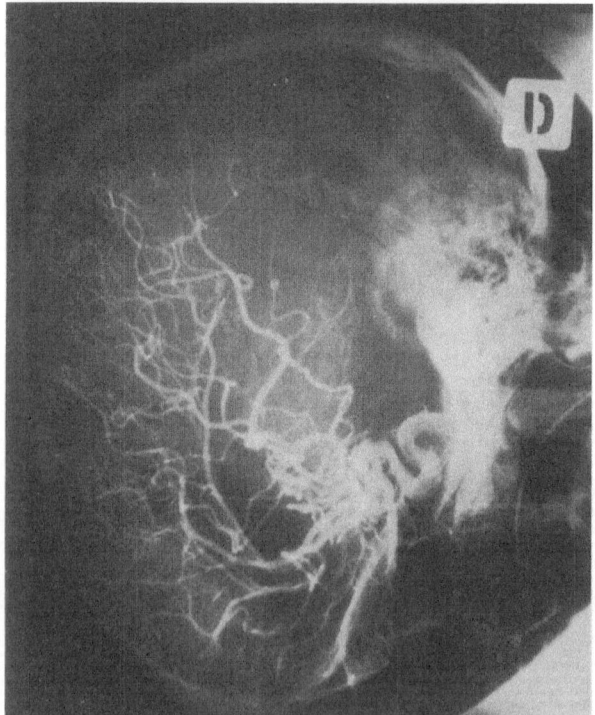

Fig. 11b

bleeding origin and the receiving vein can play a part in prolonging the bleeding. To be visualized, these aspects need the vizualitation of the external carotid, which is not always the case.

The EDH angiographic diagnosis is above all linked to subdural hematomas and some brain contusion-dilacerations[38, 47, 60, 152, 220]: *The sub-*

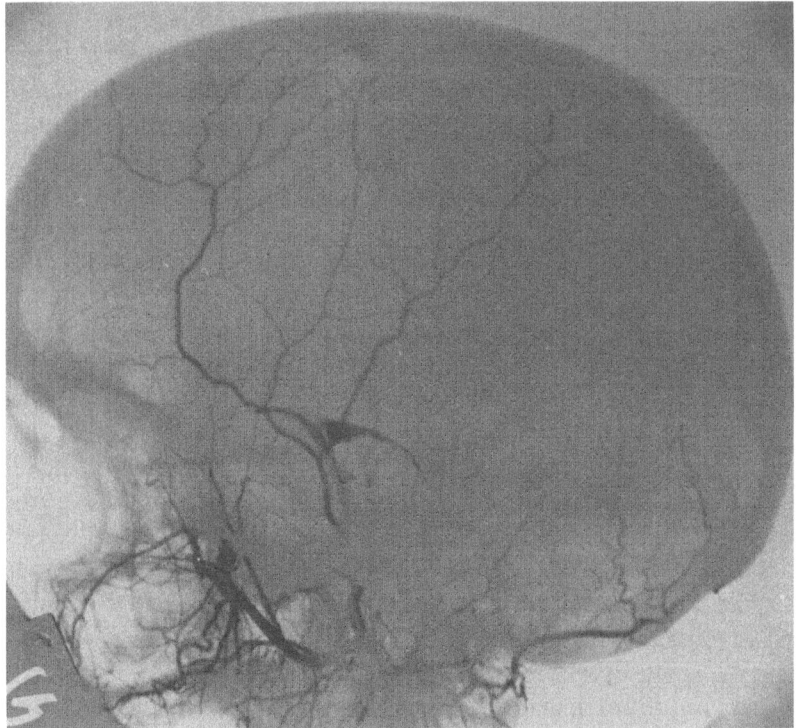

Fig. 12. Extravasation and false aneurysm of the middle meningeal artery

*dural hematoma* is detected because of the image of a spreading detachment which has a crescent shape. Peripheral small cortical arterial analysis can contribute to the diagnosis because they are fully perceptible in subdural hematomas, whereas they are distorted or stretched in extradural ones[8, 63, 220]. Anyway, the interest of the diagnosis of sub- or extradural location of hematomas is negligible for the existence of an important detachment systematically leads to surgery.

*Some brain contusion-dilacerations* can arouse as many difficulties in a diagnosis especially in their frontopolar, subfrontal and temporo-basilar localizations as a lack of peripheral vascularization can simulate a detachment. In that case, the analysis of the meningeal artery anterior branches or of ethmoidal arteries[37] and the arterial and venous analysis of the temporal pole[33] can contribute to the diagnosis of an oblique or Hirtz incidence. If there is doubt, the burr hole will enable knowledge of the exact nature of the lesion.

This diagnosis is more difficult when there are:

*b) EDH associated* with intracranial lesions which are usually concealed by the extradural collection and most often detected during surgery or during the next examination when the EDH has been removed. However, we must remember a small shift of vessels contrasting with an important detachment or on the contrary, a small detachment with an important shifting of vessels must make us try to detect an associated lesion either homo- or contralaterally. This will emphasize the importance of angiographies with compression of the opposite side, that we prefer to a bilateral angiography[223].

*3. CT scan:* In fact, it is the only examination that immediatly allows a lesional check-up, a precise topographical diagnosis and that corroborates the nature of the lesions and their repercussions on the brain. Since its use, several articles have been devoted to it and EDH have been described[2, 44, 52, 57, 110, 118, 127, 143, 164, 205, 209, 224].

*a) The hematoma*, its shape and location are characteristic (Fig. 13): well delineated biconvex or lenticular area, immediately adjacent to the cranial vault, with a sharp inner margin, linked to the skull with an obtuse angle[110]. Atypical forms have been reported, among others, by Cordobes[30]: he described in 41 cases, 2 double biconvex hematomas, 2 round-shaped hematomas with irregular outlines and 4 crescent lens-shaped hematomas as seen in subdural hematomas.

Usually, acute EDH have a high hyperdensity (HU 64–76) linked to the organized clot. Sometimes they can be isodense[176] when the blood is fluid (few minutes old hyperacute bleeding, coagulation troubles) but in other cases there look heterogeneous[57] because there are iso- or hypodense areas in the middle of the hyperdensity, these areas corresponding with non-coagulated blood, when the blood is still partly fluid. This heterogeneity can also be explained by the presence of numerous little air bubbles, especially with an open fracture; sometimes, sedimentation phenomena may occur[110].

The longer existing EDH may be moderately hyperdense, isodense and later hypodense. Hypodensity has been regarded as characteristic of chronic hematomas by Zimmerman[224], though hyperdensity can last over the 10th day[158, 159] and isodense hematomas appear between the 3rd and the 14th day[36, 81, 89, 156]. On the whole, hypodense hematomas are described from the 7th day[158, 159, 224]. The injection of contrast material can lead to modifications of the density[57, 158, 201]: Tsai[201] has recorded in 16/48 acute EDH an increasing hyperdensity which becomes homogeneous. This iodized opacification can sometimes visualize a jet of the contrast material[158, 201]

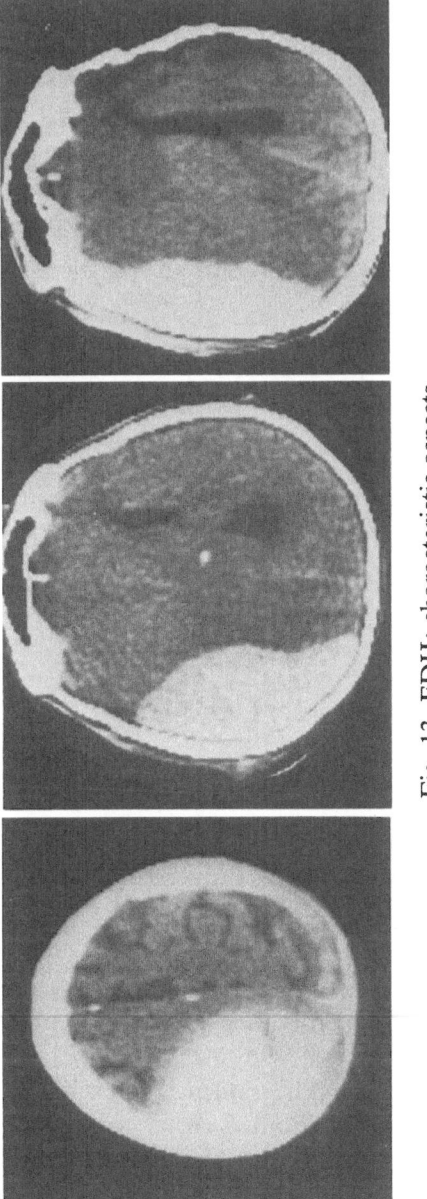

Fig. 13. EDH: characteristic aspects

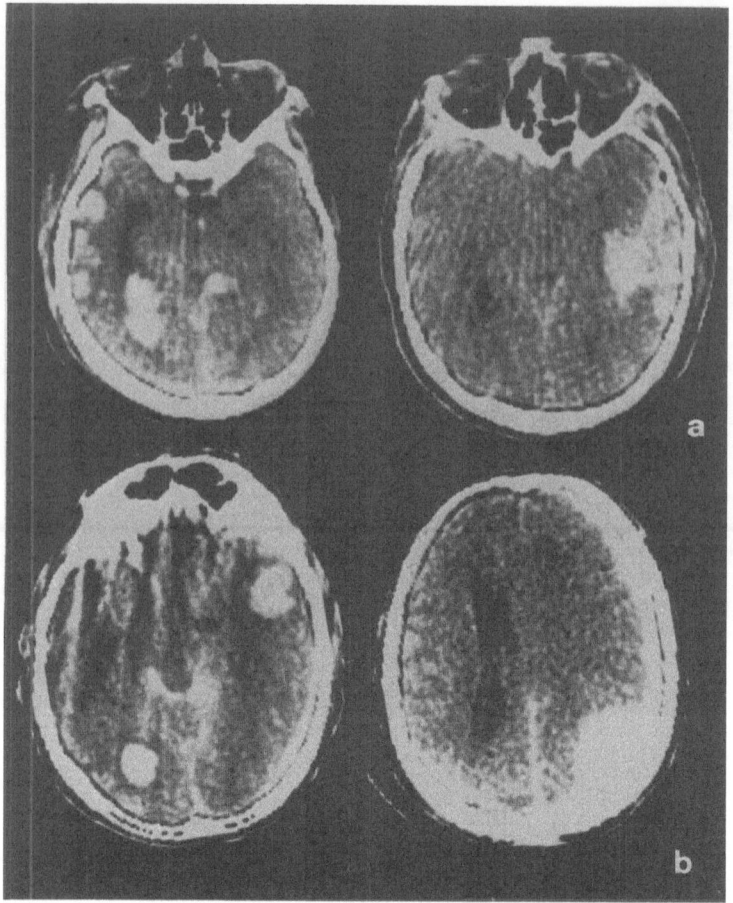

Fig. 14. EDH with associated lesions: a) intracerebral hematomas and dilaceration,
b) subdural and intracerebral hematomas

which equals on the CT scan the angiographical sign described by Lindgren. In chronic hematomas whether they are iso- or hypodense or in those whose hyperdensity is attenuated, the use of contrast material enables the visualization of the internal hematoma limit which is underlined by a rim enhancement[2, 29, 81, 153, 213] attributed either to the shifted dura[118], or to the fibro-vascular tissue which covers the dura or to the congestive cortex[81].

The rare, nonfatal and nonoperated hematomas resorb. This resorbtion, watched with iterative CT scan[94, 159, 215] is sometimes preceded by an "expansile phase" that Pang[159] notes in 5 cases/11, and occurs between the third week and three months.

On the whole, the EDH CT scan diagnosis is easy because its hyperdense biconvex "lens" shape distingues it from other hematomas. Let us

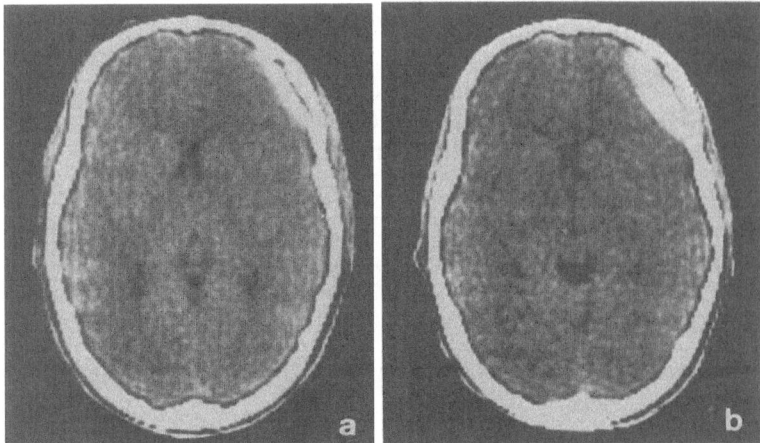

Fig. 15. CT scan 6 hours (a) and 1 week (b) after trauma showing increasing of an EDH

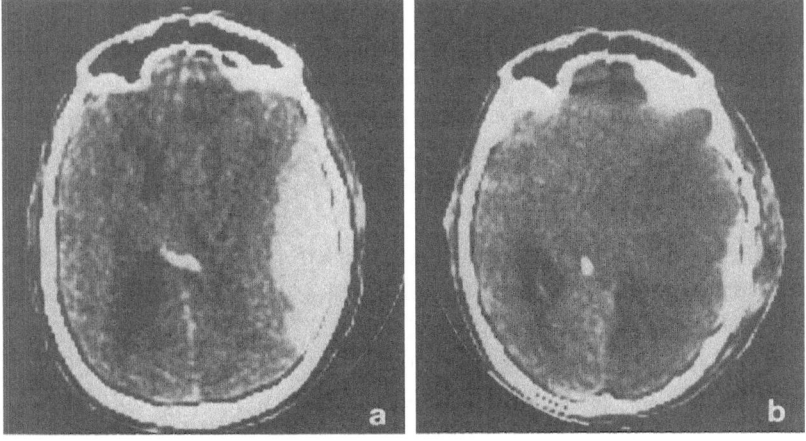

Fig. 16. CT scan in an operated patient showing large softening (a) before, (b) after intervention

remember that some crescentic forms looking like subdural hematomas have been described[30] and that we can rarely visualize hyperdense acute subdural hematomas whose shape is that of a biconvex "lens"[110]. However, the hematoma can escape notice if isodense, and this stresses the importance of the injection of a contrast material if the emergency allows it.

*b) The hematoma repercussions* on the brain (mass effect, edema, softening), and *the existence of associated lesions* (Fig. 14) must be estimated in order to set a complete lesional evaluation. Let us stress the importance of the CT scan while observing (Figs. 15, 16) brain injured[26, 189] and operated patients[39] in order to detect a late or early lesion or a recurrence.

## G. Treatment

### I. Surgical

*1. Operative indications:* In principle when dealing with EDH the operation is aimed at suppressing compression before it is too late[147].

*a) So the operative indication is absolute* in most cases, when there is trouble of consciousness and or immediate or secondary neurological signs, whether there are associated lesions or not, even if Xuxiang (Pang)[159] has successfully medically cured 9 patients with brain stem dysfunction and who had large hematomas.

*b) It may be debated in some cases* according to the hematoma and the state of consciousness.

The hematoma volume is seldom reported in the literature and it is not easily estimated exception the CT scan[43, 159, 224]. Usually, EDH are operated when their thickness exceeds 1.5 cm[150] and their volume about 40 cc (our series) though there seems to be a "critical" volume under which the hematoma can resorb[159]. Smaller EDH can be operated if they lead to a mass-effect with neurological signs, if there are associated lesions because their removal helps the intracranial pressure to decrease, if they are located in some regions: a temporal hematoma can lead to compression signs more rapidly and with a smaller volume than others[50]. This applies in our opinion also to posterior fossa hematomas and the need, according to us, to evacuate them.

State of consciousness: the CT scan used systematically for cranially traumatized patients enables the detection of intracranial lesions, particularly EDH, in conscious patients[51, 54, 167, 199] and besides, many EDH, particularly in chronic forms, are operated on asymptomatic patients or patients suffering from headaches. That is why some authors have wondered whether surgery was necessary or not in these cases[16, 54, 67, 200]. Because the CT scan enables one to follow the evolution of the hematoma and particularly its spontaneous resorption, some cases of diagnosed and nonoperated EDH are reported in the literature[43, 67, 94, 159, 215, 224], some criteria allowing one to delay surgery (Pang)[159], under CT scan observation are: a normal state of consciousness, absence of neurological signs, of an associated intradural lesion and of a large temporal hematoma with a mass effect. Surgery must be faced as soon as possible if the clinical state is changing, if headaches, vomiting or obnubilation persist after the third week (for hematomas start resorbing from that date) or if there is no signs of resorption three months after the trauma (most EDH having resorbed by that time).

In fact, we think we must be careful regarding this aspect because we all observed patients who were fulfilling these conditions, suddenly deteriorating and operated too late when in coma. This can lead to death or to serious sequelae. So we prefer operating in these cases.

*2. Surgical approach:* The burr hole is still actual, its indications depend on the impossibility to obtain, in emergency cases, an angiography or a CT scan for a patient who is quickly deteriorating. It must be done just where the injured patient has been hospitalized, even if he is to be later taken to a specialized department. Indeed it is better for the patient to be decompressed under bad conditions than perfectly, but when decerebrated and in a coma.

As Gudeman describes[73] the evacuation of the hematoma needs a bone flap. The enlarged burr hole or the trephine hole are not enough to evacuate a clotted hematoma and to control the origin of the bleeding. Moreover, the need to open the dura in order to drain a subdural hematoma, to do temporal decompression or to achieve the hemostasis of an attrition justifies a large craniotomy whose advantage is to be found in the results. Nielsen[150] has observed that the death rate was of 28% with an enlarged burr hole or a trephine, whereas it was only 17% with a larger craniotomy.

When the hematoma is evacuated, the brain can remain collapsed, in which case a ventricular filling by puncture is required. Most often, it recovers, but sometimes marked cerebral swelling can lead to a large opening of the dura with or without extensive reconstruction, or to a large decompressive flap. Finally, the existence of a temporal herniation needs its decompression by the usual technique. Associated lesions detected during the intervention will be treated, the subdural hematoma with the EDH, dilacerations or intracerebral hematomas according to individual operative indications.

## II. Medical

The EDH medical treatment depends on two elements: the brain's state and the patient's situation. If the brain has remained collapsed in spite of the ventricular filling, saline serum and corticoids can be used, but their effectiveness is not certain. On the contrary, when the brain has become turgescent and, or, when there are associated lesions, all means able to reduce intracranial hypertension will be used.

In a conscious patient, no special treatment is necessary, except the prevention of post-traumatic epilepsy. In contrast, in a comatose patient, the treatment is at of every serious cranial trauma, the description of which has recently been done[137,144,175], and the treatment checked by ICP monitoring. However, two points should be noted: the need for new investigations in order to detect a recurrence or unnoticed associated lesions when no improvement is recorded after evacuation of the hematoma, and the role of hyperosmotic treatment when it is done with no control of the ICP on an observed traumatized patient because it can promote or maintain the bleeding.

## H. Outcome and Results

*I. Death rate:* The death rate in EDH can change according to the series: 30 to 40% [35,55,77,105,168,228], 20 to 30% [30,91,114,117,133,199], 10 to 20% [83,101,217]. Because of improved reanimation methods for cranial traumas and the CT scan, this rate is about 20% [30,114,116]: thus, in our series, the death rate which was of about 33% before the CT scan is now of 22%. However, we are still far from the "ideal" mortality: 10% [90] or 12% [133,199] obtained when the EDH are diagnosed and treated as soon as possible.

*II. The prognosis factors* are well known in neurotraumatology, so they will be briefly mentioned. Some are common to all cranial traumas: general factors [84,102,104,197,206], clinical status [21,78,155,161,203], others depend on the lesion itself [30,101,107,217].

*1. General factors:* The age can interfere with the prognosis: the death rate is lower for children than for adults: 8 to 12% [18,24,55,65,83,101], 14.5% in our series. The death rate is higher for adults: 37% in our series although it goes from 30 to 45% between 15 and 50 years, from 50 to 90% when 50 to 90 years. Teasdale *et al.* [199] noticed that under 20, the death rate is half as much as that between 20 and 40 years. Frequent associated lesions and eventual diseases (vascular, alcoholism, diabetes) are involved in these bad results for adults.

Polytrauma adds its own severity to the hematoma and when lesions have been serious we have noted 33 deaths/44 cases in our series.

*2. Clinical factors:* They depend on the state of consciousness. We must take into account the evolution process and particularly the existence or not of coma. Thus, EDH evolving without coma, whether the evolution is quick or not, are a good prognosis. It is not the same with forms evolving with a coma (Fig. 7): 90 to 95% of dead patients have been operated when in coma and the death rate increases with the gravity of coma. Some clinical signs are said to have a bad prognosis: bilateral mydriasis 75 (our results) to 100% [30] death, decerebration: 50 [30] to 100% [150] death, neurovegetative, respiratory, cardio vascular disorders...

*3. Hematoma factors:* They occur in an obvious way whether there are associated lesions to the hematoma or not.

*a) The existence of associated lesions* considerably worsen the EDH prognosis: the death rate is higher than for pure EDH, from 26 to 40% [30,43,101,117,199], and we thought it was particularly important in our series (51%) and Zuccarello's (50%) [228].

*b) Pure EDH:* They have a better prognosis since the death rate is from 6 to 20% [30,43,101,117,134,199], 21% in our series, 24% in Zuccarello's. Three points must be taken into account in the general prognosis of pure EDH:

On the one hand, the evolution rate since most deaths are to be found in hyperacute and acute forms (Fig. 8). This stresses the importance of an early intervention[7, 142, 198]. For instance, Mendelow *et al.*[142] observed that when the intervention takes place 8 hours after the appearance of signs, the death rate is 33% though it is 9% if the delay is reduced to one hour.

On the other hand, the volume of the hematoma and the death rate increases according to its volume: about 50 cc: 12% dead, about 50 to 100 cc: 33% dead, more than 100 cc: 66% dead in our series.

Lastly, its localization: lateral hematomas which are likely to evolute in an acute way have a higher death rate than other hematomas which have a subacute or chronic evolution (see topographic forms).

*III. Sequelea:* Among alive patients, most authors[172, 223] observed 70% recoveries with good results, 30% recoveries with sequelae, which corroborates with our series. To us, sequelae are as frequent in children as in adults but the most serious and persistant ones are to be found more often when the hematoma is associated with a cerebral lesion than when pure[67], us. Considering the results, the balance may be still found heavy. Badly reported results are mostly linked to the way patients are recruited, indeed they are most often transferred from a peripheral hospital when there is clinical deterioration and then they are hospitalized, investigated and operated too late. In fact the patient with an extradural hematoma leads to a full recovery if operated in time or does not survive.

## I. How to Do It

We envisage in this section the course to follow according to the clinical state and to the management.

### I. Course to Follow According to the Clinical State

Clinically, the EDH can take different aspects (according to the age, the associated lesions or to its localization): there are some forms with an immediate coma, others, with a free interval or with minor trouble of consciousness, forms which are not specific to the EDH and which are found in other cranial trauma complications, which are difficult to detect and must be treated early in order to operate as soon as possible before it is too late. This implies the course to follow with all cranial traumatized patients depends chiefly on the state of consciousness and we consider operating on the conscious patient, when the trauma leads to immediate trouble of consciousness, or deteriorating patient.

*1. The conscious patient:* has the most likely good prognosis. Nevertheless, the possible appearance of secondary deterioration needs supervision. When there is no fracture, the patient will be kept under observation after loss of consciousness. An EEG and an ophthalmological investigation will be required and if they are normal it will not be necessary to continue the observation period over 48 to 72 hours.

If there is a fracture, the hospitalization will be necessary for about ten days: an EEG and on ophthalmologic investigation will be requested on the patient's admission and discharge. The existence or appearance in a conscious patient of neurological, electroencephalographic signs or of a papillar edema require complementary investigations (angiography or CT scan) and if an EDH is detected, he will be operated.

2. *Patient with immediate trouble of consciousness:* We have to be certain that all neurological signs have been immediate and have not followed a free interval, even the shortest one. Anyway, investigations will be required (angiography or CT scan) and a detected EDH on an obnibulated or comatose patient automatically needs to be evacuated.

3. *Deteriorating patient:* Any deterioration in a cranial traumatized patient must make us think of a hematoma and then, all must be done to operate this hematoma before irreversible brain lesions appear. Everything depends on the speed of the evolution. If there is a hyperacute evolution, the burr hole is needed. If there is no way to get an emergency angiography or a CT scan. The burr hole must be performed right away where the patient is hospitalized, even if he is to be taken to a specialized ward later, after decompression has been made. With a slower deterioration, a brain angiography or a CT scan can be carried out; the choice depending on the equipement available.

4. *An already operated patient:* if there is no improvement after surgery or if the patient is deteriorating after improvement, an angiography or a CT scan should be done in order to detect a possible recurrence of the EDH or an associated lesion.

5. *Polytraumatized patient:* he sets a serious problem, difficult to solve in some cases, particularly when there is an abdominal or thoracic emergency. Polytrauma requires the presence of several specialist near the patient, which unfortunately does not always happen since patients are too often taken from one specialized ward to another. Furthermore, in our experience the possibility of the formation of a hematoma during general anesthesia prohibits all interventions unmotivated by a vital emergency at least during 24 hours.

## II. Course to Follow According to the Management

1. *Operative treatment:* If the patient is not hospitalized in a specialized ward, the need for a burr hole can be discussed. A burr hole is generally made on the mydriasis side, opposite to the hemiplegia, facing the fracture. The skin incision is initiated 1 cm anterior to the tragus, 2 cm above the zygomatic arch and carried vertically on 4 cm. A possible enlargement superiorly and posteriorly over the ear will be ensured with a scalp revealing the temporal region. The hemostasis is often obtained with the use of

beckman's erin type, which separates muscles and skin. The trepanning is achieved with the use of a manual trepan first with a starting drill and then with a spherical drill; the hole can be enlarged with a gouge after enlarging the scalp incision if necessary. The hematoma comes out under pressure generally looking like "currant jelly" blending fluid blood with clots. It is removed with hot serum irrigation, suction and a carefully handled spoon. A drain is slipped into the epidural space, the skin is sutured and the patient taken to a specialized ward. When the preauricular burr hole has revealed nothing particular, others will be made the same way in the posterior temporal, frontal or parietal regions, knowing that the EDH is usually located in sloping ares. If during operation the dura appears to be tense and bluish, it is probably because of a subdural hematoma. So, a small incision carefully achieved in the dura will enable draining of a part of the hematoma.

When arrived in a specialized ward, an angiography or a CT scan will be required and if the hematoma removal has been uncomplete, the intervention will be followed by a boneflap. The hematoma evacuation and particularly its basal extension will be completed according to the same principles, while respecting the thinness of clots which insure the surface hemostasis. The removal of the collection leads to the cause of bleeding which is generally the middle meningeal artery and which can either be coagulated or ligatured. If the artery bleeds in the bone, hemostasis will be achieved with wax, and this applies also to the edges of the fracture if they are responsible for the bleeding. On the whole, the hemostasis is never perfect and an oozing of the dura or of the bone may persist. The hematoma recurrence must be avoided first by suspending the dura with stitches which will hold it to the epicranium and, secondly, by placing a drain in the epidural space. If the brain seems to be collapsed and if it does not recover after removal of the collection, intraventricular or intrathecal injections of physiological serum could help, together with intravenous saline serum and corticoids. In some cases the opening of the dura can be discussed and if there is an associated subdural hematoma, it must be removed by soft suction and warm serum irrigation. If there is temporal herniation, in that case an erin is slipped under the carefully lifted temporal lobe; the decompression being efficient when the LCR comes to the surface. A major cerebral swelling can lead to a decompressive bone flap with a large opening of the dura which will be left open or close after reconstruction. When the operation is over, the flap will be set back and the suture is done on three levels: muscular, epicranial and skin.

*2. Medical treatment:* The medical treatment is managed according to two possibilities:

If the hematoma has not been diagnosed and the patient is being observed we must not trust an innoportune antiedema treatment which could help or maintain a bleeding. That is why the intracranial pressure needs to be controlled.

If the hematoma has been operated and the patient is recovering, no particular treatment is required except prevention of posttraumatic epilepsy owing to barbiturates. If the patient remains in a grave state, other investigations will be required to look for a reccurrence or for unnoticed intracranial lesions. The treatment will be that of any severe cranial trauma: control of vital functions and of metabolic problems, respiratory assistance, prevention of neurovegetative disorders (lytic cocktails, barbiturates) and of intracranial hypertension (steroids, diuretics, hypertonic solutions) under ICP monitoring. All these stress the need of intensive care.

## References

1. Alexander, G. L., 1961: Extradural haematoma at the vertex: J. Neurol. Neurosurg. Psychiat. *24*, 381—384.
2. Allen, J. H., 1977: Computed tomographic scan findings in closed head trauma. Computed Axial Tomography *1*, 115—120.
3. Andreoli, A., Bollini, C., Calbucci, F., Frattarelli, M., Grossi, C., Munari, C., 1977: Extradural haematoma of the anterior cranial fossa (23 cases). Acta Neurochir. (Wien) *36*, 148.
4. Araki, C., Handa, H., Handa, J., Yoshida, K., 1964: Traumatic aneurysm of the intracranial extradural portion of the internal carotid artery. J. Neurosurg. *36*, 64—67.
5. Arkins, T. J., McLennan, J. E., Winston, K. R., Strand, R. D., Suzuki, Y., 1977: Acute posterior fossa epidural hematomas in children. Amer. J. Dis. Child. *131*, 690—692.
6. Arseni, C., Oprescu, I., 1972: Traumatologie Cranio-cerebrala. Editura Medicala Bucureşti.
7. Bartlett, J. R., Neil-Dwyer, G., 1979: Extradural haematoma: effect of delayed treatment. Brit. Med. J. *II*, no. 6187, 440—441.
8. Baumgartner, J., Woringer, E., Braun, J. P., Abara, M., Maistre, H., 1965: HED Diagnostique Angiographique. Neurochirurgie *11*, no. 3, 225—232.
9. Ben Hassine, K., 1971: Contribution à l'étude des HED occipitaux. Thèse médecine Lyon.
10. Besson, G., Leguyader, J., Bagot, D-arc, M., Garré, H., 1978: L'hématome extradural de la fosse postérieure. Problèmes diagnostiques (10 observations). Neurochirurgie *24*, 53—63.
11. Billet, R., 1959: L'aspect artériographique des épanchements extra-cérébraux précoces en Neuro-chirurgie d'urgence. Neurochirurgie *5*, 344—348.
12. Bonnal, J., 1951: Hématome chronique de la fosse postérieure. Revue Neurol. *85*, 439—443.
13. Borzone, M., Gentile, S., Perria, C., Rosa, M., Vertex epidural hematomas. Surg. Neurol. *11*, 277—284.

14. Bourhis, R., 1962: Contribution à l'étude clinique, radiologique, et théra-peuthique de l'HED traumatique (à propos de 177 cas). Thèse médecine Rennes.
15. Bullock, R., van Dellen, J. R., 1982: Chronic extradural hematoma. Surg. Neurol. *18*, 300—302.
16. Burres, K. P., Hamilton, R. D., 1979: Chronic extradural hematoma: case report. Neurosurgery *4*, 60—62.
17. Calbucci, F., Andreoli, A., Bollini, C., Frattarelli, M., Grossi, C., Munari, C., 1977: Extradural haematoma of the posterior fossa. Acta Neurochir. (Wien) *36*, 147.
18. Campbell, J. B., Cohen, J., 1951: Epidural haemorrhage and the skull of children. Surg. Gynec. Obstet. *92*, 257—280.
19. Campiche, R., 1962: Hématome épidural subaigu de localisation inhabituelle avec son image artériographique. Radiol. clin. *31*, 95—100.
20. Carcassonne, M., Choux, M., Grisoli, F., 1977: Extradural haematoma in infants. J. Pediatric Surg. *12*, 1 (69−73).
21. Carlsson, C. A., von Essen, C., Löfgren, J., 1968: Factors affecting the clinical course of patients with severe head injuries. Part 1: Influence of biological factors. Part 2: Significance of posttraumatic coma. J. Neurosurg. *29*, 242−251.
22. Cervantes, L. A., 1983: Concurrent delayed temporal and posterior fossa epidural hematomas. J. Neurosurg. *59*, 351−353.
23. Chodkiewicz, J. P., Creissard, P., Redondo, A., Vedrenne, C., 1972: Étude anatoma-clinique de 150 traumatismes crânio-encéphaliques. Neurochirurgie *18*, 77−86.
24. Choux, M., Grisoli, F., Peragut, J. C., 1975: Extradural haematoma in children. 104 cas. Child's Brain *1*, no. 6, 337−347.
25. Clavel, M., Onzain, I., Gutierez, P., 1982: Chronic epidural hematomas. Acta Neurochir. (Wien) *66*, 71−81.
26. Clifton, G. L., Grossman, R. G., Makela, M. E., *et al.,* 1980: Neurological course and correlated computerized tomography findings after severe closed head injury. J. Neurosurg. *51*, 611—624.
27. Columella, F., Delzanno, G. B., Nicola, G. C., 1959: L'ematoma epidurale al vertice. Sist. nerv. *2*, 104−118.
28. Columella, F., Gaist, G., Piazza, G., *et al.,* 1968: Extradural haematoma at the vertex. J. Neurol. Neurosurg. Psychiatry *31*, 315−320.
29. Cordobés, F., Lobato, R. D., Amor, T., *et al.,* 1980: Epidural haematoma of the posterior fossa with delayed operation. Report of a "chronic" case. Acta Neurochir. (Wien) *53*, 275−281.
30. Cordobés, F., Lobato, R. D., Rivas, J. J., *et al.,* 1981: Observations on 82 patients with extradural hematoma. Comparison of results before and after the advent of computerized tomography. J. Neurosurg. *54*, 179−186.
31. Cronqvist, S., Koher, R., 1963: Angiography in epidural haematoma. Acta Radiologica (Diag.) *1*, 42−52.
32. Cros, J., 1983: L'Hématome sous dural traumatique de l'adulte. Thèse médecine, Marseille.

33. Dahlstrom, L., Fagerberg, G., Lanner, L., Stattin, S., 1969: Anatomical and angiographic studies of arteries supplying anterior part of the temporal lobe Acta Radiol. (Diag.) *9*, 257.

34. Da Pian, R., Benati, A., Bricolo, A., Tomasi, A., Perbellini, D., dalle Ore, G., 1963: Ematomi extradurali traumatici del terzo medio del seno longitudinale superiore. Ospᴊdal. Ital. Chir. *8*, 667 − 676.

35. Dapian, R., dalle Ore, G., Bricolo, A., Benati, A., Buffatti, P., 1967: Ematomi extradurali traumatici considerazioni su 72 casi operati. Minerva Neurochirurgica *11*, no. 3 − 4, 181 − 186.

36. Davis, C. H. G., Nichols, R. W. T., 1980: Late diagnosis by computerized tomography of unsuspected extradural haematoma (letter). Lancet *2*, 416 − 417.

37. Dee, D., Woesney, M. E., Sanders, J., 1974: Frontal epidural hematoma. The angiographic diagnosis with a new finding. Amer. J. Roentgenol. *122* (3), 525 − 530.

38. Dettori, P., Giovanni, R., 1966: Angiographic technique and diagnosis in brain lacerations and extradural hematomas. Acta radiologica: Diagnosis *5*, 100 − 109.

39. Dolinskas, C., Zimmerman, R. A., Bilaniuk, L. T., Bruce, D., Uzell, H., 1978: The course of mass effect following surgical evacuation of extracerebral hematomas: computed tomographic demonstration. Neuroradiology *15*, 127, 68.

40. Duret, H., 1919: Traumatismes cranio-cérébraux. Félix Alcan édit.

41. Ericson, K., Håkansson, S., Löfgren, J., Zwetnow, N. N., 1978: Arteriovenous shunting—the basis pathophysiological mechanism in epidural hematoma. Acta Neurochir. (Wien) *42*, 257 − 258.

42. Ericson, K., Håkansson, S., Löfgren, J., Zwetnow, N. N., 1979: Extravasation and arteriovenous shunting after epidural bleeding—a radiological study. Neuroradiology *17*, 239 − 244.

43. Ericson, K., Håkansson, S., 1981: Computed tomography of epidural hematomas. Association with intracranial lesions and clinical correlation. Acta Radiol. (Diag.) *22*, 513 − 519.

44. Espagno, J., Manelfe, C., Bousigue, J. Y., *et al.,* 1980: Intérêt et valeur pronostique de la T.D.M. en traumatologie cranio-cérébrale. J. Neuroradiol. *70*, 121 − 132.

45. Fenelon, J., 1965: Contribution à l'étude des hématomes extra-duraux. Thèse Médecine Bordeaux, no. 119.

46. Ferris, E. J., Kirch, R., Shapiro, J. H., 1967: Epidural haematomas. Varied angiographic signs. Amer. J. Roentgenol. *101*, 100 − 106.

47. Ferris, E. J., Lehrer, H., Shapiro, J. H., 1967: Pseudosubdural hematoma. Radiology *88*, 75 − 84.

48. Fincher, E. J., 1951: Arteriovenous fistula between the middle meningeal artery and the greater petrosal sinus. Ann. Surg. *133*, 886 − 888.

49. Fisher, R. G., Kin, J. K., Sachs, E., Jr., 1958: Complications in posterior fossa due to occipital trauma; their operability. J.A.M.A. *167*, 176 − 182.

50. Ford, L. E., McLaurin, R. L., 1963: Mechanisms of extradural hematomas. J. Neurosurg. *20*, 760 − 769.

51. Frankhauser, H., Kiener, M., 1982: Delayed development of extra dural haematomas. Acta Neurochir. (Wien) 60, 29 – 35.

52. French, B. N., Dublin, A., 1977: The value of computerized tomography in the management of 1,000 consecutive head injuries. Surg. Neurol. 7, 171.

53. Freytag, E., 1963: Autopsy findings in head injuries from blunt force statistical evaluation of 1, 3, 6, 7 cases. Arch. Path. 75, 402 – 413.

54. Galbraith, S., Teasdale, G., 1981: Predicting the need for operation in the patient with an occult traumatic intracranial hematoma. J. Neurosurg. 55, 75 – 81.

55. Gallagher, J. P., Browder, E. J., 1968: Extradural hematoma. Experience with 167 patients. J. Neurosurg. 29, 1 – 12.

56. Galligioni, F., Bernardi, R., Pellone, M., Iraci, G., 1968: Angiographic signs of rupture of the middle meningeal artery without epidural hematoma. Amer. J. Roentgenol. 104, 71 – 74.

57. Gardeur, D., Metzger, J., 1982: Tomodensitometrie intracranienne. Livre IV: pathologie traumatique cranio-cérébrale, Vol. 1, p. 190. Ed. Marketing Paris.

58. Garza-Mercado, R., Rangel, R. A., 1979: Extradural hematoma associated with traumatic middle meningeal artery pseudoaneurysm: report of two cases. Neurosurgery 5, 500 – 503.

59. Garza-Mercado, R., 1983: Extradural hematoma of the posterior cranial fossa. J. Neurosurg. 59, 664 – 672.

60. Gentile, S. L., Gentilomo, A., Perria, L., Rossi, G. F., Viale, G., 1967: Su alcuni problemi di diagnostica angiographica nella patologia endocranica traumatica di interesse chirurgico. Minerva Neurochirurgica 11, 3, 4, 171.

61. Gerlach J., 1957: Erkennung, Behandlung und Prognose der intrakraniellen Blutungen und Hämatome. I. Einleitung und Epiduralhämatome. Med. Klin. 52, 1914 – 1916.

62. Giordano, C., Zito, F., 1981: Chronic evolution of an acute epidural haematoma. A case report. J. Neurosurg. Sci. 25, 109 – 111.

63. Glickman, M. G., Handel, F., Hoff, J. T., Coulson, W., 1976: Cerebral cortical arteries in the diagnosis of epidural hematoma. Neuroradiology 10 (4), 187 – 195.

64. Goodkin, R., Zahniser, J., 1978: Sequential angiographic studies demonstrating delayed development of an acute epidural hematoma. J. Neurosurg. 48, 479 – 482.

65. Goutelle, A., Lapras, Cl., Dechaume, J. P., Chadensson, O., 1970: Djordje-vitch, L'hématome extradural traumatique de l'enfant. Pédiatrie 25, 21 – 30.

66. Grant, W. T., 1944: Chronic extradural hematoma: Report of a case of hematoma in anterior cranial fossa. Bull. Los Angeles Neurol. Soc. 9, 156 – 162.

67. Grevsten, S., Pelletieri, L., 1982: Surgical decision in the treatment of extradural haematoma. Acta chirurg. Scand. 148, 97 – 102.

68. Grisoli, F., 1971: Contribution à l'étude des hématomes extra-duraux du nourrisson et de l'enfant (à propos de 86 observations). Thèse Médecine de Marseille.

69. Gros, C., Vlahovitch, B., Frerebeau, P., Ouakine, G., Aussilloux, C., Godlewski, G., 1967: Les hématomes extra-duraux atypiques. Critères diagnostiques. Montpellier chirurgical *XIII*, no. 5, 657 – 669.

70. Grusckiewicz, J., 1972: Ipsilateral exophthalmos in subfrontal epidural haematomas. J. Neurosurg. 613 – 615.

71. Gruszkiewicz, J., Platt, H., 1973: Subfrontal epidural hematomas. Neurochirurgica *16*, 54 – 59.

72. Gudeman, S. K., Kishore, P. R., Miller, J. D., *et al.*, 1979: The genesis and significance of delayed traumatic intracerebral hematoma. J. Neurosurg. *5*, 309 – 313.

73. Gudeman, S. K., Ward, J., Becker, D. P., 1982: Operative treatment in head injury. Clin. Neurosurg. *29*, 326 – 345.

74. Guillaume, J., Pecker, J., 1951: Une forme particulière d'épanchement traumatique intracrânien: l'Hématome basilaire. Presse Médicale *59*, 345 – 346.

75. Guillermain, P., Gomez, A., 1979: Les hématomes extraduraux traumatiques. Livre jubilaire en hommage au Pr. J. E. Paillas, Marseille, 153 – 182.

76. Guillermain, P., Lena, G., Reynier, Y., *et al.*, 1982: Les hématomes intracérébraux post traumatiques: à propos de 38 cas. Neurochirurgie *28*, 309 – 314.

77. Gurdjian, E. S., Webster, J. E., 1958: Head injuries, mechanisms, diagnosis and management, p. 482. Boston: Little Brown Ed.

78. Gutterman, P., Shenkin, H. A., 1970: Prognostic features in recovery from traumatic decerebration. J. Neurosurg. *32*, 330 – 335.

79. Habash, A. H., Sortland, Q., Zwetnow, N. N., 1982: Epidural hematoma pathophysiological significance of extravasation and arteriovenous shunting. An analysis of 35 patients. Acta Neurochir. (Wien) *60*, 7 – 27.

80. Håkansson, S., Löfgren, J., Zwetnow, N. N., 1977: The intracranial pressure course in experimental epidural haemorrhage. Acta Neurochir. (Wien) *37*, 294 – 295.

81. Handa, J., Handa, H., Nakano, Y., 1979: Rim enhancement in computed tomography with chronic epidural hematoma. Surg. Neurol. *11*, 217 – 220.

82. Hawkes, C. D., Ogle, W. S., 1962: Atypical features of epidural hematoma in infants, children, and adolescents. J. Neurosurg. *19*, 971 – 980.

83. Heiskanen, O., 1975: Epidural hematoma. Surg. Neurol. *4* (1), 23 – 26.

84. Heiskanen, O., Sipponen, P., 1970: Prognosis of severe brain injury. Acta Neurol. Scand. *46*, 343 – 348.

85. Helmer, F. A., Sukoff, M. H., Plaut, M. R., 1968: Angiographic extravasation of contrast medium in an epidural hematoma. Case report. J. Neurosurg. *29*, 652 – 654.

86. Heyser, J., Weber, G., 1964: Die epiduralen Hämatome. Schweiz. Med. Wschr. *94*, 1 (2 – 3), 2 (46 – 52).

87. Higazi, I., El-Banhawy, A., El-Nady, F., 1969: Importance of angiography in identifying false aneurysm of the middle meningeal artery as a cause of extradural hematoma. Case report. J. Neurosurg. *30*, 172 – 176.

88. Hirsch, J. F., David, M., Borne, G., 1962: Un signe angiographique des

hématomes extra duraux (le décollement de l'artère méningée moyenne). Neurochirurgie 5, 91 – 99.

89. Hirsh, L. F., 1980: Chronic epidural hematomas. Neurosurgery 6, 508 – 512.

90. Hooper, R. S., 1954: Extradural hematoma of the posterior fossa. Brit. J. Surg. 42, 19 – 26.

91. Hooper, R., 1959: Observations an extradural haemorrhage. Brit. J. Surg. 47, 71 – 87.

92. Huber, P., 1962: Die Verletzung der Meningealfasern beim epiduralen Hämatom im Angiogramm. Fortschr. Gb. Röntgenstr. 96, 207 – 220.

93. Huber, P., 1964: Zerebrale Angiographie beim frischen Schädel-Hirntrauma. Stuttgart: G. Thieme.

94. Illingworth, R., Shawdon, H., 1983: Conservative management of intracranial extradural haematoma presenting late. J. Neurol. Neurosurg. Psychiat. 46, 558 – 560.

95. Imler, R. L., Jr., Skultety, F. M., 1954: Subacute extradural hematomas. Ann. Surg. 140, 194 – 196.

96. Ishii, R., Ueki, K., Ito, J., 1976: Traumatic fistula between a lacerated middle meningeal artery and a diploic vein. J. Neurosurg. 44, 241 – 244.

97. Iwakuma, T., Brunngraber, C. V., 1973: Chronic extradural hematomas. A study of 21 cases. J. Neurosurg. 38, 488 – 493.

98. Iwata, K., 1964: Sagittal sinus hematoma. Angiographic demonstration and clinical pathology. Pac. Med. Surg. 72, 340 – 342.

99. Jackson, I. J., Speakman, T. J., 1950: Chronic extradural hematoma. J. Neurosurg. 7, 444 – 447.

100. Jackson, D. C., du Boulay, G. H., 1964: Traumatic arteriovenous aneurysm of the middle meningeal artery. Brit. J. Radiol. 37, 788 – 789.

101. Jamieson, K. G., Yelland, J. D. N., 1968: Extradural hematoma. Report of 167 cases. J. Neurosurg. 29, 13 – 23.

102. Jane, J. A., Rimel, R. W., 1982: Prognosis in head injury. Clin. Neurosurg. 29, 346 – 352.

103. Jennett, B., Carlin, J., 1978: Preventable mortality and morbidity after head injury. Injury 10, 31 – 39.

104. Jennett, B., Teasdale, G., Braakman, R., et al., 1979: Prognosis of patients with severe head injury. Neurosurgery 4, 283 – 289.

105. Jonker, C., Oosterhuis, H. J., 1975: Epidural hematoma. A retrospective study of 100 patients. Clin. Neurol. Neurosurg. 78 (4), 233 – 245.

106. Josephson, S., 1962: Epidural haematoma a 10 year series. Acta chir. Scand. 124, 26 – 35.

107. Khatib, R., Cook, A. W., Sparacio, R. R., 1967: Mortality in epidural hematoma. Surg. Gynec. Obstet. 125, 591 – 594.

108. Khatib, R., Gannon, W. E., Cook, A. W., 1968: Cerebral angiography in supratentorial epidural hematoma. N.Y. State J. Med. 68, 2547 – 2549.

109. Koch, R. L., Glickman, M. G., 1971: The angiographic diagnosis of extradural haematoma of posterior fossa. Amer. J. Roentgenol. 112, 2, 289 – 295.

110. Koo, A. H., Laroque, A. L., 1977: Evaluation of head trauma by computed tomography. Radiology 123, 345 – 350.

111. Kothandaram, P., Shetty, K. R., 1979: Delayed extradural haematoma. Review of 10 cases. Acta Neurochir. (Wien) *46*, 176.
112. Koulouris, S., Rizzoli, H. V., 1980: Acute bilateral extradural hematoma: Case report. Neurosurgery *7*, 608–610.
113. Krayenbühl, H., Yaşargil, M. G., 1965: Die zerebrale Angiographie, 2. Aufl. Stuttgart: Thieme.
114. Kretschmer, H., 1981: Verlaufsdynamik und Frühprognose traumatischer intrakranieller Blutungen: 1. Epidurale Hämatome. Aktuel. Traumatol. *11*, 1, 17–23.
115. Kuhn, R. A., Kugler, H., 1964: False aneurysms of the middle meningeal artery. J. Neurosurg. *21*, 92–96.
116. Kushner, M. J., Luken, M. G., 1983: Posterior fossa epidural hematoma. Neuroradiology *24*, 169–171.
117. Kvarnes, T. L., Trumpy, J. H., 1978: Extradural hematoma. Report of 132 cases. Acta Neurochir. (Wien) *41*, 223–231.
118. Lanksch, W., Grumme, Th., Kazner, E., 1979: Computed tomography in head injuries, pp. 17–21. Berlin-Heidelberg-New York: Springer.
119. Larghero, P., 1955: Hématomes intra-crâniens d'origine traumatique. Paris: Masson et Cie.
120. Lazorthes, G., 1952: Les hémorragies intra-crâniennes traumatiques spontanées et du 1er âge, p. 1 (256). Paris: Masson et Cie.
121. Lebeau, J., Gruner, J., Minuit, P., 1955: Remarque sur une série de 400 traumatismes crâniocérébraux graves. Neurochirurgie *1*, 117–126.
122. Lebeau, T., Feld, M., Tavernier, J. B., 1959: L'angiographie cérébrale dans les traumatismes crâniens cérébraux fermés. E.M.C.: neurologie 17585 (6.10).
123. Leclercq, I. A., Rozycki, T., 1979: Chronic calcified epidural hematoma in a child. RI Med. J. *62*, 97–99.
124. Lecount, E. R., Apfelbach, C. W., 1920: Pathological anatomy of traumatic fractures of cranial bones and concomittant brain injuries. J.A.M.A. *74*, 501–511.
125. Lecuire, J., Lapras, A., Goutelle, A., Gacon, G., Dechaume, J. P., 1967: Les hématomes extra-duraux préfontaux à propos 18 observations. Neurochirurgie *13*, no. 3, 431–443, 9.
126. Leguyader, J., Besson, G., Blain, F., 1980: Aspects angiographiques des hématomes extra-duraux de la fosse postérieure. SEM. Hop. Paris *56*, 837–841.
127. Levander, B., Stattin, S., Svendsen, P., 1975: Computer tomography of traumatic intra- and extracerebral lesions. Acta Radiol. (suppl. 346), 1–7.
128. Levy, A., 1980: Contribution à l'étude des H.E.D. post-traumatiques. A propos de 507 observations. Thèse Médecine Marseille.
129. Liliequist, B., 1967: Roentgenologic appearances of traumatic lesions of middle meningeal artery. Acta Radiol. *6*, 513–518.
130. Lindgren, E., 1954: Röntgenologie. In: Handbuch der Neurochirurgie, Zweiter Band (Olivecrona, H., Tönis, W., eds.), p. 221. Berlin-Göttingen-Heidelberg: Springer.
131. Loew, F., Wuestner, S., 1960: Diagnose, Behandlung und Prognose der

traumatischen Hämatome des Schädelinneren. Acta Neurochir. (Wien), (Suppl. 8).

132. Löfgren, J., Zwetnow, N. N., 1972: Experimental studies on the dynamic course of intracranial arterial bleeding. Acta neurol. scand. *48*, 252.

133. McKissock, W., Taylor, J. C., Bloom, W. H., *et al.,* 1960: Extradural haematoma. Observations on 125 cases. Lancet *2*, 167−172.

134. McLaurin, R. L., Ford, L. E., 1964: Extradural hematoma. Statistical survey of 47 cases. J. Neurosurg. *21*, 364−371.

135. MacRea, D. L., 1966: The role of radiology in the management of the head injuried patient. "Head injury" conference proceedings. Caveness and Walker Ed. (1.6).

136. Mansuy, L., Lecuire, T., 1955: Les traumatismes crânio-cérébraux fermés récents. Paris: Masson Ed. (122).

137. Marshal, L. F., Bowers, S. A., 1982: Medical management of head injury. Clin. Neurosurg. *29*, 312−325.

138. Mathur, P. P., Dharker, S. R., 1980: Fluid chronic extradural haematoma. Surg. Neurol. *14*, 81−82.

139. Matwijecky, C., Steinbol, P., 1982: Hemianopsia: a presenting feature of acute epidural hematomas. Neurosurgery *11*, 247−249.

140. Mazza, C., Pasqualin, A., *et al.,* 1982: Traumatic extradural haematomas in children; experience with 62 cases. Acta Neurochir. (Wien) *65*, 67−80.

141. Mealey, X., 1960: Acute extra dural hematomas without demonstrable skull fractures J. Neurosurg. *17*, 27−34.

142. Mendelow, A. D., Karmi, M., Paul, K., *et al.,* 1979: The importance of immediate surgery in patients with extradural haematoma. Acta Neurochir. (Wien) *46*, 174.

143. Merino de Villasante, J., Taveras, J. M., 1976: Computerized tomography (C.T.) in acute head trauma. Amer. J. Roentgenol. *126*, 765−778.

144. Miller, J. D., Butterworth, J. F., Gudeman, S. K., *et al.,* 1981: Further experience in the management of severe head injury. J. Neurosurg. *54*, 289−299.

145. Moris, I. S., King, R. B., 1973: Extravasation of angiographic contrast material from a torn middle meningeal artery into the dipliae. J. Neurosurg. *38*, 89−91.

146. Morley, J. B., Langford, K. H., 1970: Abnormal brain scan with subacute extradural haematomas. J. Neurol. Neurosurg. Psychiatry *33*, 679−686.

147. Munro, D., Maltby, G. L., 1941: Extradural hemorrhage. A study of forty-four cases. Ann. Surg. *113*, 192−203.

148. Nakazawa, S., Yamakawa, K., 1981: Traumatic posterior fossa epidural hematoma. Neurol. Surg. *9*, 3 (401, 406).

149. Nicola, N., Dietrich, U., Seibert, H. K., 1981: Value of computerized tomography in setting the indication for surgical treatment of extradural haematomas with a delayed course (abstract). Acta Neurochir. (Wien) *56*, 255.

150. Nielsen, S., Voldby, B., 1977: Epidural haematomas during 30 years. Acta Neurochir. (Wien) *37*, 294.

151. Nora, P. F., Rosenbluth, P. R., 1957: Chronic extradural hematoma. Amer. J. Surg. *94*, 628–631.
152. Norman, O., 1956: Angiographie différenciation between acute and chronic sub dural and extra dural haematomas. Acta Radiologica *46*, (1), 2 (379).
153. Omar, M. M., Binet, E. F., 1978: Peripheral contrast enhancement in chronic epidural hematomas. J. Comput. Assist. Tomogr. *2*, 332–335.
154. Ommaya, A. K., Grubb, R. L., Naumann, R. A., 1971: Coup and contre-coup injury: observations on the mechanics of visible brain injuries in the Rhesus monkey. J. Neurosurg. *35*, 503–516.
155. Pagni, C. A., 1973: The prognosis of head injured patients in a state of coma with decerebrated posture. J. Neurosurg. Sci. *17*, 289–294.
156. Paillas, J. E., Sedan, R., 1959: Les formes atypiques des hématomes extraduraux. Marseille chirurgical *11*, no. 3, 370–373.
157. Paillas, J. E., Bonnal, J., Lavieille, J., 1964: Angiographic images of false aneurysmal sac caused by rupture of median meningeal artery in the course of traumatic extradural hematomata. Report of 3 cases. J. Neurosurg. *21*, 667–671.
158. Palmieri, A., 1981: Extravasation of contrast enhanced blood in epidural hematoma. Neuroradiology *21*, 163–164.
159. Pang, D., Horton, J. A., Herron, J. M., *et al.*, 1983: Non surgical management of extradural hematomas in children. J. Neurosurg. *9*, 958–971.
160. Parkinson, D., Reddy, V., Taylor, J., 1980: Ossified epidural hematoma: case report. Neurosurgery *7*, 171–173.
161. Pazzaglia, P., Frank, G., Frank, F., *et al.*, 1975: Clinical course and prognosis of acute post-traumatic coma. J. Neurol. Neurosurg. Psychiatry *38*, 149–154.
162. Pecker, J., Javallet, Lemen, N. G., 1959: L'HED. Réflexion sur une série de 111 cas personnels. Neurochirurgie *51*, 428–449.
163. Pellet, W., Vittoni, F., Dufour, M., Paillas, J. E., 1971: Visualisation artériographique de la fuite vasculaire lors des hématomes juxta-duraux traumatiques. Sem. Hop. Paris *47*, 935–943.
164. Perini, S., Maschio, A., Beltramello, A., Benati, A., Bricolo, A., 1978: The role of computed tomography in the diagnosis and management of head injuries. Review of 442 cases. J. Neurosurg. Sci. *22*, 51–62.
165. Petit-Dutaillis, D., Pertuiset, B., Verley, R., 1955: Les hématomes extraduraux subaigus. Neurochirurgie *1*, 321–323.
166. Phonprasert, C., Suwanwela, C., Hongsaprabhas, C., Prichayudh, P., O'Charoen, S., 1980: Extradural hematoma: Analysis of 138 cases. J. Trauma *20*, 679–683.
167. Pierron, D., George, B., Ouahes, O., *et al.*, 1981: Tomodensitometrie et hématomes intracraniens post-traumatiques sans manifestation clinique. Neurochirurg. *27*, 4, 213–216.
168. Pouyanne, H., Salles, M., Leman, P., Fenelon, J., 1965: L'hématome extradural. Samii Edit. Bordeaux, 175.
169. Pozzati, E., Frank, F., Frank, G., *et al.*, 1980: Subacute and chronic extradural hematomas: a study of 30 cases. J. Trauma *20*, 795–799.

170. Punt, J., 1978: Chronic extradural hematoma presenting 33 years after penetrating cranial trauma. Case report. J. Neurosurg. *49*, 103 – 106.

171. Queloz, J. M., 1967: L'Hematome epidural infantile. Thèse Médecine Genève.

172. Rakotobe, A., 1964: Considérations sur les suites éloignées des hématomes juxta-duraux opérés. Thése médecine Marseille.

173. Rappaport, Z. H., Shaked, I., 1982: Delayed epidural hematoma demonstrated by computed tomography: case report. Neurosurgery *10*, 487 – 489.

174. Reight, E. E., O'Connell, T. J., 1962: Extradural hematoma of the posterior fossa with concomitant supratentorial subdural hematoma. Report of a case and review of the literature. J. Neurosurg. *19*, 359 – 364.

175. Reulen, H. J., Schurman, K., 1981: Nonsurgical management of severe head injury Prog. Neurol. Surg. vol. 10, p. 291 – 322. Basel: Karger.

176. Rieth, K. G., Schwartz, F. T., Davis, D. O., 1979: Acute isodense epidural hematoma on computed tomography. J. Comput. Assist. Tomogr. *3*, 691 – 693.

177. Roberson, F. C., Kishore, P. R. S., Miller, J. D., Lipper, M. H., Becker, D. P., 1979: The value of serial computerized tomography in the management of severe head injury. Surg. Neurol. *12*, 161 – 167.

178. Robertson, J. H., Clark, W. C., 1982: Bilateral occipital epidural hematomas. Surg. Neurol. *17*, 468 – 472.

179. Romano, A., Walzer, I., 1983: Ipsilateral exophthalmos due to subfrontal epidural hematoma. Surg. Neurol. *19*, 77 – 79.

180. Rowbothan, G. F., 1949: Acute injuries of the head. Edinburgh: E. S. Livingstone.

181. Rowbotham, G. F., Whalley, N., 1952: Prolonged compression of the brain resulting from an extradural haemorrhage. J. Neurol. Neurosurg. Psychiat. *15*, 64 – 65.

182. Rumbaugh, C. L., Bergeron, R. T., Kurze, T., 1972: Intracranial vascular damage associated with skull fractures. Radiology *104*, 81 – 87.

183. Saba, M. I., King, R. B., 1973: Extravasation of angiographic contrast material from a torn middle meningeal artery into the diploi. J. Neurosurg. *38*, 89 – 91.

184. Saeki, N., Hinokuma, K., Uemura, K., *et al.,* 1979: Subacute bilateral epidural hematomas in an infant. Surg. Neurol. *11*, 67 – 69.

185. Schechter, M. M., Zingesser, L. H., Rayport, M., 1966: Torn meningeal vessels: An evaluation of a clinical spectrum through the use of angiography. Radiology *86*, 686 – 695.

186. Schechter, M. M., 1966: Angiography in head trauma. Clin. Neurosurg. *12*, 193 – 225.

187. Schorstein, J., 1944: Intracranial haematoma in missile wounds. In: Cairns, H. (ed.): Brit. J. Surgery, War Supplement, no. 1, pp. 96 – 111. Bristol: John Wright.

188. Sicat, L. C., Brinker, R. A., Abad, R. M., Rouit, R. L., 1975: Traumatic pseudoaneurysm and arteriovenous fistula involving middle meningeal artery. Surg. Neurol. *3*, 97 – 103.

189. Sichez, J. P., Melon, E., Metzger, J., 1981: Intérêt de la tomodensitométrie dans le diagnostic lesionnel et la surveillance précoce des traumatisés dans le coma. Nelle Presse Med. *10*, 971−973.

190. Sparacio, R. R., Khatib, R., Chiu, J., *et al.*, 1972: Chronic epidural hematoma. J. Trauma *12*, 435−439.

191. Stevenson, G. C., Brown, H. A., Hoyt, W. E., 1964: Chronic venous epidural hematoma at the vertex. J. Neurosurg. *21*, 887−891.

192. Stone, J. L., Schaffer, L., Ramsey, R. G., Moody, R. A., 1979: Epidural hematomas of the posterior fossa. Surg. Neurol. *11*, 419−424.

193. Stroobandt, G., 1963: L'HED préfrontal, étude d'une série personnelle. Acta Neurol. Psych. Belg. *63*, 569−576.

194. Svendsen, V., 1972: Epidural hematoma in children. Excerpta Medica Neurol. Neurosurg. *25*, no. 2627, 462−463.

195. Szapiro, J., Jagodzinski, Z., Wiervszewska, A., Lebski, J., 1968: Symptomes trompeurs dans les hématomes intra-crâniens post-traumatiques. Acta Neurochir. (Wien) *19*, 32.

196. Tawfik, M. E., 1976: Subacute extradural haematoma. J. Egypt. Med. Assoc. *59*, 551−556.

197. Teasdale, G., Galbraith, S., Jennett, B., 1976: Traumatic intracranial haematomas—detection, prognosis and management. J. Neurol. Neurosurg. Psychiat. *39*, 918.

198. Teasdale, G., Galbraith, S., 1979: Extradural haematoma: effect of delayed treatment. Brit. Med. J. *i*, 1793.

199. Teasdale, G., Galbraith, S., 1981: Acute traumatic intracranial hematomas. Progr. Neurol. *10*, 252−290.

200. Trowbridge, W. V., Porter, R. W., French, J. D., 1954: Chronic extradural hematomas. Arch. Surg. Chicago *69*, 824−830.

201. Tsai, F. Y., Huprich, J. E., 1978: Further experience with contrast enhanced CT in head trauma. Neuroradiology *16*, 314−317.

202. Tsai, F. Y., Teal, J. S., Itabashi, H. H., 1980: CT of posterior fossa trauma. J. comp. Asst. tomog. *4*, 201−305.

203. Turazzi, S., Alexandre, A., Bricolo, A., 1975: Incidence and significance of clinical signs of brain stem traumatic lesions. Study of 2,600 head injured patients. J. Neurosurg. Sci. *19*, 215−222.

204. Vance, B. M., 1927: Fractures of the skull, complications and causes of death. A review of 512 necropsis and of 61 cases studical clinically. Arch. Surg. *14*, 1023−1092.

205. Van Dongen, K., Braakman, R., 1981: Computed tomographies in head injury. Progr. Neurol. Surg. *10*, 198.

206. Vapalathi, M., Troupp, H., 1971: Prognosis for patients with severe brain injuries. Brit. Med. J. *3*, 404−407.

207. Vigouroux, R., Sedan, R., Choux, M., Baurand, C., 1963: Les hématomes extraduraux frontaux post-traumatiques. Neurochirurgie *9*, no. 2, 197−218.

208. Vigouroux, R. P., Choux, M., Baurand, C., Naquet, R., Guillermain, P., Guidicelli, G., 1969: Les hématomes extra-duraux occipitaux post-traumatiques. Neurochirurgie *15*, 91−106.

209. Vigouroux, R. P., Baurand, C., Gomez, A., et al., 1976: Intérêt de la tomographie axiale commandee par ordinateur (tacographie) dans les traumatismes craniocérébraux. Neuro-chirurgie 22, no. 3, 281–291.

210. Vigouroux, R. P., Guillermain, P., Gomez, A., 1979: Étude d'une série de 400 hématomas extra-duraux. Conférence internationale de Neurotraumatologie lors du XVIIIe Congresso latino-americano de Neurocirurgia, Buenos Aires.

211. Vigouroux, R. P., Guillermain, P., 1981: Post-traumatic hemispheric contusion and laceration. Progr. Neurol. Surg. 10, 49–163.

212. Vigouroux, R. P., Guillermain, P., Diaz-Vasquez, P., 1982: Traumatismes craniens chez le sujet du 3ème âge. Société de Médecine du Trafic-Lille.

213. De Vries, J., Wattendorff, A. R., Hekster, R. E. M., 1981: Chronic epidural haematoma with partial rim enhancement. A case report. Neuroradiology 22, 167–168.

214. Wackenheim, A., 1962: Le diagnostic radiologique des lésions traumatiques intracrâniennes. Strasbourg Méd. 13, 311–394.

215. Weaver, D., Pobereskin, L., Jane, J. A., 1981: Spontaneous resolution of epidural hematomas. Report of two cases. J. Neurosurg. 54, 248–251.

216. Weinman, D. F., Jayamane, D., 1966: The role of angiography in the diagnosis of extra-dural haematomas. Brit. J. Radiol. 39, 350–357.

217. Weinman, D. E., Muttukumaru, B., 1968: The mortality from extradural haematoma. Aust. NZ J. Surg. 38, 104–107.

218. Wertheimer, P., Levy, A., Lapras, C., Tunisi, G., 1958: Les aspects angiographiques des épanchements intra-crâniens traumatiques. Lyon chirurgical 54/4, 481.

219. Wilson, C. B., Cronic, F., 1964: Traumatic arteriovenous fistulas involving middle meningeal vessels. J.A.M.A. 188, 953–957.

220. Winter, T. O., Glickman, M. G., 1975: The lateral angiogram in the differentiation of extracerebral hematomas. Radiology 116, 3, 661–666.

221. Wright, R. L., 1966: Traumatic hematomas of the posterior cranial fossa. J. Neurosurg. 25, 402–409.

222. Young, T. W., 1972: Chronic extradural hematoma. Brit. J. Chir. Pract. 26, 38–41.

223. Zander, E., Campiche, R., 1974: Extra-dural hematoma. In: Advances and Technical Standards in Neurosurgery, Vol. 1 (Krayenbühl, H., et al., eds.), pp. 121–139. Wien-New York: Springer.

224. Zimmerman, R. A., Bilaniuk, L. T., 1982: Computed tomographic staging of traumatic epidural bleeding. Radiology 144, 809–812.

225. Zingesser, L. H., Schechter, M. M., Rayport, M., 1965: Truths and untruths concerning the angiographic findings in extradural haematomas. Brit. J. Radiol. 38, 835–847.

226. Zuccarello, M., Pardatscher, K., Andrioli, G. C., et al., 1981: Epidural hematomas of the posterior cranial fossa. Neurosurgery 8, 434–437.

227. Zuccarello, M., Fiore, D. L., Trincia, et al., 1982: Epidural haematoma at the vertex. Acta Neurochir. (Wien) 66, 195–206.

228. Zuccarello, M., Fiore, D. L., Trincia, G., Andrioli, G. C., 1982: Extradural Hematoma: statistical analysis of 413 cases. Advances in Neurotraumatology. Milano abstracts, 49.
229. Zuccarello, M., Fiore, D. L., Pardatsche, K., et al., 1983: Chronic extradural haematomas. Acta Neurochir. (Wien) 67, 57–66.
230. Zwetnow, N. N., Habash, A. H., et al., 1983: Comparative analysis of experimental epidural and subarachnoid bleeding in dogs. Acta Neurochir. (Wien) 67, 67–101.

# Acute Subdural Hematomas

D. P. Becker

Division of Neurosurgery, Department of Surgery, University of California
Los Angeles School of Medicine, Los Angeles, California (U.S.A.)

With 18 Figures

## Contents

## Introduction and General Principles

Acute subdural hematoma (ASDH) is a common occurrence following severe head injury. Early diagnosis and rapidly executed treatment for acute subdural hematomas strikingly improve outcome. It is a misconception that an operation is rarely necessary in head injury. In most large series of patients with severe head injury, *i.e.,* patients unable to speak or follow commands, the incidence of intracranial mass lesions treated operatively is in the range of 40 to 60% (Becker *et al.* 1977, Jennett *et al.* 1976, Pagni 1973, Pazzaglia *et al.* 1979, Rossanda *et al.* 1973). In close to half of patients requiring operation, the primary diagnosis is acute subdural hematoma. Untreated, these lesions give rise to an extremely high mortality rate. It follows that neurological surgeons should be actively involved in the critical management of these patients, or at least readily available. Since an emergency operation is often required in the care of a patient with severe brain injury, the surgeon should have a working knowledge of all aspects of the operative techniques required for treating head injury (Becker *et al.* 1982).

An understanding of the causes of death and morbidity in head injury is a prerequisite for providing proper patient care. After a head injury, patients who die usually do so for one of three reasons: prolonged apnea at the scene of the accident; severe uncontrolled intracranial hypertension; or an undesirable systemic medical event (myocardial infarction, pneumonia, sepsis, blood loss, or the like). Morbidity also is the result of these secondary concomitants of trauma (Becker *et al.* 1982).

Patients who develop an acute subdural hematoma almost always have had a major underlying brain injury. The amount of brain movement required to cause a brain surface contusion which bleeds into the subdural space, or to lacerate a bridging vein usually also causes diffuse neuronal and axonal injury extending throughout the neuraxis. This underlying primary brain injury is exclusive of the mass lesion effect, brain shift and elevated intracranial pressure that result from the subdural blood accumulation. But it is important to know that many of the underlying brain-injured cells have the potential for recovery—that is, they have not been disrupted and destroyed. They are in a precarious dysfunctional state, more vulnerable than normal cells to a second insult such as ischemia brought on by arterial hypotension or elevated intracranial pressure and brain shift or hypoxemia from respiratory insufficiency (Jenkins *et al.* 1984, Mauls Conference). To give the injured brain the best possible environment to heal, one must prevent elevated intracranial pressure or brain compression from causing a secondary brain injury. Therefore, early evacuation of extracerebral masses is advocated and there is strong evidence that this is indeed beneficial (Seelig *et al.* 1981).

**Prognosis**

The mortality rate reported in comatose patients with traumatic ASDH has been appallingly high: 60 to 90% (Browder 1943, Cooper *et al.* 1976, Gutterman and Shenkin 1970, Harris 1971, Ransohoff *et al.* 1971, Richards and Hoff 1974, Talalla and Morin 1971). The ASDH is usually accompanied by associated primary brain damage and the high mortality has previously been ascribed to this (Chambers 1951, Cooper *et al.* 1976). This belief has fostered a fatalistic attitude among many physicians and has

Table 1. *Reported Studies of Acute Subdural Hematoma in Comatose Patients*[88]

| Series (year) | Number of patients | Mortality | Functional recovery % |
|---|---|---|---|
| Browder (1943) | 51 | 82 | — |
| McLaurin and Tutor (1961) | 74 | 73 | 16 |
| Gutterman and Shenkin (1970) | 14 | 65 | 35 |
| Ransohoff *et al.* (1971) | 35 | 60 | 28 |
| Jamieson and Yelland (1972) | 207 | 63 | — |
| Richards and Hoff (1974) | 100 | 75 | 14 |
| Cooper *et al.* (1976) | 50 | 90 | 4 |
| Bricolo and Turazzi (1980)* | 94 | 67 | 26 |
| Seelig and Becker (1981) | 82 | 57 | 34 |

* Bricolo, A., Turazzi, S.: Personal communication, June, 1980.

frustrated modern neurosurgery in its attempts to deal effectively with the problem (Seelig *et al.* 1981).

A few studies (Becker *et al.* 1977, Chambers 1951, Gutterman and Shenkin 1970, Rose *et al.* 1977, Shigemori *et al.* 1979) have suggested that prompt surgical evacuation of the traumatic ASDH might reduce this high mortality rate, as has been the experience with epidural hematomas (Mendelow *et al.* 1979). Earlier investigators (Browder 1943, Jamieson and Yelland 1972, McLaurin and Tutor 1961, Rosenbluth *et al.* 1962, Talalla and Morin 1971) reported that comatose patients with an ASDH who had the operation within 24 hours of injury had a very high mortality rate. According to Browder (1943) and Cooper (1976), little progress had been made in recent times to improve the mortality rate of more than 80% observed in patients with ASDH.

In 1981, the Richmond Head Injury group reported a major mortality reduction in comatose patients with acute subdural hematoma when the hematoma was evacuated within four hours of injury. The overall mortality rate in 82 patients with ASDH was 57%, with good to moderate recoveries in 34% (Seelig *et al.* 1981). These data compared favorably with the results of other investigators (Browder 1943, Cooper *et al.* 1976, Gutterman and

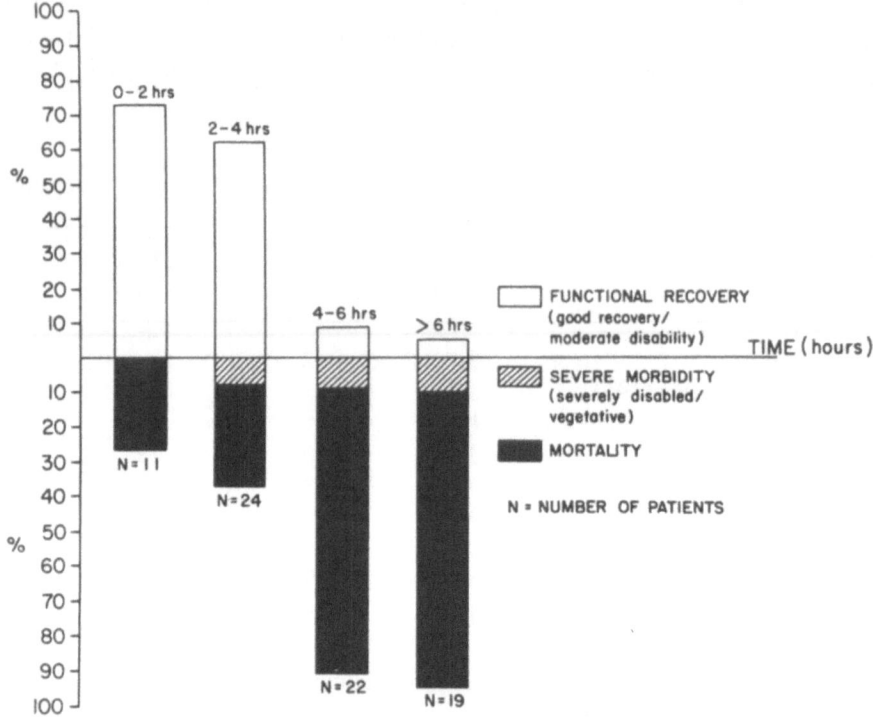

Fig. 1. Influence of time relay from injury to surgical intervention on outcome in 76 patients with acute subdural hematoma. There was a significant increase in mortality when the delay exceeded four hours (p < 0.0001). The range of time delay in the group who underwent surgery more than six hours after injury was 6.2 to 18.3 hours. (From Seelig *et al.* 1981. Reprinted by permission)

Shenkin 1970, Jamieson and Yelland 1972, McLaurin and Tutor 1971, Ransohoff *et al.* 1971) (Table 1).

Of most practical importance was the finding that comatose patients with ASDH who underwent rapid surgical decompression (within four hours of injury) had decreased mortality: 30% (Fig. 1). The mortality rate of 30% in patients with ASDH treated within four hours approaches the rate of 29% in patients with other severe head injuries who do not have a subdural hematoma (Table 2). Thus, rapid transport to a hospital that is capable of providing prompt diagnosis and surgical decompression within

Table 2. *Variables Influencing Outcome in Acute Subdural Hematoma (ASDH) as Compared with all Other Severe Head Injuries (from Seelig, Becker, Miller et al., Richmond Series)*[88]

| Variable | Severe head injuries excluding ASDH | ASDH | Significance of difference* |
|---|---|---|---|
| Number of patients | 284 | 82 | — |
| Age (year) | 26 | 41 | $p < 0.01$ |
| Sex (%) | | | |
|   Male | 76 | 75 | NS |
|   Female | 24 | 25 | NS |
| Mortality (%) | 29 | 57 | $p < 0.0001$ |
| Severe morbidity | | | |
|   (severe disability/vegetative) (%) | 9 | 9 | NS |
| Functional recovery | | | |
|   (good recovery/moderate disabilty) (%) | 62 | 34 | $p < 0.0001$ |
| Mode of injury | | | |
|   (vehicular accident) (%) | 79 | 55 | $p < 0.0001$ |
| Postoperative intracranial pressure (%) | | | |
|   < 20 mm Hg | 59 | 53 | NS |
|   Uncontrollable | 15 | 24 | NS |
| Initial neurologic examination (%) | | | |
|   Bilaterally absent pupillary light reflexes | 29 | 45 | $p < 0.01$ |
|   Absent or impaired oculomotor function | 33 | 60 | $p < 0.0001$ |
|   Decerebrate or flaccid | 32 | 47 | $p < 0.02$ |
| Time from injury to surgical decompression | | | |
|   Number of patients | 47** | 76*** | — |
|   Mean time lapse | $326 \pm 34.1$ | $325 \pm 27.3$ | NS |

  * NS denotes not significant.

  ** Forty-seven of the 61 craniotomies performed for intracerebral hemorrhage contusions or epidural hematoma. In 14 patients, the period between injury and surgical decompression could not be determined.

  *** Seventy-six of the 82 patients with ASDH. In six patients, the onset of injury could not be determined.

four hours of the injury will substantially reduce mortality in patients with traumatic ASDH. Since ASDH develops in approximately 25% of patients who are admitted while comatose from head injury, this information is critically important for rescue squads, emergency-room physicians, and

Table 3. *Comparison of Variables Influencing Outcome in Acute Subdural Hematoma (from Seelig, Becker, Miller et al., Richmond Series)*[88]

| Variable | Death | Functional recovery | Significance of difference* |
|---|---|---|---|
| Number of patients | 47 | 28 | — |
| Age (year) | 41 | 41 | NS |
| Sex (%) | | | |
|   Male | 85 | 54 | $p < 0.01$ |
|   Female | 15 | 46 | $p < 0.01$ |
| Mode of injury | | | |
|   (vehicular accident) (%) | 62 | 43 | NS |
| Postoperative intracranial pressure (%) | | | |
|   < 20 mm Hg | 30 | 79 | $p < 0.001$ |
|   Uncontrollable | 43 | 0 | $p < 0.0001$ |
| Cerebral contusion or hematoma (%) | | | |
|   Present | 67 | 53 | NS |
|   Absent | 33 | 47 | NS |
| Multimodality evoked potentials (number of patients) | | | |
|   Normal | 4 | 19 | $p < 0.001$ |
|   Abnormal | 15 | 0 | |
| Initial neurologic examination (%) | | | |
|   Bilaterally absent pupillary light reflexes | 57 | 25 | $p < 0.02$ |
|   Absent or impaired oculomotor function | 70 | 43 | $p < 0.05$ |
|   Decerebrate or flaccid | 56 | 29 | $p < 0.05$ |
| Time from injury to surgical decompression | | | |
|   Number of patients | 44 | 26 | — |
|   Mean time lapse ± SEM (minutes) | $390 \pm 38.5$ | $170 \pm 18.3$ | $p < 0.0001$ |

\* NS denotes not significant.

tertiary physicians who are directly involved in the transport, diagnosis and treatment of the patients.

In the Richmond series, the patients with less severe neurologic deficits on admission and low postoperative ICP had significantly better outcomes. Age did not significantly affect outcome among the 82 comatose patients with ASDH, but older patients were more prone to ASDH; therefore, age may have predisposed this group of patients to a higher mortality rate than that of patients with other head injuries. This possibility has been previously recognized (Becker *et al.* 1977, Cooper *et al.* 1976, Greenberg *et al.* 1977, Jamieson and Yelland 1972, Richards and Hoff 1974), as have the facts that men have worse outcomes than women and are more prone to ASDH, and that motor-vehicle-related accidents are a less common cause of ASDH than of other types of head injuries (Table 3) (Seelig *et al.* 1981).

Chambers (1951) was one of the first to emphasize that prompt surgical removal of a traumatic intracranial hematoma, whether extradural or intradural, was beneficial even if the patient's neurologic condition appeared terminal. Gutterman and Shenkin (1970) demonstrated that patients with traumatic decerebration associated with either an extradural or intradural hematoma had 40% mortality when craniotomy began within four hours of the onset of decerebration but had 100% mortality when the procedure began after six hours. Cooper *et al.* (1976), in a retrospective analysis of 50 cases of traumatic ASDH, reported that in 45 fatalities an average of six hours elapsed from admission to operation, as compared with 4.4 hours in the five survivors.

Richards and Hoff, in 1974, recorded a 75% mortality rate in 100 patients with an ASDH who had surgery an average of seven hours after injury. Emergency air ventriculostomy and computed tomography allowed the Richmond group to reduce the time from injury to operation to 5.4 hours in the average patient with an intracranial hematoma, including patients with an ASDH (see Table 1). Functional recovery from ASDH, however, was associated with an average of only 2.8 hours of delay (Table 2) (Seelig *et al.* 1981).

Patients who underwent surgery for an ASDH within four hours of the injury had a 60 to 70% functional recovery rate, as compared with only 10% in those who had the operation more than four hours after the injury ($p < 0.0001$). Severe morbidity and mortality were three times greater in patients who underwent surgery after four hours from the injury. Rapid removal of the ASDH prevents prolonged preoperative increased ICP and brain shift and therefore diminishes the probability of subsequent focal-tissue ischemia or brain-stem compression or both.

Several investigators (Becker *et al.* 1977, Braakman *et al.* 1980, Brendler and Selverstone 1970, Bricolo *et al.* 1977, Jamieson and Yelland 1972, Price and Knill-Jones 1979, Rosenbluth *et al.* 1962) have noted that younger patients have better quality of survival, tolerate longer periods of coma or decerebration and have fewer life-threatening medical or surgical complications of head injury (*i.e.,* gastric ulcer or pneumonia). Richards and Hoff (1974) described 100 patients with ASDH, with an average age of 47 years and contrasted the average age of 36 years in survivors with that of 51 years in non-survivors. The average age of survivors in the Richmond series was 44 years, and that of non-survivors was 51 (Seelig *et al.* 1981).

In most reports, intracranial hypertension has been defined as mean pressure in excess of 15 to 20 mm Hg (Fleischer *et al.* 1976, Johnston *et al.* 1970, Lundberg 1960, Shigemori *et al.* 1979). McKissock reported that five of six patients with ASDH had lumbar pressure over 15 mm Hg (McKissock *et al.* 1960). Shigemori *et al.* (1979) found in 15 patients with ASDH that five had ICP levels above 70 mm Hg 24 to 48 hours after the operation and all five died. Only two of seven patients with ICP between 35 and 70 mm Hg survived. Three of their patients with ICP below 35 mm Hg survived to have a functional recovery. Sustained, uncontrollable intracranial hypertension over 60 mm Hg occurred in 15% of the Richmond patients with head injuries, 24% of all patients with an ASDH, and 43% of those who died after an ASDH. The ICP of patients who had functional recovery from an ASDH was less than 20 mm Hg in 79% of the cases. Only 30% of the non-survivors had a peak ICP of less than 20 mm Hg. Postoperative elevation of ICP was associated with poor outcome in the Richmond series and that of Shigemori *et al.* (1979).

Of the several factors that influence mortality, the neurologic status present before surgical decompression of a traumatic intracranial mass lesion can be a major determinant of outcome. This point has been well documented by Jennett (1976, 1979). McLaurin and Tutor (1961) stated that level of consciousness was the most important guide to the need for surgical intervention and was of considerable prognostic value. Eighteen percent of their 90 patients were conscious up to the time of operation; they had only 6% mortality. The remaining 82% of their patients were comatose and had 77% mortality. McLaurin and Tutor (1961) and Richards and Hoff (1974) found a 75% mortality rate associated with pupillary abnormalities, as compared with 35% in patients whose pupils were normal. Jamieson and Yelland (1972) noted 85% mortality in patients with bilateral pupillary abnormalities. In the Richmond series, 25% of the patients with bilaterally absent pupillary light reflexes had a functional recovery.

The presence of decerebrate rigidity before operation also has a devastating effect on outcome. Mortality in patients with ASDH and decerebration has been reported to range from 65 to 90% (Browder 1943, Cooper *et al.* 1976, Gutterman and Shenkin 1970, Harris 1971, Jamieson and Yelland 1972, Ransohoff *et al.* 1971, Richards and Hoff 1974, Talalla and Morin 1971). Only 29% of our patients with decerebrate rigidity had a functional recovery (Seelig *et al.* 1981).

## Etiology of Acute Subdural Hematoma

Just as in most cases of severe head injury some subarachnoid blood is present, so also is subdural blood common after major injury. This subdural bleeding may, however, become extensive enough to act as an extra-axial compressive lesion and pose a threat to life. Sizeable subdural hematomas can develop under two circumstances, each of which may have different implications for the patient (Miller and Becker 1982).

Bleeding may accumulate around a brain laceration, often a polar laceration of the temporal or frontal lobe. Frequently, such patients have also sustained severe diffuse primary brain injury and have been unconscious from the start. The subdural hematoma forms adjacent to damaged and necrotic brain and is often continuous with an intracerebral hematoma, formed in the depths of the brain laceration. This complex of hematoma and lacerated necrotic and swollen brain is aptly termed "burst temporal (or frontal) lobe". Patients with this lesion may show delayed neurological deterioration around the third or fourth day after injury, and some such cases may be labeled subacute subdural hematoma. This term probably is erroneous because computed tomography (CT) or other studies performed on admission in such patients show that hematoma is present soon after the injury in nearly all cases. Probably the reason for the later deterioration is delayed swelling of the damaged brain. The advent of computed tomographic X-ray scanning has shed new light on this area by revealing developing areas of luceny in the temporal lobe of such cases over a period of days following injury.

The second circumstance in which subdural hematoma may rapidly form is when a surface or bridging vessel (usually a vein) is torn during the movement of the brain that accompanies head acceleration or deceleration at impact. In some cases the actual brain damage is mild, so a dramatic clinical picture results in which there is a brief, lucid interval following injury, followed by rapid neurological deterioration. The same picture may develop after a direct blow to the skull in which a surface artery is ruptured. In these cases the threat to the patient's life is entirely due to the hematoma. The speed of the neurological deterioration may be such that these patients can fare no better than those in whom the hematoma is merely an extension of severe primary brain damage (Miller and Becker 1982).

Reports in which both forms of hematoma are included show a very high mortality rate ranging to over 90% (Cooper *et al.* 1976, Fell *et al.* 1975, Harris 1971, Jamieson and Yelland 1972, Landig *et al.* 1941, Lewin 1949, Loew and Wüster 1960, McKissock *et al.* 1960, Moiel and Caram 1967, Ransohoff *et al.* 1971, Richards and Hoff 1974, Talalla and Morin 1971). This high mortality rate relates to the major underlying diffuse brain injury that many of these patients have sustained, which is then compounded by rapid brain compression as a result of the subdural or intracerebral hematoma. Because many of these patients are unconscious when first seen in the hospital, further neurological deterioration, which prompts the search for an intracranial mass lesion, all too often takes the patient to the point at which operative decompression cannot reverse the secondary brain stem damage.

## Pathophysiology

Three broad concepts are important in comprehending the nature of head injury. First, in a severe injury many brain cells are functionally impaired but not disrupted by the initial impact, and if conditions are favorable, the cells can recover after minutes, or even after hours or days. The next concept is that secondary pathophysiological processes, both biochemical and structural (mass lesions), may result in further major cellular damage, both to the previously injured neurons and even to uninjured cells; a major goal of therapy is to avert these secondary processes. Finally, an understanding of the loci, extent, and types of brain injury in each patient is necessary because the entire management program should center on an understanding of the patient's intracranial disorder in structural and functional terms (Becker *et al.* 1982).

Consequent on the brain's mobility within the cranium, its poles sustain the greatest deformation. Holbourn postulated that the poles are particularly stressed during rotational injuries, and that shearing forces, especially at the frontal and temporal tips, cause most of the damage (Holbourn 1943) (Fig. 2). The more popular view is that the brain's poles forcibly impinge on the interior of the skull with sudden deceleration or acceleration: the frontal poles against the anterior fossa, the temporal tips against the sphenoid bones. Since most forces applied to the head contain a lateral rotational element, there is usually more damage on one side than on the other, but it is common to have damage on both sides of the brain. This bilateral damage is an important factor in the determination of outcome (Sweet *et al.* 1978). Demonstration of midline brain shift may only be an indication of which is the more severely damaged side. It is the location of the damage that characterizes polar lesions. In brain contusion there is subpial extravasation of blood and swelling of the affected area; if the lesion is severe much of the damaged area may be necrotic, soft and hemorrhagic. When the pia mater is torn, cerebral laceration is present by definition, but the borderline between contusion and laceration may not be very clear. Contusions and laceration of the brain both produce appropriate signs of neurological dysfunction when located in eloquent areas of the brain, *e.g.,* the motor, and are important in the differential diagnosis of hemisparesis after head injury (versus intracranial hematoma). There are not any immediate specific neurological signs to indicate the more common lesions of the frontal or temporal tips, and old scars in these areas may be seen as incidental findings at autopsy in patients who made recoveries from head injuries years earlier and had no focal neurological signs. The clinical importance of polar lesions in the immediate or early post-injury period derives from their propensity to swell or to bleed, or both, and thereby to act as intracranial expanding lesions potentially responsible for secondary brain dysfunction (Miller and Becker 1982).

TRAUMA

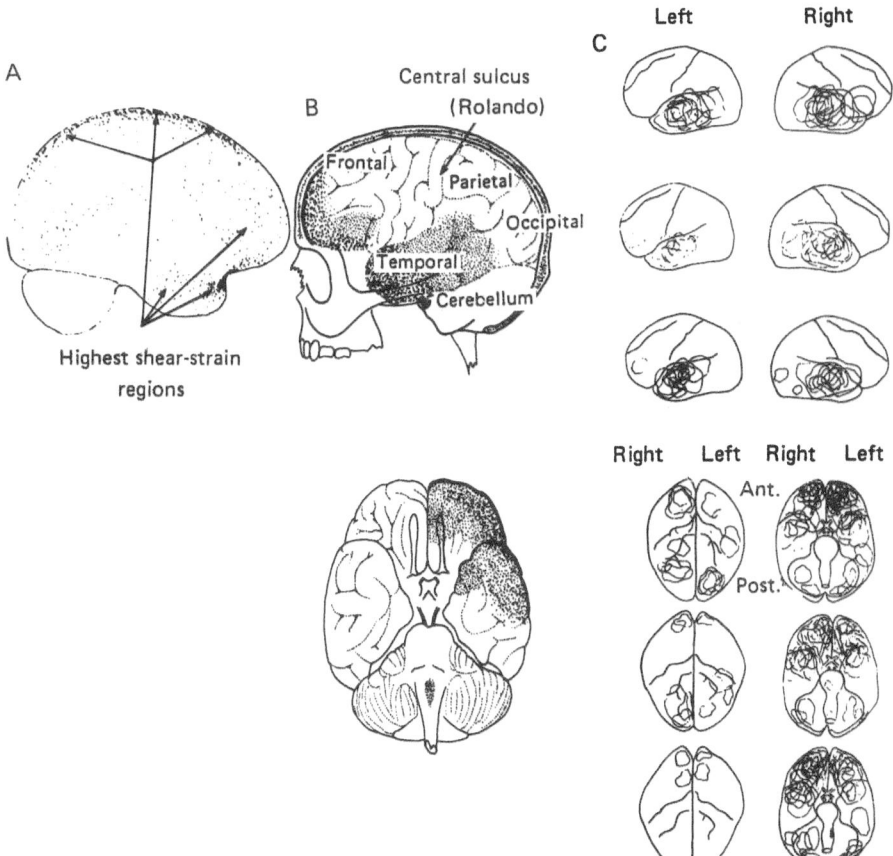

Fig. 2. Composite drawing showing the theoretical model used by Holbourn to predict the shear-strain relationships that occur when a rotational acceleration is induced. The density of the stippling is proportional to the degree of shear-strain observed in the model. Compare the regions of dense stippling, *i.e.,* regions of high stress, to the observed loci of contusion in the human as shown in B and the composite C, drawn from 152 consecutive autopsies after fatal head injuries in humans. Holbourn also predicted a narrow band of severe strain along the superior margin of the hemisphere, which correlates well with the frequently observed avulsion of cortical-sinus anastomotic veins. (From Holbourn, A. H. S.: The mechanics of brain injuries. Brit. Med. Bull. *3*, 147 − 149, 1945, and Gurdjian, E. S.: Recent advances in the study of impact injury of the head. Clin. Neurosurg. *19*, 1 − 42, 1972. Reprinted by permission)

## Secondary Brain Displacement

Any discrete expanding intracranial mass, whatever its nature and site, will usually produce brain shift and distortion together with increased intracranial pressure, which will ultimately lead to herniation of brain out of the bony-dural compartment in which the mass originates. The relationship between volume of mass, the rate at which it expands, the intracranial pressure, the degree of distortion and herniation of the brain, and the neurological dysfunction that results therefrom is subtle and influenced by antecedent factors such as the cerebrospinal fluid volume and the shape of the tentorial hiatus (Corsellis 1958, Miller and Adams 1972). Broadly speaking, the faster a mass expands, the higher is the intracranial pressure relative to the degree of brain distortion produced. This is clearly illustrated by comparison of acute and chronic subdural hematoma. In the former case the intracranial pressure is often over 50 mm Hg on admission to the hospital in patients who have 10 mm of midline shift, whereas in a patient with chronic subdural hematoma that has developed over a longer time interval, a midline shift of 20 mm may be associated with normal pressure (Miller *et al.* 1977, 1982).

There is, however, a close intertwining of brain shift and increased intracranial pressure. Many of the neurological signs that occur with major mass lesions and are attributed to raised pressure are more probably due to brain displacement. Increases in pressure, particularly differential changes in pressure across the tentorium and foramen magnum, are often related to the process of brain shift and herniation from one compartment to another. In head injury the great majority of expanding mass lesions are supratentorial. The infratentorial lesions, posterior fossa-epidural or subdural hematoma, cerebellar hematoma, or contusion are rarities. Supratentorial lesions, which in patients with head injury may not infrequently be bilateral, produce characteristic types of brain displacement, distortion, and herniation according to the site or sites of the mass lesions. An extra-axial mass depresses underlying brain, flattening the gyri and compressing surface vessels (Shapiro *et al.* 1966). Elsewhere the subarachnoid space becomes obliterated, and the gyri flatten against the dura. The subarachnoid cisterns decrease in size, and the lateral ventricle on the side of the lesion also becomes narrowed. When the mass is intra-axial, gyri are also flattened, and the subarachnoid space and cisterns become obliterated (Miller and Becker 1982).

The decrease in intracranial cerebrospinal fluid volume is important in relation to the regulation and transmission of intracranial pressure. Displacement of the fluid is one factor responsible for spatial compensation in which intracranial pressure can remain close to normal despite expansion of the mass lesion (Langfitt 1969). As the fluid spaces around the midbrain at the tentorial hiatus become occluded, however, the mechanisms for bulk flow and absorption of cerebrospinal fluid are interfered with, and transmission of pressure across the tentorium becomes progressively impaired so that the true level of supratentorial pressure is no longer reflected in measurements taken from the spinal subarachnoid space (cistern or lumbar). As the block becomes more complete, lumbar pressure deviates more from supratentorial pressure until lumbar subarachnoid pressure may return to normal at a time when intraventricular pressure is over 50 mm Hg (Kaufmann and Clark 1970 a, Langfitt *et al.* 1964 a, Leech and Miller 1974). When this stage has been reached, the outlook for the patient is poor unless decompression is immediately effected (Miller and Becker 1982).

When the expanding mass lesion is predominantly unilateral, the midline structures are shifted to the opposite side. The interventricular septum and the third ventricle, which are detectable by echoencephalography, and the pineal gland which, if calcified, will be visible on plain X-rays, can define the degree of midline shift. The internal cerebral vein and anterior cerebral-pericallosal artery complex also shift and can be visualized by angiography. As this shifting process proceeds, the cingulate gyrus herniates under the free edge of the falx cerebri, pressing the corpus callosum downward on the side of the mass lesion; this produces the characteristic "tilted gull-wing" appearance on angiography (in the anteroposterior view). The falx may also be tilted or shifted away from the mass. The medial portion of the temporal lobe on the side of the lesion (uncus and hippocampal gyrus) becomes pressed against the side of the midbrain; this is part of the process of obliteration of the cistern ambiens, and the whole process of midline brain shift can be viewed as a prelude to tentorial herniation. Nonetheless, in patients with head injury, there is a correlation between the occurrence of significant midline shift and the incidence of signs of severe neurological dysfunction (Miller and Becker 1982).

## Tentorial Herniation

A major landmark in neurological surgery was the recognition of the clinical features of tentorial herniation and the identification of the pathological processes leading to it. In patients with head injury it allowed the differentiation of primary and secondary lesions of the brain. The primary lesions were due to the impact forces at the time of injury, and the secondary lesions are due to the effects of a secondary space-occupying lesion such as a hematoma or swollen contusion (Meyer 1920, Miller and Becker 1982, Sunderland 1958).

Following clinical descriptions of the tentorial pressure cone by Vincent and coworkers (1936) and Jefferson (1938), it was linked with ipsilateral oculomotor palsy and medial occipital (posterior cerebral artery) infarction (Jefferson 1938, Moore and Stern 1938, Reid and Cone 1939). Later the association between disturbances of consciousness and tentorial herniation was elucidated (Cairns 1939, McNealy and Plum 1962). Detailed experimental studies further explained the correlation between tentorial coning, pupillary dilation, changes in pulse and blood pressure, and brain stem hemorrhages (Hoff and Reis 1970, Jennett and Stern 1960, Klintworth 1966).

In the best-known form of tentorial herniation, there occurs bulging and herniation of the uncus and medial portion of the hippocampal gyrus between the free edge of the tentorium and the midbrain. The midbrain is compressed from side to side and elongated in its anterior-posterior diameter, and the opposite cerebral penduncle may be compressed against the tentorial edge on the other side sufficiently hard to create a detectable lesion. This mechanism is invoked to explain ipsilateral hemiparesis in chronic subdural hematoma (Gurdjian and Thomas 1974). The herniating brain also causes distortion of the oculomotor nerve by compression between the posterior cerebral artery and the petroclinoid ligament, and the posterior cerebral artery may be so compromised as to produce infarction in its territory of distribution. In the acute stage visible grooving of the undersurface of the temporal lobe can be seen at autopsy. In certain patients, hemorrhage occurs into the ipsilateral oculomotor nerve where it crosses the posterior cerebral artery.

The clinical correlates of this process are depression of consciousness, possibly due to distortion or deafferentation of the upper part of the reticular activating system; contralateral (or sometimes ipsilateral) hemiparesis progressing to decerebrate rigidity; and ipsilateral pupillary dilation with loss in the affected eye of the direct and consensual light response and external movements other than abduction. By the time occipital infarction occurs, the patient is not sufficiently conscious to be tested for visual field deficits (Miller and Becker 1982).

### Intracranial Hypertension

Raised intracranial pressure is the rule in patients with acute mass lesions complicating head injury (Fig. 3). Even after artificial ventilation or operative decompression or both, elevated intracranial pressure still remains a problem in many patients, requiring further therapy—in 50% of those with mass lesions and in 33% of those with diffuse brain injury. Many of the neurological signs attributed to increased intracranial pressure— headache, vomiting, drowsiness, bradycardia, arterial hypertension, and irregular respiration—are likely to be due to brain stem shift or distortion. It is important to try to relate increased intracranial pressure to brain distortion and herniation rather than to any particular neurological symptom or sign (Miller *et al.* 1977, Miller and Becker 1982). Brain herniation at the tentorial or foramen magnum level clearly has an influence on intracranial pressure in that there is loss of the free transmission of pressure between the cranial and spinal compartments (Kaufmann 1970 a, Langfitt 1964 a). In addition, since the distribution of the compliance of the

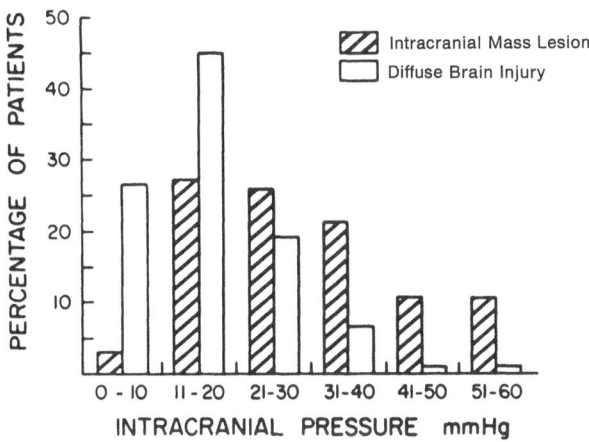

Fig. 3. Distribution of intracranial pressure levels recorded on admission in 160 patients with severe head injury (62 patients with intracranial mass lesions requiring operative removal or decompression and 98 patients with diffuse brain injury). (From Miller, J. D., Becker, D. P., Ward, J. D., Sullivan, H. G., Adams, W. E., and Rosner, M. J.: Significance of intracranial hypertension in severe head injury. J. Neurosurg. *47*, 503 – 516, 1977. Reprinted by permission)

entire craniospinal axis is 50% supratentorial, 20% infratentorial, and 30% spinal, it may be expected that when tentorial herniation occurs secondary to a supratentorial mass lesion, compliance would decrease and the pressure-volume curve in the supratentorial compartment would become much steeper (Löfgren and Zwetnow 1972, Marmarou and Shulman 1976, Pasztor *et al.* 1975) (Fig. 4). It appears that changes in neurological status that are associated with alterations in intracranial pressure are in fact often mediated by the influence of intracranial pressure on brain shift. This relationship would explain the paucity of neurological signs despite severely elevated pressures that are seen in patients with benign intracranial hypertension, a condition in which brain shift does not occur (Johnston and Paterson 1974).

Intracranial pressure may affect neurological function by increasing to an extent that it becomes a factor limiting cerebral blood flow. This is most obvious in those critically ill patients in whom angiography shows nonfilling of the intracranial portion of the internal carotid artery (Balslev-Jorgenson *et al.* 1972, Heiskanen and Vapalahti 1964, Troupp 1963). In such patients, the intracranial pressure has attained the level of arterial pressure, with the result that cerebral perfusion pressure has fallen to zero.

In most patients with head injury, neurological and neurophysiological dysfunction becomes markedly more frequent when intracranial pressure is

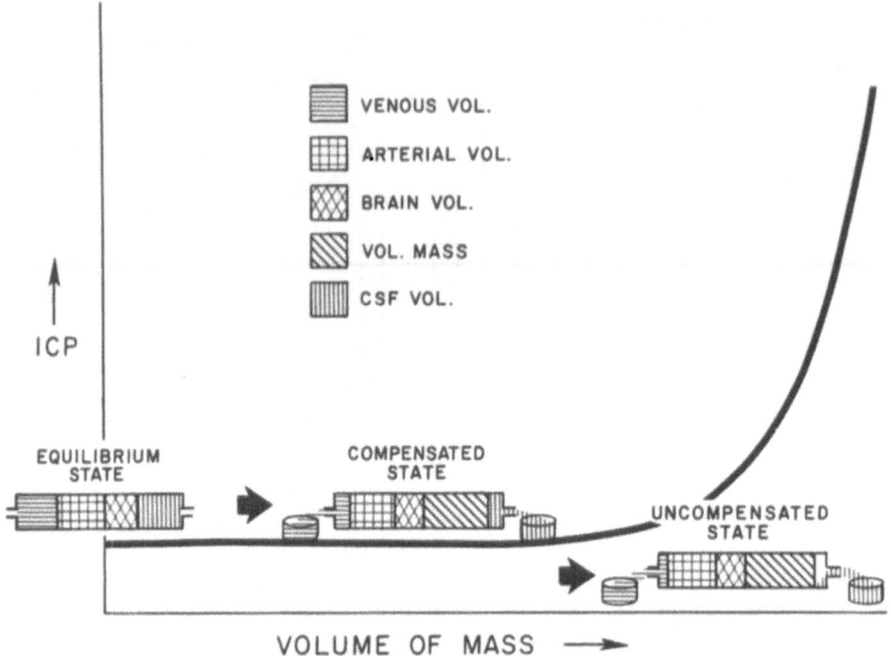

Fig. 4. Curve reflecting the relationship between pressure and volume

persistently over 40 mm Hg (Greenberg *et al.* 1976). It is clear now that an important link between intracranial pressure and brain function is the level of cerebral blood flow. Under controlled experimental conditions, if cerebral blood flow can be maintained, intracranial hypertension causes no impairment of cortical neurophysiological function up to intracranial pressure levels of 50 mm Hg and more. If the cerebral blood flow decreases, then lesser degrees of intracranial hypertension impair cortical electrical activity and it fails altogether when the flow falls below 40% of normal (Grossman *et al.* 1975). This relationship of neuronal function and perfusion pressure may form the basis for the sudden neurological deterioration that can occur precipitately in patients with no brain shift or mass lesion when intracranial pressure rises over 30 or 40 mm Hg (Becker 1976).

## Diagnosis of Acute Subdural Hematoma

A prompt and orderly analysis of the nature and magnitude of all damage sustained by patients with head injury is necessary for appropriate and definitive emergency management. The most immediate requirement is to determine the intracranial damage. The surgeon must define the presence or absence of intracranial hematomas, contusions, and major zones of diffuse or focal edema. The urgency of a given situation can be quickly determined by testing the ability of the patient to follow a simple-stage command, which serves as a measure of a considerable degree of neurological function. Although inability to follow such a command is not necessarily associated with impending neurological deterioration, should deterioration occur in such a patient, he will immediately be in a critical neurological state. For this reason *loss of this ability should indicate prompt diagnostic testing*. This principle must be adhered to in all patients, since successful therapy must take place *before* herniation syndromes occur or are permitted to progress. Criteria for operative intervention needs to be established in each patient promptly, *before* clinical signs of herniation (deepening coma, dilating pupil, progressive paresis, posturing limbs, and the Cushing response) appear. Intracranial pressure associated with impending herniation syndromes is usually above 40 to 50 mm Hg. While delayed but technically satisfactory operations performed after these signs occur may salvage the patient, the final outcome is always less satisfactory. A better recovery for the patient can be achieved by earlier recognition and evacuation of mass lesions (Becker *et al.* 1977, 1982).

### Computed Tomography

Prior to the advent of computed tomography in 1972, radiological investigation in acute head injury consisted primarily of radiography of the skull, cerebral angiography, and encephalography. The radiographs of the skull were helpful in the detection of fractures, scalp injury, foreign bodies and pneumoencephalus. Evaluation of intracranial lesions was limited to the detection of mass effects as shown by displacement of the pineal body or choroid plexus if they were calcified. Contrast procedures such as angiography and to a lesser degree encephalography were necessary to localize the traumatic intracranial lesions as shown by the displacement of either vascular structures or the ventricular system. Computed tomography has revolutionized the diagnostic evaluation of traumatic intracranial lesions. With its unique ability to detect the subtle differences in soft-tissue density, computed tomography is valuable in detecting various traumatic intracranial lesions: intra- and extracerebral hematomas, infarctions, edema, contusions, and the like. Computed tomography has replaced cerebral angiography as the primary radiological method of investigation in head injury (Becker *et al.* 1982).

The patient should be handled with caution to avoid further injury during the procedure. Associated injuries, especially those involving the cervical spine, should be considered before the patient is moved or manipulated. A transtable lateral radiograph of the cervical spine may

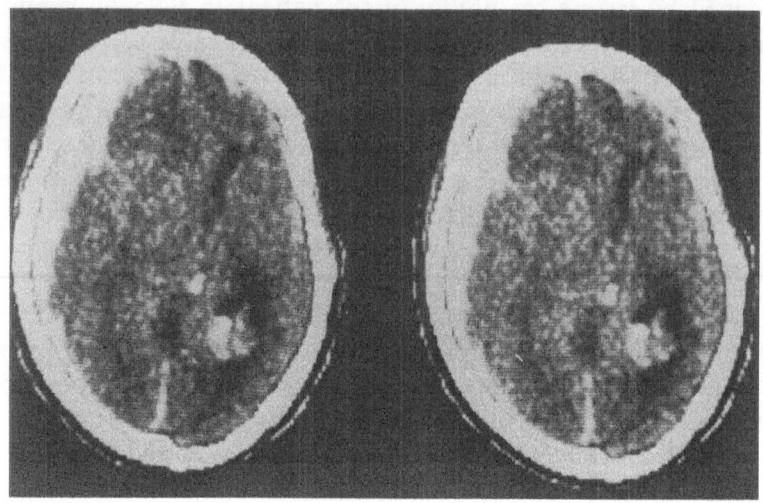

Fig. 5. A single scan at the level of the lateral ventricles revealing a large subdural hematoma on the left side with appropriate left-to-right midline displacement. The patient was immediately taken to the operating room for craniotomy without performing a complete computed tomographic examination, thus saving time. A subsequent examination revealed the full extent of the right-sided intracerebral hematoma, which did not require operative removal. (From Ref. 7, p. 1953, reprinted by permission)

detect the presence of a fracture before the patient is transferred for computed tomographic examination. If a fracture is present, depending upon its severity and extent, the cervical spine should be adequately immobilized before the scan is performed. If necessary, a physician should be with the patient throughout the scanning to assure immobilization. Whenever possible, the examination should include the posterior fossa structures.

In patients with multiple injuries and in whom hemorrhage is suspected in other parts of the body that may require an immediate operative procedure, the cranial CT examination can be modified to save time. In such instances only a single scan through the level of the lateral ventricles should be obtained. This view is adequate to evaluate the supratentorial structures and will reveal the presence of midline displacement or a large extra- or intracerebral hematoma that would require immediate craniotomy (Fig. 5). A complete examination can be performed subsequently for the detection of additional intracranial lesions. However, a significant hematoma may be present over the high convexity bilaterally and still escape detection if only a single scan is obtained. The majority of acute subdural hematomas are seen

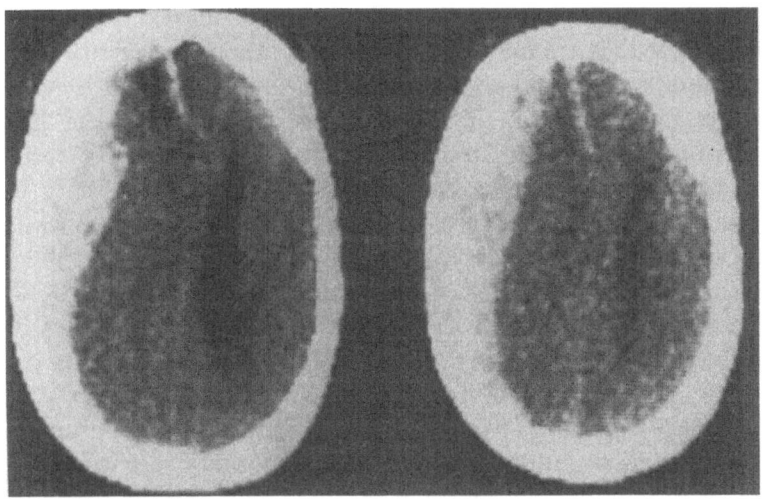

Fig. 6. Acute subdural hematoma follows the surface of the brain, thus having a concave inner margin. (From Ref. 7, p. 1969, reprinted by permission)

as zones of increased density following the surface of the brain, thus having a concave inner margin and convex outer margin adjacent to the inner table of the skull (Fig. 6). The typical subdural hematoma tends to be more diffuse than an epidural hematoma, the peripheral expansion of which is limited by firm dural attachment to the inner table. A subdural hematoma measuring 5 to 6 mm in depth is usually clearly seen on computed tomography. Smaller lesions, however, may not be seen because of the close proximity of the hematoma to the bony calvarium, and even a significant hematoma along the high convexity and displacing the ventricle may be missed (Becker *et al.* 1982).

### Angiography

The major limitations of computed tomography in head injury are in visualizing traumatic isodense lesions and its inability to demonstrate adequately the vascular damage resulting from head injury. While one may see the result of vascular injury on computed tomography, the exact location and nature of the vascular injury itself can be adequately evaluated only by angiography. The presence of an aneurysm may be suspected on computed tomography following contrast infusion. Small traumatic aneurysms of the cortical arteries are difficult to visualize, however, and if they are associated with extracerebral hematomas, it may be impossible to detect the aneurysm without angiography.

Subfacial herniations are generally well seen on CT scan, but transtentorial herniation, a well-known secondary complication of head injury, may not be detected. As shown by Osborn, if there is narrowing of the subarachnoid space around the brain stem on one side with evidence of brain stem distortion and in the presence of supratentorial mass, the diagnosis of transtentorial herniation may be suggested (Osborn 1977). Angiography may be required to detect the displacement of such vascular structures as the anterior choroidal artery, posterior communicating and cerebral arteries, and basilar vein of Rosenthal to make the radiological diagnosis of impending transtentorial herniation. Vertebral angiography can detect the presence of upward herniation, but marked distortion of the quadrigeminal plate cistern associated with a posterior fossa mass may be evident on computerized tomography. Vertebral angiography is also valuable in the detection of tonsillar herniation. Thus angiography should be considered in situations when 1. vascular injury is suspected, 2. the findings on computed tomography are not consistent with the patient's neurological status, and 3. isodense lesions are suspected either clinically or because of mass effect seen on the CT scan (Becker et al. 1982).

### Ventriculography and Intracranial Pressure Measurement

Ventriculography with intracranial pressure measurement in acute head injury provides information that will effectively guide appropriate early management. This test can be done rapidly and in experienced hands carries minimal risk to the patient (Becker et al. 1976a, Kaufmann 1970b). It provides two critical bits of information for the treating physician: the degree of supratentorial brain shift and the level of intracranial pressure. Prior to the advent of computed tomography, this test and angiography were the most useful emergency radiological studies for patients who were not following commands after head injury. In a few clinics, ventriculography and intracranial measurement was the emergency procedure of choice because of the speed with which it could be obtained (Becker et al. 1975). In comparison with ventriculography, computed tomography and angiography both define the degree of brain shift at least as well and are certainly better for determining locations of injury. But knowledge of the patient's intracranial pressure soon after injury is of benefit in overall diagnosis and management.

The test still has an important role in emergency diagnosis. If the hospital has no computed tomography available, and angiography cannot be obtained quickly, this test should be used in patients who are unable to speak or follow commands. Other indications include conditions in which patients with severe brain injuries have other extracranial injuries that require immediate operation or that prevent transfer for computed tomography or angiography. A delay in diagnosis of intracranial damage until after the patient has had operative treatment for an extracranial lesion should not be permitted.

If the procedure is performed in a methodical and standardized fashion, the ventricle can almost always be cannulated to provide a satisfactory intracranial pressure measurement and air study, even when there is major ventricular shift or the ventricles are tiny, or both. If there are no focal signs that favor a unilateral mass lesion, the right side should be chosen for the study. If the clinical examination suggests the presence of a right-sided intracranial mass lesion, the left side of the skull is entered, for it is easier to cannulate the ventricle on the side opposite the lesion. The technique described here has been used by the author and his associates in well over 500 patients, many with acute brain injury, with a morbidity rate of less than 0.5% and a failure rate of 3% (Fig. 7) (Becker *et al.* 1982).

The scalp is shaved in the region of the coronal suture, and a twist drill hole is made with a small drill, 4 cm off the midline and approximately 1.5 cm anterior to the coronal suture. The hole is directed toward the nasion and in the sagittal plane 2 cm anterior to the external auditory canal. The dura is penetrated with no. 18 needle. A no. 16 brain cannula is directed first toward the nasion. If the ventricle is not hit, the cannula is next directed toward the ipsilateral pupil, and if this fails, a third pass is made toward the contralateral pupil. If three passes fail, the procedure is repeated in a similar fashion on the other side. If three passes on the second side also fail, the procedure should be abandoned. When the ventricle is entered, care must be taken to lose as little cerebrospinal fluid as possible. A manometer previously filled with sterile saline to a level of 300 mm of water and extended by flexible tubing is then connected via a stopcock on the end of the tubing to the ventricular cannula. A resting intracranial pressure is obtained from the level of the foramen of Monro with the patient laying flat. At the time of measurement, the arterial blood pressure should not be below normal and any hypercarbia or hypoxia should have been corrected. With these abnormalities, intracranial pressure readings can be misleading, for arterial hypotension may falsely lower the pressure and hypercarbia and hypoxia may raise it.

After measuring the pressure, approximately 7 cc of air are carefully exchanged for cerebrospinal fluid, the head in tilted from side to side, and a brow-up anteroposterior Towne's position skull X-ray is obtained after the

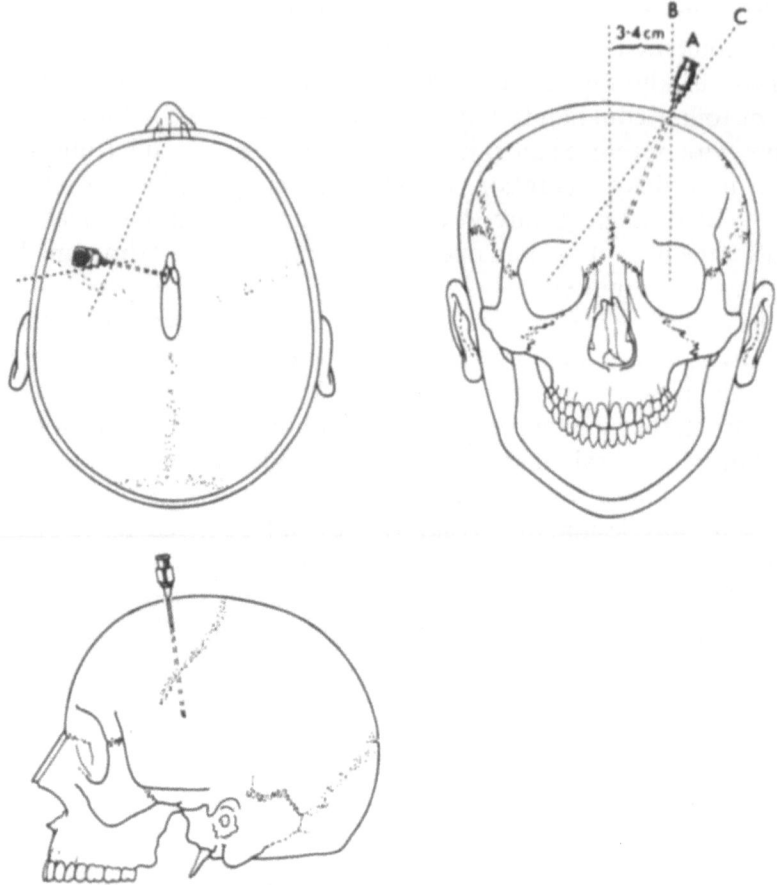

Fig. 7. Precoronal suture method for performance of twist drill ventriculostomy. The hole is directed toward the nasion and in the sagittal plane 2 cm anterior to the external auditory canal. No more than three passes per side should be made (the first toward the nasion, *A*; the second toward the ipsilateral inner canthus, *B*; and the third toward the contralateral inner canthus, *C*). If three passes on the opposite side also fail, the procedure should be abandoned. With this method, the ventricle can almost always be cannulated, even when it is compressed or shifted. (From Ref. 7, p. 1991, reprinted by permission)

cannula is removed (Fig. 8). Normal intracranial pressure in the relaxed patient who is neither hypotensive, hypercarbic, nor hypoxic is 10 mm Hg or less (Lundberg 1960). Elevations above this level are abnormal. While pressure in the range of 10 to 15 mm Hg may occur with only minor shifts of intracranial volume, when pressures are over 15 mm Hg a major intra-cranial alteration has occurred (Miller 1975). When pressures are recorded in the range of 20 mm Hg or more, this implies either a major intracranial hematoma, a serious diffuse brain injury, or both (Becker *et al.* 1975). A sizable change in intracranial volume and pressure-volume dynamics is required to raise intracranial pressures to this level.

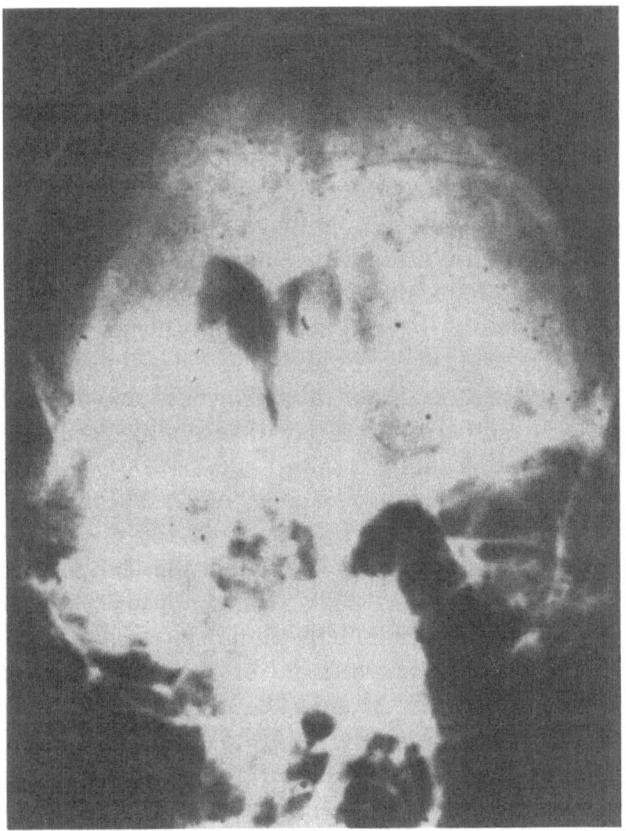

Fig. 8. Brow-up anteroposterior limited ventriculogram performed in the emergency room via a precoronal twist drill ventriculostomy. The combination of information on intracranial pressure level and degree of supratentorial midline brain shift and ventricular compression greatly aids in defining the type of immediate management required. (From Ref. 7, p. 1992, reprinted by permission)

Most dangerous acute traumatic unilateral intracranial mass lesions will shift the midline 5 mm or more. This will invariably be associated with an elevated intracranial pressure unless a cerebrospinal fluid leak is present (Becker *et al.* 1975). Serious temporal lobe lesions may cause only minimal shift of the midline, but in this case the intracranial pressure will be elevated, and if the third ventricle is seen on the air study, it will often be shifted more than the lateral ventricles. If there is little or no midline shift, the pressure is elevated and the patient is not hypercarbic, then there are either bilateral mass lesions or a serious diffuse brain injury. In this case, if the pressure is above 20 mm Hg, the patient should have angiography or computed tomography to rule out bilateral hematomas or contusions that might require operative intervention (Becker *et al.* 1982).

### Diagnostic or Exploratory Burr Holes

Prior to the availability of angiography and computed tomography, diagnostic or exploratory burr holes were a useful initial procedure, but they now have a limited role in the modern diagnosis and management of acute head injury. If a patient shows a progressive deficit that can be temporarily arrested or reversed with osmotic agents such as mannitol, operative treatment should be preceded by computed tomography, ventriculography, or angiography to define the location of the intracranial lesions. If a particularly urgent operation is required, one can get a single-level CT cut across the midsupratentorial space, a rapid ventriculogram, or a single-injection, single X-ray, anteroposterior carotid angiogram in the emergency room or on the operating table.

An exploratory burr hole should be considered as the primary diagnostic procedure only if computed tomography and angiography are not promptly available, the ventricle cannot be cannulated and the patient is rapidly deteriorating with the signs of unilateral progressive brain shift and tentorial herniation. If this rapid deterioration occurs, the side to be explored first should be determined by the following signs in order of importance: 1. the side of the dilating pupil, 2. the side of any unilateral skull fracture, and 3. the side contralateral to any progressive motor sign such as weakness or posturing. Almost all major *acute hematomas* causing tentorial herniation will be on the side of the dilating pupil (Kennedy and Wortis 1931). Similarly, if there is a unilateral skull fracture, most progressively growing acute intracranial hematomas will be on the side of the fracture (Lewin 1976). False localizing signs, such as pupillary dilation developing contralateral to the clot, are seen more often in association with chronic subdural hematoma (Browder 1943, Sunderland 1958). Rarely, the pupil ipsilateral to an acute developing hematoma may initially constrict because of impending medial temporal lobe herniation (Gurdjian 1974, Sunderland 1958).

In acute closed head injury, the initial burr hole should be in the temporal region. It should be enlarged to a small craniectomy so the area under the dura is clearly visible and can be inspected and an initial decompression can be performed (see Fig. 12). If an acute extradural clot is not identified and *the patient has clearly shown the clinical signs of unilateral supratentorial mass development,* further multiple ipsilateral or contralateral burr holes should *not* be done, as this will delay diagnosis and treatment. Rather, one should proceed with the trauma craniotomy in Fig. 10, as this will most rapidly provide for an accurate intraoperative diagnosis and permit adequate therapy.

Only in the rare situation in which one might be operating upon a patient who is showing progressive deterioration without local signs, such as from a frontal or occipital hematoma, and no other diagnostic test could be performed, might the use of multiple diagnostic holes be useful. Similarly, exploratory burr holes contralateral to a completed craniotomy are indicated only if the surgeon strongly suspects a contralateral previously undiagnosed mass, for example, when there is acute intraoperative swelling of a normal-looking hemisphere that might be due to an enlarging contralateral hematoma.

## Management

All patients who are not verbalizing *and* cannot any commands should be intubated promptly (Maciver *et al.* 1958, Rose *et al.* 1977). The recommendation for early and prompt endotracheal intubation of the patient with a severe brain injury is, in part, based on observation of the high incidence of hypoxemia occurring in these patients. While the arterial oxygen tension can often be brought into the normal range with oxygen delivered by nasal catheter or mask, endotracheal intubation and positive-pressure ventilation usually are required to reverse atelectasis, and normo-xemia can then be maintained with an inspired oxygen concentration of less than 40%, which is in the nontoxic range. There are other reasons why prompt intubation is wise. Aspiration prior to arrival at the hospital and even after arrival is common. Aspiration of saliva or gastric contents may occur unobserved in patients with depressed pharyngeal and laryngeal reflexes. Even though frank clinical pulmonary edema with frothy fluid coming from the trachea is unusual after head trauma, there may be subclinical pulmonary edema that may, along with atelectasis, account for early hypoxemia in these patients. In any event, intubation and positive-pressure ventilation are effective therapy for both conditions. When positive-pressure ventilation is initiated early, progressive respiratory failure is seen only rarely, though the ventilation frequently must be maintained for several days (Becker *et al.* 1976 b). Additionally, respiratory insufficiency in the comatose patient can occur suddenly owing to upper airway obstruction, generalized seizure activity, or soft-tissue swelling in the neck, and intubation will prevent the problem. Acute respiratory insuffici-ency is especially important as a potential problem during in-hospital transportation or during computed tomography, angiography, or other diagnostic procedures. CT scanning is improved by keeping the patient immobile, and an intubated ventilated patient can easily be temporarily paralyzed with pancuronium (Pavulon) (Becker *et al.* 1982).

The arterial blood pressure should be measured promptly in the emergency room. If the patient is hypotensive, the pressure should, of course, be brought to normal range. The neurological examination is misleading in the hypotensive patient following head injury, and the patient who is "comatose" when his arterial blood pressure is 40 to 50 mm Hg may become responsive, even to verbal stimuli, when the arterial blood pressure is brought to a normal range. Likewise, intracranial pressure measurements are invalid during arterial hypotension; low or mildly elevated intracranial pressure can be observed in a hypotensive patient, but as soon as arterial blood pressure is brought up to normal, the intracranial pressure can rise dramatically (Becker *et al.* 1982).

## Operative Treatment of Acute Closed Head Injuries

Two sets of factors define whether a patient with an acute closed head injury requires an operation: the clinical status of the patient, and the findings on X-ray studies of the head. Since an operation is advocated herein when a major intracranial mass is identified, whether or not signs of tentorial herniation have yet emerged, the criteria for considering a mass as "operative" are dealt with in detail.

### Clinical Status as an Indication for Operation

A patient who *progressively* deteriorates from being able to talk to showing signs of tentorial herniation should have prompt operative therapy. Progressively diminishing responsiveness, development of uni-lateral pupillary dilation, associated flexor or extensor posturing, and increasing arterial hypertension and bradycardia associated with periodic breathing indicate third nerve and brainstem compression from tentorial herniation. While such clinical pictures will inevitably occur and require immediate operation, progressive deterioration should ideally be re-cognized earlier and the masses should be evacuated. It is incumbent, then, upon nurses and physicians evaluating such patients to be able to recognize the more subtle changes that develop while intracranial pressure is rising and brain shift is occurring. Even in fine neurosurgical units, early subtle signs of deterioration may escape recognition, and signs of brain com-pression and shift are discovered too late for reasonable salvage of the patient (Reilly *et al.* 1975, Rose *et al.* 1977).

Just as the shape of the pressure-volume intracranial pressure curve shows that the intracranial pressure may suddenly rise enormously with only a small increment of additional mass, so in the clinical situation patients may be doing reasonably well, only to deteriorate very suddenly and develop decerebrate posturing and a unilateral fixed and dilated pupil. This course is easily recognized in patients with a "lucid interval" who harbor an epidural hematoma, but may also be seen in patients with a large unilateral frontal or temporal contusion and hematoma or subdural hematoma. Brain function may remain surprisingly *good* in the face of a growing mass lesion and then *rapidly* deteriorate as intracranial spatial compensation is exceeded. In this situation, intracranial pressure rises suddenly and rapidly, impairing cerebral perfusion, and brain shift reaches a critical point at which signs of major upper brain stem compression suddenly appear. The more subtle signs of neurological impairment must be attended to. Not only progressive depression in a wakeful state, but a slight increase in disorientation and especially increasing restlessness are often seen with growing mass lesions. If it is already known that a mass exists, and profound disorientation, marked sleepiness, or increasing restlessness is occurring, serious consideration should be given to prompt evacuation of the mass. The development of mild or moderate contralateral weakness may be another early sign resulting from the cortex being compressed, but decorticate or decerebrate posturing is a late and advanced sign of brain compression. Hypertension and bradycardia associated with periodic breathing are *very late* signs of severe brain compression or torque or both. Theoretically, unilateral pupillary dilation should occur before the signs of upper brain stem compression, early enough to allow time for orderly diagnosis and treatment. Unfortunately, in acute head injury, development of a unilateral dilated and unreactive pupil from temporal lobe herniation is usually followed shortly by motor posturing (Goodkin 1978). In fact, decerebrate posturing may occur simultaneously with or even precede the pupillary abnormality (Becker *et al.* 1982).

## Radiographic Indications of a Mass Requiring Operative Treatment

*Computed Tomographic Indications.* In unresponsive patients with acute head injury, five variations of lesions seen in the CT scan are considered as potential operative mass lesions:

1. Extraaxial mass with a definite shift of the midline. If there is a clearly identifiable extraxial lesion of increased or decreased density and the midline shift is seen with the naked eye naked eye on a standard size CT scan, the lesion should be evacuated. Any shift of the midline evident on computed tomography (1 mm on the print) is equivalent approximately to a 4 mm true shift seen on ventriculography, and these lesions are almost always associated with high intracranial pressure in the early state after injury (Miller *et al.* 1977). If a small extraaxial lesion is seen, but there is no midline shift and no contralateral balancing lesion, the patient may be managed initially without operation.

2. Midline shift with no extra- or intraaxial clot seen on CT scan. If the midline is clearly shifted in an amount consistent with an actual shift of 5 mm or more and one ventricle is compressed, the patient should have an early follow-up scan if no high-density masses are seen on the CT scan. Often, the delayed scan will demonstrate that the patient has an acute subdural hematoma. Even if the shift is not due to an acute extraaxial clot, then a contusion will usually be discovered in the frontal or temporal lobe that was not seen in the CT scan. More often, a small extraaxial or intracerebral dense lesion is seen on the scan, with a large midline shift, and at operation one finds that the extraaxial mass is much larger than expected from the CT scan.

3. Intraaxial mass with midline shift. The same principles hold true here, and if there is a supratentorial intracerebral dense lesion with midline shift equivalent to 5 mm or more true shift, then the patient should have the contusion and hematoma evacuated. This is particularly important with intracerebral lesions because they almost always develop more surrounding edema and increased mass effect over several days, and if an initial midline shift of 5 mm or more is seen, any further brain swelling can be devastating. Even if the lesion is in the anterior portion of the dominant hemisphere, operative evacuation should be done if the mass or the shift or both are large. Without operation death will almost certainly occur, and with operative evacuation of the mass an occasional good result can be obtained, depending on the location and extent of the irreversible damage. The indications for operation when there is less than 5 mm of midline shift are not clear. In these situations, it is best to individualize treatment on the basis of the patient's clinical course and intracranial pressure.

4. Multiple intraaxial lesions with midline shift. Even when multiple unilateral or bilateral intracerebral lesions are present, if there is a major shift of the midline, the major shift-producing lesion or lesions should be evacuated. It is not advisable to extend the operation across the midline except very rarely for large bifrontal contusions. Bilateral temporal lobe operation for intracerebral contusion and hematoma is also not advisable. If there is no shift of the midline, the patients can often be managed successfully without operative intervention. But intracranial pressure monitoring and frequent neurological examinations must be performed in order to guide therapy and determine whether operative mass evacuation is ultimately required.

5. Bilateral extraaxial dense lesions without shift. Small bilateral extraaxial hematomas may often be managed satisfactorily without operation. Large lesions, especially if they are causing clear brain compression with ventricular impingement, should be evacuated. While even the larger lesions may occasionally disappear without operation, the evidence of brain compression on computed tomography suggests the possibility of real or

potential secondary brain injury, and this is best handled by evacuating the mass.

The foregoing indications for operation on computed tomographic criteria are defined for comatose patients. Patients who are in better neurological condition can more often be safely watched without operation, even with an intra-axial mass and some shift. These patients must be monitored very closely neurologically, and if their condition deteriorates, then the mass should be evacuated (Becker *et al.* 1982).

*Angiographic Indications.* In general, the angiographic guidelines used are the degree of midline shift and the estimated size and location of any intra-axial or extra-axial mass lesion (Hancock 1961). If the patient is not obeying commands, the following findings should be considered as indications for management by operation:

1. Extra-axial mass lesions more than 5 mm from the inner table, *if* they are associated with any degree of middle or anterior cerebral artery displacement. If there is associated major vessel displacement, this is a sign of brain compression, which should be relieved.

2. Bilateral extraaxial mass lesions more than 5 mm from the inner table. Except for patients who have prominent brain atrophy, intracranial masses of this size will usually summate to cause a major elevation of intracranial pressure.

3. Temporal lobe intraaxial mass lesions causing a major elevation of the middle cerebral artery or any degree of midline shift. These patients are in a most precarious position, as only slight swelling can cause a tentorial herniation syndrome that progresses very rapidly.

4. Intraaxial mass lesions causing shift of the midline vessels of 5 mm or more.

If patients are following one or more commands and any of the preceding criteria are present, nonoperative management may suffice. But very close neurological monitoring, perhaps coupled with intracranial pressure monitoring, is in order (Becker *et al.* 1982).

## Preparations for Operation and Anesthesia

Once operative therapy is decided upon, the surgeon should proceed with dispatch. Blood should be sent for cross-matching, and two units brought to the operating room as soon as available. Prior to anesthesia, the patient should virtually always be given intravenous mannitol in a dose that will elevate serum osmolarity by 10 to 12 mOsm. This requires at least 1 gm per kilogram; in an adult 500 ml of a 20% solution will suffice. Smaller amounts should not be used in this preoperative situation. The rationale for this maneuver is that the intracranial pressure is already dangerously high in almost all patients with large mass lesions, and serious further brain injury can occur in the 15 to 30 minutes prior to evacuation of the mass lesion. Even if the patient appears reasonably stable on the way to the operation, mannitol should be given before or during endotracheal intubation and induction of anesthesia, as during these maneuvers the brain may be further insulted by increasing brain shift or increase in intracranial pressure, and some time will elapse before the dura can be opened (Becker *et al.* 1975, 1976 a, 1982).

Volatile anesthetics such as halothane should not be used because of their well-known cerebral vasodilator effect. This will cause increased intracranial blood volume and, in a patient with a mass lesion, a dangerous rise in intracranial pressure toward blood pressure levels together with a reduction in blood pressure. Various combinations of nitrous oxide, barbiturates, narcotics, and tranquilizers are favored because of their minimal effect on intracranial pressure. Blood gases should be measured during the operation and arterial oxygen tension maintained above 80 mm Hg. Arterial carbon dioxide tension should be quickly brought to levels between 25 and 30, but intraoperative ranges as low as 15 to 20 mm Hg are usually well tolerated clinically. Intraoperative hyper-ventilation should be accomplished with a large tidal volume and a slow to normal respiratory rate, rather than by increasing ventilatory rate much above normal levels, to allow time for good venous return (Becker *et al.* 1976 a, 1982).

## Positioning of the Patient

The patient is generally placed in a mildly flexed position. All pressure points are padded and anesthesia personnel should have access to the patient. In addition, there should be sufficient room for the surgical team. If the CT has shown that the lesion is unilateral, then the head can be placed in a donut and turned in the appropriate position. If there is evidence of bilateral lesions or involvement of the midline structures or if there is any doubt as to extent of the lesion, then provisions should be made to gain access to both sides of the head. We accomplish this by the use of the subdural headrest and the Mayfield head holder. This enables one to do either unilateral or bilateral scalp and skull flaps and to reposition the head during surgery if necessary (Ward and Becker 1983) (Figs. 9 and 10).

### *Operative Technique for Traumatic Intracranial Mass Lesions*

Because most patients with acute subdural hematomas also have an underlying brain contusion, the two entities must be considered together in any discussion of the operation. The most skillful operative technique and the best surgical judgment should be brought to bear on traumatic intracranial mass lesions. Just as neurosurgeons accept that superior

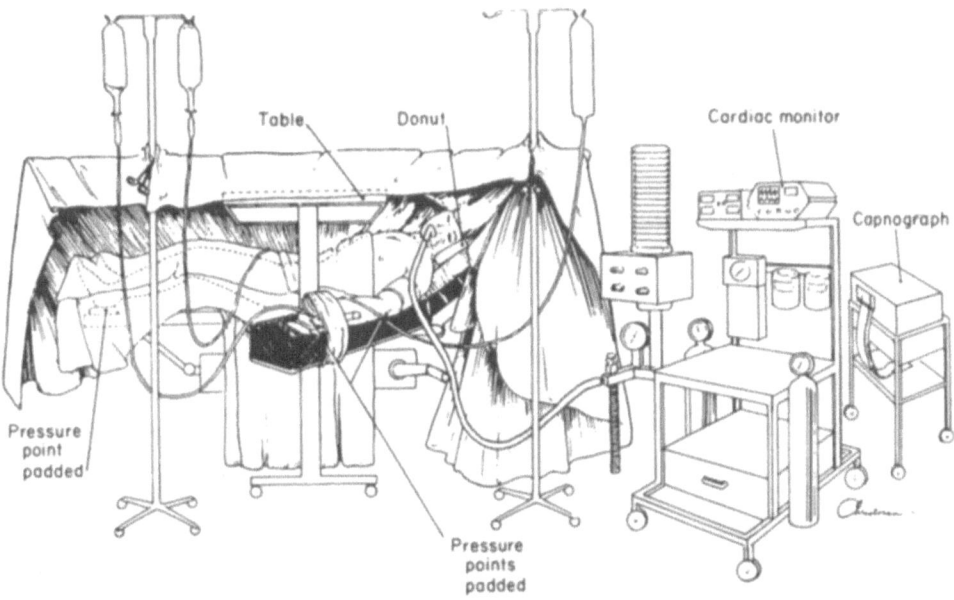

Fig. 9. Positioning of the patient from anesthesia viewpoint. Note that there is good access to the patient and his airway and that all pressure points are padded. (From Ref. 97, reprinted by permission)

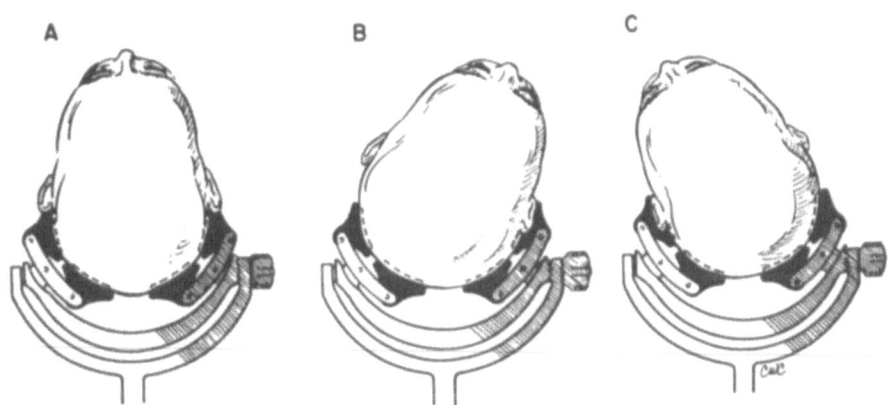

Fig. 10. Position of head in Mayfield head holder to gain access to both sides of head. (From Ref. 97, reprinted by permission)

surgical skill and judgment will yield improved results in aneurysm, arteriovenous malformation, and benign brain tumor operations, these same efforts will also improve results in the operative treatment of trauma. In performing the "decompression", gentle handling of the brain is imperative, and firm brain retraction should not be done, as acutely injured brain tissue is quite vulnerable to this type of insult. The immediate goals of operation are reduction of intracranial pressure and brain shift, control of hemorrhage, and prevention of secondary delayed elevation in intracranial pressure and brain shift from brain swelling, inadequately evacuated clot or contusion, or recurrent clot. Judgment regarding extent of brain contusion excision may be a critical determinant of ultimate outcome. Likewise, meticulous hemostasis and maneuvers to prevent postoperative intracranial hematoma or brain herniation through bony defects can be expected to reduce the ultimate morbidity.

### Rationale for Use of the Basic Large Craniotomy Trauma Flap

There is a high incidence of temporal and frontal contusions and tearing of midline bridging veins in severe brain injury associated with mass lesions requiring operation. The frontal and temporal contusions may not be demonstrable on angiography, and will of course not be seen on ventriculography. Likewise, smaller multifocal contusions may not be seen on computed tomography, particularly soon after injury, before progressive edema develops around the contusion. Since adequate decompressive operations may require debridement of these lesions, the frontal and temporal poles should be accessible in the field of exposure. While the temporal tip and pole are the sites usually involved in temporal lobe contusion, the frontal lesions commonly begin at the tips and extend over the inferior surface, involving the orbital gyri and inferior frontal lobe. Thus, the inferior frontal lobe should be accessible down the floor of the anterior fossa.

With severe rotational brain injuries, one or more midline bridging veins may have been torn. This is a common cause of the acute subdural hematoma, and when the hematoma is evacuated, major intraoperative hemorrhage can occur from these vessels when the pressure tamponade is released (Gurdjian and Thomas 1974, Becker *et al.* 1979). Severe bleeding from these midline vessels may develop after the internal decompression, and if only a limited temporal craniotomy is done for temporal lobe swelling and contusion, great difficulty can be encountered in controlling the hemorrhage that is coming from a distance away from the bone flap (Chambers 1951). To anticipate this potential problem, the craniotomy flap should also expose the area close to the midline. The basic craniotomy flap, therefore, should be generous enough and placed so as to permit one to deal quickly with the most frequently found disorder without further operative extension for additional exposure (Fell *et al.* 1975). The exposure should provide adequate access to decompress the epidural and subdural space; to debride contused cerebral tissue (anterior temporal and frontal lobes and orbital gyri) and remove associated intracerebral hematomas as necessary;

to control hemorrhage from avulsed bridging veins to the sagittal sinus and from temporal lobe to transverse sinus and petrosal sinuses; to control hemorrhage from the skull base, to pack sinuses as necessary, and to repair potential cerebrospinal fluid fistulae; and to explore and manage lesions of vascular and neural elements at the base as necessary (Becker *et al.* 1982).

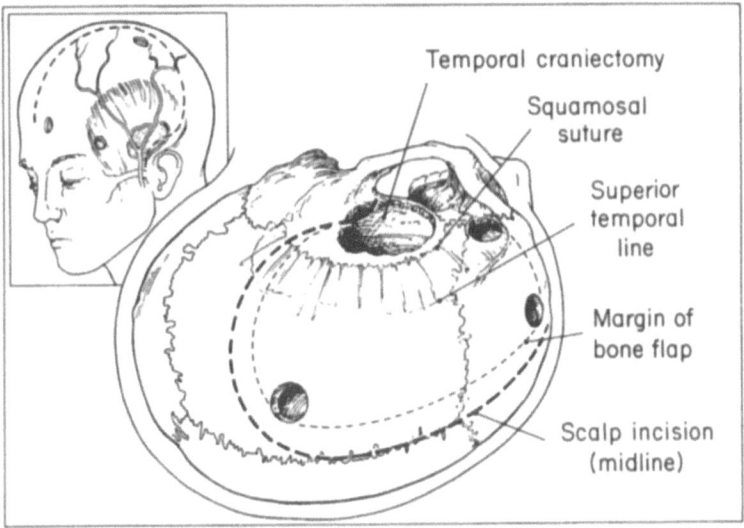

Fig. 11. Outline of the standard craniotomy flap recommended for evacuation of acute epidural, subdural, and intracerebral hematomas and contusions. This exposure will provide access to the critical areas commonly injured in acute acceleration or deceleration "rotational" injuries. Through this flap the surgeon will be able to decompress the epidural and subdural spaces, debride contused anterior temporal and frontal lobes and orbital gyri and control hemorrhage from midline avulsed bridging veins or the basal dural or skull areas. (From Ref. 7, p. 2027, reprinted by permission)

## Technique of Basic Large Trauma Craniotomy

*Scalp Incision.* The skin incision is outlined as shown in Fig. 11. It is begun 1 cm anterior to the tragus at the temporal portion of the zygomatic arch, carried superiorly and posteriorly over the ear, posteriorly around the parietal bone to the midline, where it is brought anteriorly on the midline down to the midforehead. The forehead incision, which comes below the hairline, can be closed by using plastic surgical techniques, and the minimal visible scar is small sacrifice for the added exposure of the frontal lobe gained by this flap.

*Immediate Temporal Decompression.* If the patient has been deteriorating rapidly prior to operation, a quick decompression is the immediate goal. In this situation the portion of the incision just anterior to and above the ear should be opened first down through the temporalis muscle to bone (Fig. 12). A burr hole and small craniectomy should be accomplished quickly, and the dura opened in cruciate fashion. Most often this maneuver will

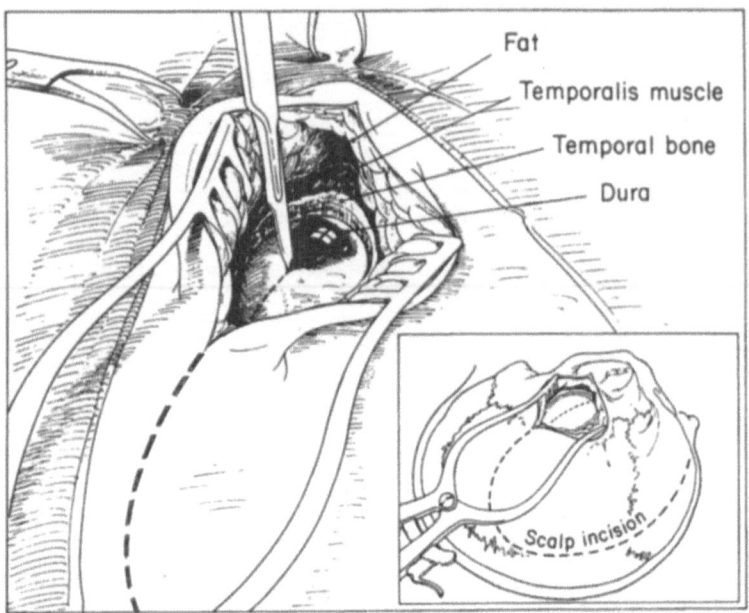

Fig. 12. If the patient has been deteriorating prior to operation or if the intracranial pressure is known to be very high and there is a major shift, an initial quick subtemporal decompression should be done. One should then proceed with the formal craniotomy. (From Ref. 7, p. 2027, reprinted by permission)

afford some immediate relief of elevated intracranial pressure when a small amount of extraaxial clot or contused temporal lobe herniates out through the craniectomy site. One should then proceed to perform the formal craniotomy, and not be satisfied with this small decompression (Chambers 1951, Davis 1946, Fell *et al.* 1975, Gibbs 1970, McKissock *et al.* 1960).

*Bone Flap.* Either a free bone flap or one based on the temporalis muscle can be raised. The medial portion of the craniotomy should be approximately 2 to 3 cm from the midline. The bone flap should be brought low across the frontal bone, across the sphenoid wing, below the pterion to the temporal bone. The opening is further enlarged by resection of the lateral portion of the sphenoid wing (Fig. 13).

*Dural Opening.* The incision is begun in the temporal region, a continuation of the dural temporal opening if an initial temporal craniectomy and dural incision have been made, or the anterior frontal region (Fig. 14). With this approach, if the brain herniates through the dura because of mass effect, the herniated cerebral tissue will be part of a relatively silent

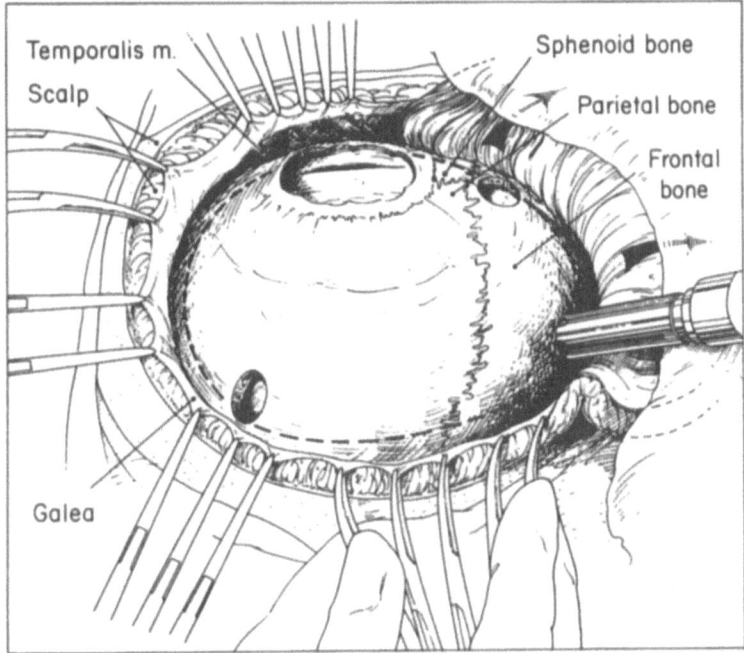

Fig. 13. Either a free bone flap or one based on the temporal muscle can be raised. The medial portion of the bone flap should be 2 to 3 cm from the midline. Far anterior placement of the forward holes permits easy access to anterior temporal lobe and orbital gyri. (From Ref. 7, p. 2028, reprinted by permission)

lobe. This herniation usually occurs only when the temporal or frontal tip is severely contused. The remainder of the dural opening can then be completed with little further herniation of tissue. If intact cortex begins to herniate, further maneuvers to reduce brain swelling should be instituted immediately: additional mannitol, increased hyperventilation, barbiturates, and perhaps even transient reduction of arterial blood pressure to reduce and relieve cerebrovascular engorgement. The dural opening should be curved gently as it is carried anteriorly, up to the anterior medial border of the bone flap. An incision from the center of this dural flap, directed posteromedially, will complete the opening. This dural opening provides access to the frontal and temporal lobes and the anterior and middle fossae.

The vast majority of unilateral intracranial hemorrhages and contusions can now be dealt with. The lateral parietal and occipital cortex may be inspected, but is not fully exposed. The orbital gyri are readily accessible, as are the inferior temporal gyrus and more basal structures. Inspection of the basal structures can be accomplished, if necessary. Hemorrhage from the

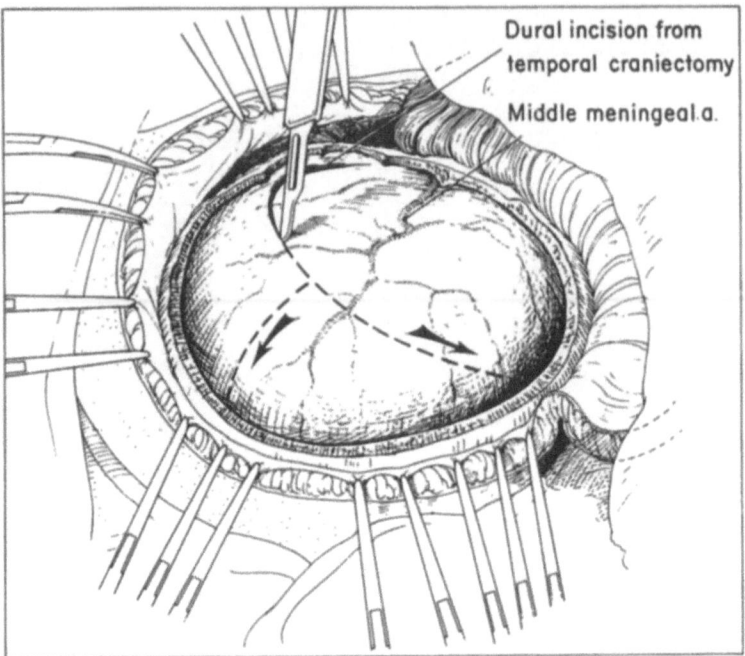

Fig. 14. The dural opening shown here provides safe access to basal, midline, and anterior regions. (From Ref. 7, p. 2028, reprinted by permission)

middle meningeal artery is readily controlled, even down to the foramen spinosum. The intracranial surface of the sagittal sinus is exposed, and hemorrhage from avulsed emissary cortical veins can be controlled without further bone resection or undue retraction on the brain.

*The Acute Subdural Hematoma.* Acute subdural hematoma should always be dealt with via the large craniotomy, never through burr holes or a limited temporal craniectomy (Richards and Hoff 1974, Whaley 1948). In fact, a rule to follow in all subdural hematomas, regardless of the age of the lesion, is that if any clotted blood is present, a craniotomy flap should be turned down (Bucy and Oberhill 1968). Once the dura is opened, the clot should be gently removed from the cortical surface (Fig. 15). Removal of the clot is best done with a combination of irrigation, cup forceps evacuation, and gentle suction. Large fragments of clot that are over the occipital lobe or on the floor of the anterior or middle fossae can be gently washed and teased out. These large fragments can be exposed by placing a brain retractor over the appropriate lobe and allowing the clot to extrude slowly to be extracted with forceps. Tiny bits of clot under the dura and bone should not be vigorously pursued.

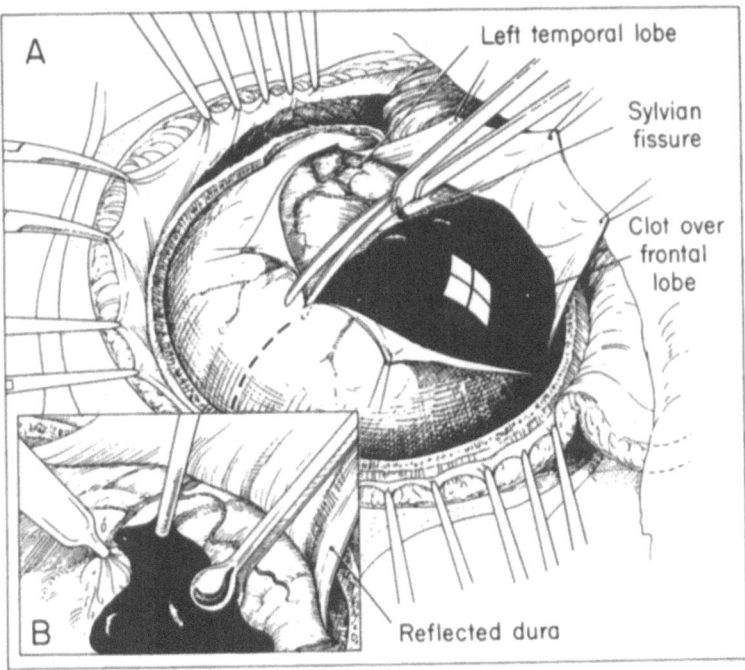

Fig. 15. A) A typical acute subdural hematoma is shown here. B) After the dura is open, the clot should be gently removed by means of irrigation, forceps extraction, and careful suctioning. (From Ref. 7, p. 2031, reprinted by permission)

A bleeding major surface artery or vein will often be identified after the clot is removed (Chambers 1951). It can usually be sealed by bipolar coagulation. If the bleeding is coming from a midline bridging vein, a middle fossa vessel, or a vessel that is located under the intact dura and bone, great care must be taken in exposing and controlling the bleeding vessel. In the management of an avulsed bridging vein, the cortical open end is usually easily controlled with bipolar coagulation. The sinus side of the vessel may be troublesome, and if bipolar coagulation or Gelform or operative packing fails, a small piece of beaten muscle carefully placed directly over the venous opening will usually produce satisfactory hemostasis (Fig. 16).

*Cerebral Contusion in Association with the Acute Subdural Hematoma.* Contusions usually appear on the surface of the anterior and inferior frontal

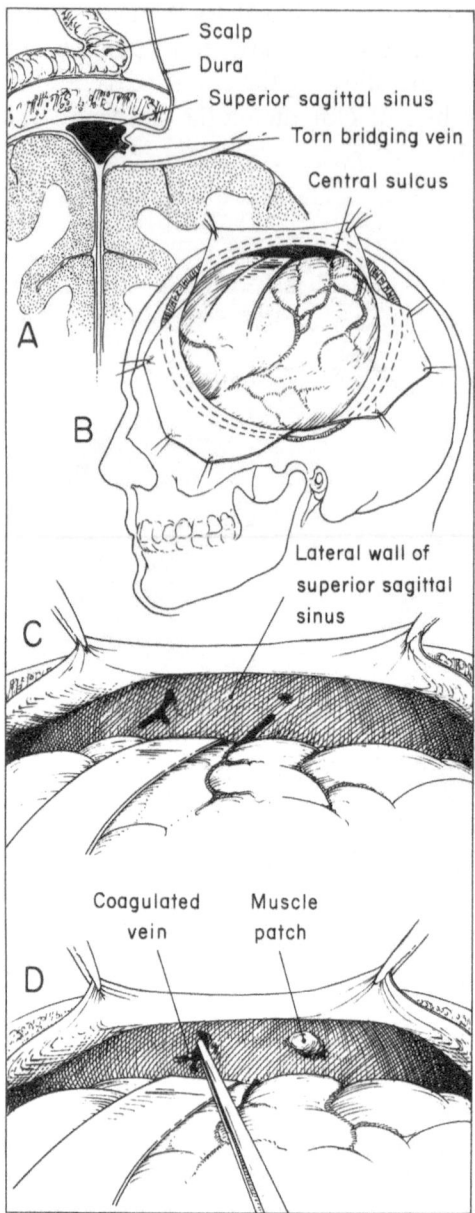

Fig. 16. A) Bleeding from avulsed midline bridging veins commonly occurs after evacuation of the hematoma or contusion. B, C, D) Simple coagulation will often suffice, but a patch of beaten muscle is still the finest hemostatic agent when sinus bleeding from an avulsed draining vein is not easily controlled with coagulation or synthetic hemostatic agents. (From Ref. 7, p. 2032, reprinted by permission)

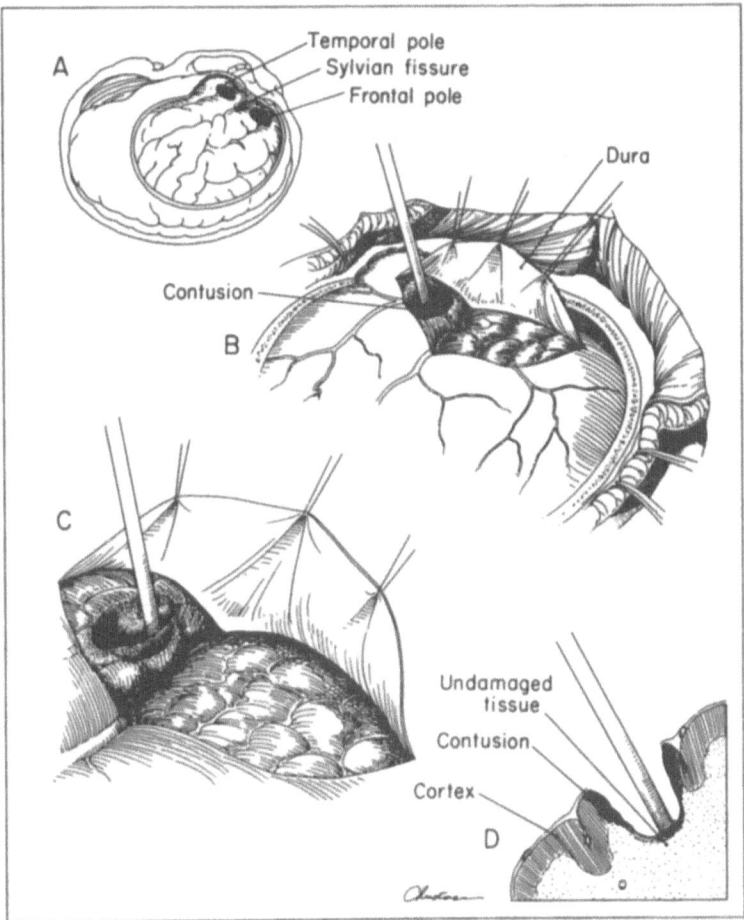

Fig. 17. A) Visual location of traumatic contusions. B) Dural opening. C, D) Removal of the contused brain only. (From Ref. 7, p. 2033, reprinted by permission)

lobes and the temporal lobes (Fig. 17). They are composed of necrotic brain tissue that is infiltrated with blood. The brain tissue in a confluent contusion is irreversibly and irreparably destroyed and not only serves as a primary mass lesion but may go on to cause further major brain swelling in and around itself; for this reason necrotic contusions should be removed when exposed at operation. Surface contusions larger than 2 cm in diameter should be removed. Often a surface contusion 2 cm in diameter will extend several centimeters or more deep into the hemisphere, and the cortical edge of the contusion is only the "tip of the iceberg".

Once the contusion is exposed it should be gently sucked out. The soft, friable, wet, purple-blue necrotic tissue can be easily aspirated. Suction should continue until a circumferential margin of healthy brain tissue is reached. One should not hesitate to aspirate all necrotic tissue, even in multiple sites, over the anterior temporal and frontal lobes. Contusions over the more posterior-superior temporal lobe, or in the region of the central sulcus or the parietal or occipital lobes, should be carefully evaluated, and if they are clearly large necrotic contusions, they should also be removed. Removing contusions in these areas will *not increase* the neurological deficit if one works entirely within the contusion, and ultimate postoperative neurological function may be surprisingly good even when contusions are removed from areas near the primary motor cortex and surface speech centers. The secondary brain edema that occurs around the contusions can be reduced by operative removal, and the postoperative clinical status and ultimate result may be improved (Becker *et al.* 1979, Heiskanen and Vapalahti 1972).

*Acute Brain Swelling During Operation.* Occasionally, sudden and rapid massive brain swelling will occur during an operation. The swelling may occur immediately after dural opening, or sometimes moments or even many minutes after a large clot or contusion has been excised. A probable cause is defective cerebral autoregulation. With the sudden decrease of extravascular pressure that occurs at dural opening or mass lesion evacuation, the cerebrovascular bed distends passively from the arterial blood pressure head, and a sizable increase in cerebral blood volume results (Kobrine *et al.* 1977). The other less common cause is from new acute intraoperative hemorrhage and the rapid accumulation of a clot contralateral to the craniotomy or in an ipsilateral area hidden from the operative exposure. True brain edema occurring as rapidly as this is only rarely the cause of such intraoperative swelling, and even then is probably associated with cerebral vasodilatation.

Intraoperative brain swelling must be dealt with promptly and aggressively. Thiopental (500 mg in an adult) will often produce dramatic detumescence of the swollen brain and permit brain relocation (Ward *et al.* 1984). The barbiturate reduces cerebral blood flow, blood volume and often arterial blood pressure. Reduction of systolic arterial blood pressure to 60 to 90 mm Hg will almost always permit the brain to return to its normal position. Simultaneously, the anesthesiologist should rapidly administer even more mannitol and increase the tidal volume to further lower the arterial carbon dioxide tension. After two to four minutes the blood pressure should be allowed to seek its own level naturally again. Often, this combination of maneuvers will capture and reverse the acute swelling. The induced hypotension may have to be repeated until the mannitol further shrinks the brain or while autoregulation improves, but prolonged induced hypotension must be avoided or severe brain ischemia will ensue.

If the preceding maneuvers fail to relocate the brain within the skull, a frontal or temporal lobectomy may be necessary for internal decompression. An internal decompression by a frontal or temporal lobectomy should ordinarily be done only if one of these lobes shows some evidence of contusion or hemorrhage. All reasonable maneuvers should be considered to get the brain back into place to permit bone flap replacement (Cooper *et al.* 1976).

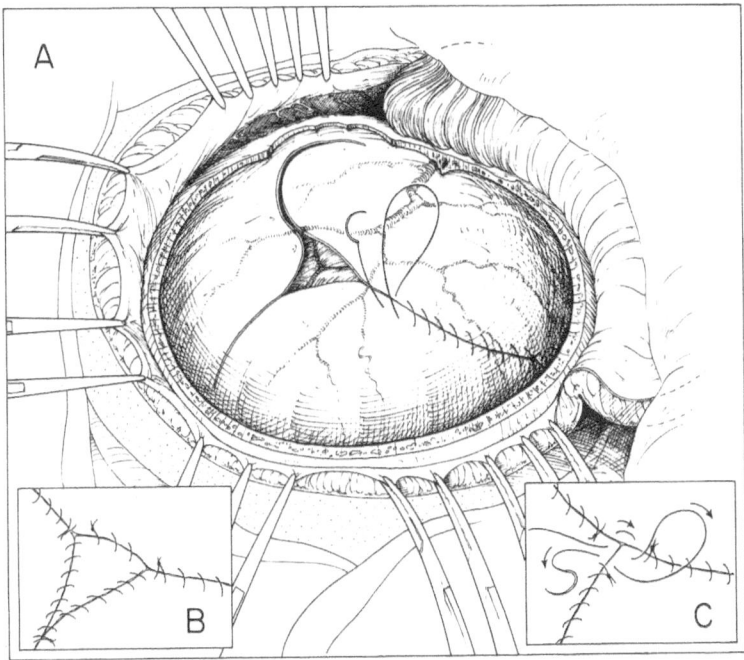

Fig. 18. A) Complete closure of the dura, using a graft if necessary, is recommended for a number of reasons, the most important being that this will help keep the brain from herniating through the craniotomy site over bony edges. The bone flap is also replaced, if at all possible, and fixed in place with nonmetallic sutures. B) The graft.
   C) Detail of suture pattern. (From Ref. 7, p. 2035, reprinted by permission)

*Closure of the Craniotomy Flap.* Complete closure of the dura and replacement of the bone flap should always be done, if possible, and may require a periosteal graft (Fig. 18). Dural closure is recommended because postoperative extradural bleeding is kept out of the subarachnoid space; cortical adhesions to soft tissues are less likely; cerebrospinal fluid wound leak or fistulae may be reduced; any wound infection that may occur will more likely be isolated to the extradural space; and dural closure, even with a graft, helps keep the brain from herniating through the craniectomy site across the bony edges.

Unless brain swelling is massive and cannot be controlled, the bone flap should be replaced and fixed in place with suture material. Brain that herniates through a bony defect usually undergoes infarction and dies, and large craniectomies have not reduced the mortality rate or morbidity (Clark et al. 1968, Cooper et al. 1976, Kjellberg and Prieto 1971, Ransohoff et al. 1971). In fact, this "herniated" brain that extends out over bony edges tends to develop progressively increasing edema that axtends deep into white matter and may go on to involve the entire hemisphere. Brain swelling and elevated intracranial pressure in the postoperative period are best managed by medical means in the intensive care unit, and the bone flap should not be left out because the surgeon anticipates delayed brain swelling (Becker et. al. 1975).

Following skin closure, the patient should not be extubated, but should be taken to the recovery room or intensive care unit and immediately connected to a volume respirator. This prevents early postanesthesia bucking and straining, and permits smooth continuation of controlled ventilation and total care of the helpless patient (Becker et al. 1982).

## Postoperative Intensive Care and Medical Management

The cornerstones of intensive care and medical management of these patients include:

1. Neurologic monitoring including;
   a. Eye opening.
   b. Verbal response.
   c. Motor response.
   d. Motor strength.
   e. Pupil size and reactivity.
   f. Oculocephalic reflexes.
2. Monitoring of vital signs including:
   a. Blood pressure.
   b. Pulse.
   c. Respiratory status.
   d. Body temperature.
3. Monitoring of central venous pressure or pulmonary wedge pressure.
4. Monitoring of intracranial pressure.
5. Recording of intake/output.
6. Recording of medications administered.
7. Recording of body weight.
8. Monitoring of serum electrolytes, especially sodium.

The goals of modern intensive neurosurgical care of the severely head injured patient include prevention or early recognition of systemic medical complications, maintenance of a safe ICP, anticipation and prevention of additional brain insults, and maintenance of the patient in a milieu that is conducive to recovery of reversibly injured brain cells. These goals are particularly crucial for patients with acute subdural hematoma after clot evacuation.

## Intensive Medical Management Protocol

Either a central venous line or pulmonary artery catheter should be inserted upon arrival in the intensive care unit if not already done. Measurements from these lines are invaluable in assisting in decisions regarding fluid management, particularly that obtained from pulmonary artery catheters which provide pulmonary wedge pressures and cardiac indices. It is, however, a more invasive technique, and we reserve its use for the more severely ill patient. Central venous pressure should be kept between 8 to 12 cm $H_2O$. Urinary output measured via an indwelling bladder catheter should be approximately 30 ml/hour. A rate either higher or lower than this figure may indicate too much or too little fluid administration. Maintenance fluid is usually begun with 2.5% dextrose and 0.45% saline plus 20 mEq KCl/liter at 75 to 100 ml/hour in adults. Hyponatremia ($Na^+ < 130$ mEq/liter) must be avoided. Brain edema may be promoted by low serum sodium. Hyponatremia is most commonly the result of inappropriate secretion of anti-diuretic hormone (ADH). If this diagnosis is made, the initial treatment is mild fluid restriction and administration of 5% dextrose and isotonic saline solution. Hypertonic saline and/or the use of sodium-retaining steroid hormones may be required (Becker et al. 1981).

Because of the danger of aspiration and possibility of abdominal injuries, care must be made not to attempt to convert the patient from intravenous fluids to nasogastric feeding too soon. If after 3 days nasogastric tube feeding cannot be initiated, parenteral alimentation with lipid, glucose and amino acids should be administered.

Controlled ventilation is done with a volume respirator initially set in adults at a slow rate of 12 breaths/minute at a tidal volume of 12 ml/kg body weight. This setting allows for adequate venous return to the heart and assists in re-expanding collapsed alveoli. Minute volume is adjusted to bring $PaCO_2$ to between 25 and 30 mm Hg. To phase the patient onto the ventilator, intramuscular chlorpromazine, intravenous morphine, or intravenous pancuronium bromide should be administered. Neurologic deterioration due to a secondary insult may sometimes occur without affecting ICP. Therefore, the patient should be evaluated neurologically at intervals every 3 to 4 hours. Ventilator control is continued until the patient begins to follow commands or his condition becomes stable with a normal ICP for 2 days. In most instances patients need to be maintained on this regimen for only 3 to 5 days, but it can be used successfully for 3 to 4 weeks. Positive end-expiratory pressure (PEEP) 2 to 10 cm $H_2O$ is added to the system when pulmonary insufficiency is detected and a clinical picture of adult respiratory distress syndrome or pulmonary contusion is present. As a rule, low values (1 to 5 cm $H_2O$) greatly improve oxygenation without affecting the intracranial or systemic pressures adversely (Becker *et al.* 1981).

The utility of corticosteroids is still much debated in head injured patients (Braakman *et al.* 1983, Faupel *et al.* 1977, Gobiet *et al.* 1976, Gudeman *et al.* 1979) and we no longer use them routinely. Additional medications include cimetidine, 300 mg every 6 hours, or antacids to inhibit gastric acid secretion and hemorrhage.

Control of body temperature is important. Hyperthermia increases brain edema, ICP, and brain and body metabolism and predisposes to skin breakdown and formation of decubiti. Hyperthermia therefore must be vigorously treated. Because induced chronic hypothermia creates a number of medical problems, it is preferable to keep the patient in a normothermic range. Temperature is controlled with rectal acetaminophen or aspirin and a cooling blanket or mattress. Chlorpromazine may be helpful in bringing the temperature down by controlling shivering when a cooling blanket is used.

Routine nursing care should include cultures of urine, twice/week; sputum, twice/week; and CSF, daily if patient is being monitored by ventricular catheter.

Other important aspects of nursing care include elevation of the head by 20°, turning every 2 hours, frequent pulmonary toilet, long-leg anti-embolic stockings, installation of artificial tears every 4 hours, oral hygiene, and range of motion exercises to all extremities. Physical and occupational therapy departments are contacted early in the patient's hospital stay for evaluation and initiation of therapy (Becker *et al.* 1981).

Nearly all monitoring systems have a bedside and/or central station display for the appropriately monitored functions. An alarm system can indicate when desired limits are violated. Computerized recording systems are available which can compile data over a period of time varying from a few minutes to 24 hours on a single page. Nursing observations may be written in as desired on the recording. Information may be gathered continuously or at desired intervals and displayed in digital or graphic form. The computer can then make desired calculations and display the results. The information can then be stored for later reevaluation. Any combination of laboratory values, intake and output, medications, treatments, and responses may be entered and processed. The potential benefits of this system are great. Changes in the patient's condition may not only be detected more quickly but treated more efficiently.

## Conclusions

The principles outlined above for management of acute subdural hematoma are directed at making the earliest possible diagnosis and removal of the mass lesion, all the while protecting the brain from hypoxia and/or ischemia. When these principles are rigidly followed, recovery from the disorder may be dramatically improved for many patients. This organized approach to the head injured victim brings rewards for the patient and his surgeon as well.

## References

1. Balslev-Jorgenson, P., Heilbrun, M. P., Boysen, G., Rosenklint, A., Jorgenson, E. O., 1972: Cerebral perfusion pressure correlated with regional cerebral blood flow and aorto-cervical arteriography in patients with severe brain disorders progressing to death. Eur. Neurol. 8, 207 – 212.
2. Becker, D. P. (In discussion of Miller, J. D.), 1976: Clinical aspects of intracranial pressure-volume relationships. In: McLaurin, R. L. (ed.), Head Injuries: Second Chicago Symposium on Neural Trauma, pp. 247 – 248. New York: Grune & Stratton, Inc.
3. Becker, D. P., Gudeman, S. K., Miller, J. D., 1981: Head injuries: In: Goldsmith, H. S. (ed.), Practice of Surgery. Philadelphia: Harper & Row.
4. Becker, D. P., Miller, J. D., Sweet, R. C., Sweet, J. D., et al., 1979: Head injury management. In: Popp, A. J., Bourke, R. S., Nelson, L. R., Kimelberg, H. K. (eds.), Neural Trauma. Seminars in Neurological Surgery, pp. 313 – 328. New York: Raven Press.
5. Becker, D. P., Miller, J. D., Ward, J. D., Greenberg, R. P., Young, H. F., Sakalas, R., 1977: The outcome from severe head injury with early diagnosis and intensive management. J. Neurosurg. 47, 491 – 502.
6. Becker, D. P., Miller, J. D., Young, H. E., et al., 1976 a: The critical importance of intracranial pressure monitoring in head injury. In: Becks, J. W. F., Bosch, D. A., Brock, M. (eds.), Intracranial Pressure III, pp. 97 – 100. Berlin-Heidelberg-New York: Springer.
7. Becker, D. P., Miller, J. D., Young, H. F., Selhorst, J. B., Kishore, P. R. S., Greenberg, R. P., Rosner, M. J., Ward, J. D., 1982: Diagnosis and treatment of head injury in adults. In: Youmans, J. R. (ed.), Neurological Surgery, Vol. 4, pp. 1938 – 2083. Philadelphia: W. B. Saunders Co.
8. Becker, D. P., Sullivan, H. G., Adams, W. E., et al., 1976 b: Controlled hyperventilation in severe mechanical brain injury. In: McLaurin, R. L. (ed.), Head Injuries: Second Chicago Symposium on Neural Trauma, pp. 157 – 159. New York: Grune & Stratton, Inc.
9. Becker, D. P., Vries, J. K., Young, H. F., et al., 1975: Controlled cerebral perfusion pressure and ventilation in mechanical brain injury: Prevention of progressive brain swelling. In: Lundberg, N., Ponten, U., Brock, M. (eds.), Intracranial Pressure II, pp. 480 – 484. Berlin-Heidelberg-New York: Springer.

10. Braakman, R., Gelpke, G. J., Habbema, J. D. F., Maas, A. I. R., Minderhoud, J. M., 1980: Systematic selection of prognostic features in patients with severe head injury. Neurosurgery 6, 362 – 370.
11. Braakman, R., Schouten, H. J., Blaauw-van Dishoeck, M., Minderhoud, J. M., 1983: Megadose steroids in severe head injury: Results of a prospective double-blind clinical trial. J. Neurosurg. 58 (3), 326 – 330.
12. Brendler, S. J., Selverstone, B., 1970: Recovery from decerebration. Brain 93, 381 – 392.
13. Bricolo, A., Turazzi, S., Alexandre, A., Rizzuto, N., 1977: Decerebrate rigidity in acute head injury. J. Neurosurg. 47, 680 – 698.
14. Browder, J., 1943: A resume of the principle diagnostic features of subdural hematoma. Bull. N.Y. Acad. Med. 19, 168 – 176.
15. Bucy, P. C., Oberhill, H. R., 1968: Subdural hematoma in adults. Arizona Med. 25, 186 – 189.
16. Cairns, H., 1952: Disturbances of consciousness with lesions of the brain stem and diencephalon. Brain 75, 109 – 146.
17. Chambers, J. W., 1951: Acute subdural hematoma. J. Neurosurg. 8, 263 – 268.
18. Clark, K., Nash, T. M., Hutchinson, G. C., 1968: The failure of circumferential craniotomy in acute traumatic cerebral swelling. J. Neurosurg. 29, 367 – 371.
19. Cooper, P. R., Rovit, R. L., Ransohoff, J., 1976: Hemicraniectomy in the treatment of acute subdural hematoma: a re-appraisal. Surg. Neurol. 5, 25 – 28.
20. Corsellis, J. A. N., 1958: Individual variation in the size of the tentorial opening. J. Neurol. Neurosurg. Psychiat. 21, 279 – 283.
21. Davis, L. E., 1946: The Principles of Neurological Surgery. Philadelphia: Lea & Febiger.
22. Faupel, G., Reuben, H. J., Muller, P., et al., 1977: Double-blind study on the effects of dexamethason. In: Becks, J. W. F., Bosch, D. A., Brock, M. (eds.), Intracranial Pressure III. Berlin-Heidelberg-New York: Springer.
23. Fell, D. A., Fitzgerald, S., Moiel, R. H., Caram, P., 1975: Acute subdural hematomas: a review of 144 cases. J. Neurosurg. 42, 27 – 42.
24. Fleischer, A. S., Payne, N. S., Tindall, G. T., 1976: Continuous monitoring of intracranial pressure in severe closed head injury without mass lesions. Surg. Neurol. 6, 31 – 34.
25. Gibbs, J. R., 1960: Middle-meningeal hemorrhage. Lancet 2, 727 – 731.
26. Gobiet, W., Bock, W. J., Liesegang, J., et al., 1976: Treatment of acute cerebral edema with high dose of dexamethasone. In: Becks, J. W. F., Bosch, D. A., Brock, M. (eds.), Intracranial Pressure III, pp. 232 – 235. Berlin-Heidelberg-New York: Springer.
27. Goodkin, R., Szhiser, J., 1978: Sequential angiographic studies demonstrating delayed development of an acute epidural hematoma. J. Neurosurg. 48, 479 – 482.
28. Greenberg, R. P., Mayer, D. J., Becker, D. P., 1976: Correlation in man of intracranial pressure and neuroelectric activity determined by multimodality evoked potentials. In: Becks, J. W. F., Bosch, D. A., Brock, M. (eds.), Intracranial Pressure III, pp. 58 – 62. Berlin-Heidelberg-New York: Springer.

29. Greenberg, R. P., Mayer, D. J., Becker, D. P., Miller, J. D., 1977: Evaluation of brain function in severe human head trauma with multimodality evoked potentials. I. Evoked brain injury potentials, methods and analysis. J. Neurosurg. *47*, 150 – 162.

30. Grossman, R. G., Turner, J. W., Miller, J. D., Rowan, J. O., 1975: The relationship between cortical electrical activity, cerebral perfusion pressure and cerebral blood flow during increased intracranial pressure. In: Langfitt, T. W., McHenry, L. C., Reivich, M., Wallman, H. (eds.), Cerebral Circulation and Metabolism, pp. 232 – 234. Berlin-Heidelberg-New York: Springer.

31. Gudeman, S. K., Miller, J. D., Becker, D. P., 1979: Failure of high-dose steroid therapy to influence intracranial pressure in patients with severe head injury. J. Neurosurg. *51*, 301.

32. Gurdjian, E. S., Thomas, L. M., 1974: Traumatic intracranial hemorrhage. In: Feiring, E. H. (ed.), Brock's Injuries of the Brain and Spinal Cord and Their Coverings, 5th Ed., pp. 203 – 267. New York: Springer Publishing Co.

33. Gutterman, P., Shenkin, H. A., 1970: Prognostic features in recovery from traumatic decerebration. J. Neurosurg. *32*, 330 – 335.

34. Hancock, D. O., 1961: Angiography in acute head injuries. Lancet *2*, 745 – 747.

35. Harris, P., 1971: Acute traumatic subdural hematomas: results of the neurosurgical care. In: Head Injuries: Proceedings of an International Symposium, pp. 321 – 326. Edinburgh: Churchill-Livingstone.

36. Heiskanen, O., Vapalahti, M., 1972: Temporal lobe contusion and hematoma. Acta Neurochir. (Wien) *27*, 29 – 35.

37. Hoff, J. T., Reis, D. J., 1970: Localization of regions mediating the Cushing response in the central nervous system of the cat. Arch. Neurol. (Chicago) *22*, 228 – 240.

38. Holbourn, A. H. S., 1943: Mechanisms of brain injuries. Lancet *2*, 438 – 441.

39. Jamieson, K. G., Yelland, J. D. N., 1972: Surgically treated traumatic subdural hematomas. J. Neurosurg. *37*, 137 – 149.

40. Jefferson, G., 1938: The tentorial pressure cone. Arch. Neurol. Psychiat. *40*, 857 – 876.

41. Jenkins, L. W., Marmarou, A., Lewelt, W., Becker, D. P., 1984: Increased vulnerability of the traumatized brain to early ischemia. Nato Advanced Research Workshop: Mechanisms of Secondary Brain Damage. In: Baethmann, A. (ed.), Mauls/Sterzing, Italy.

42. Jennett, B., Teasdale, G., Braakman, R., et al., 1976: Predicting outcome in individual patients after head injury. Lancet *1*, 1031 – 1034.

43. Jennett, B., Teasdale, G., Galbraith, S., et al., 1979: Prognosis in patients with severe head injury. Acta Neurochir. (Wien), (Suppl.) *28*, 149 – 152.

44. Jennett, W. B., Stern, W. E., 1960: Tentorial herniation, the midbrain and the pupil. J. Neurosurg. *17*, 598 – 609.

45. Johnston, I., Paterson, A., 1974: Benign intracranial hypertension II. CSF pressure and circulation. Brain *97*, 301 – 312.

46. Johnston, I. H., Johnston, J. A., Jennett, B., 1970: Intracranial pressure changes following head injury. Lancet *2*, 1365 – 1369.

47. Kaufmann, G. E., Clark, K., 1970 a: Continuous simultaneous monitoring of intraventricular and cervical subarachnoid cerebrospinal fluid pressure to indicate the development of cerebral or tonsillar herniation. J. Neurosurg. *33*, 145—150.

48. Kaufmann, G. E., Clark, K., 1970 b: Emergency frontal twist drill ventriculostomy. J. Neurosurg. *33*, 226—227.

49. Kennedy, F., Wortis, S. B., 1931: Modern treatment of increased intracranial pressure. JAMA *96*, 1248—1286.

50. Kjellberg, R. N., Prieto, A., Jr., 1971: Bifrontal decompressive craniotomy for massive cerebral edema. J. Neurosurg. *34*, 488—493.

51. Klintworth, G. K., 1966: Secondary brain stem hemorrhage. J. Neurol. Neurosurg. Psychiatry *29*, 423—425.

52. Kobrine, A. J., Timmons, E., Rajjoub, J. K., *et al.*, 1977: Demonstration of massive traumatic brain swelling within 20 minutes after injury. J. Neurosurg. *46*, 256—258.

53. Landig, G. H., Browder, E. J., Watson, R. A., 1941: Subdural hematoma: A study of one hundred and forty-three cases encountered during a five-year-period. Ann. Surg. *133*, 170—188.

54. Langfitt, T. W., 1969: Increased intracranial pressure. Clin. Neurosurg. *16*, 436—471.

55. Langfitt, T. W., Weinstein, J. D., Kassell, N. F., Gagliardi, L. J., 1964 a: Transmission of increased intracranial pressure. II. Within the supratentorial space. J. Neurosurg. *21*, 998—1005.

56. Langfitt, T. W., Weinstein, J. D., Kassell, N. F., Simeone, F. A., 1964 b: Transmission of increased intracranial pressure. I. Within the cranio-spinal axis. J. Neurosurg. *21*, 998—1005.

57. Leech, P. J., Miller, J. D., 1974: Intracranial volume/pressure relationships during experimental brain compression in primates. I. Pressure responses to changes in ventricular volume. J. Neurol. Neurosurg. Psychiatry *37*, 1093—1098.

58. Lewin, W., 1949: Acute subdural and extradural hematoma in closed head injuries. Ann. R. Coll. Surg. Engl. *5*, 240—274.

59. Lewin, W., 1976: Changing attitudes to the management of severe head injuries. Brit. Med. J. *2*, 1234—1239.

60. Loew, F., Wüstner, S., 1960: Diagnose, Behandlung und Prognose der traumatischen Hämatome des Schädelinneren. Acta Neurochir. (Wien) *8* (Suppl.), 1—158.

61. Löfgren, J., Zwetnow, N. N., 1973: Cranial and spinal components of cerebrospinal fluid pressure-volume curve. Acta Neurol. Scand. *49*, 575—585.

62. Lundberg, N., 1960: Continuous recording and control of ventricular fluid pressure in neurosurgical practice. Acta Psychiat. Neurol. Scand. *36* (Suppl.): *149*, 1—193.

63. Maciver, I. N., Frew, I. J. C., Matheson, J. G., 1958: The role of respiratory insufficiency in the mortality of severe head injury. Lancet *1*, 390—393.

64. Marmarou, A., Shulman, K., 1976: Pressure-volume relationships-basic aspects. In: McLaurin, R. L. (ed.), Head Injuries: Second Chicago Symposium on Neural Trauma, pp. 233—236. New York: Grune & Stratton, Inc.

65. McKissock, W., Richardson, A., Bloom, W. H., 1960: Subdural hematoma: a review of 389 cases. Lancet *1*, 1365 – 1369.

66. McLaurin, R. L., Tutor, F. T., 1961: Acute subdural hematoma: review of ninety cases. J. Neurosurg. *18*, 61 – 67.

67. McNealy, D. E., Plum, F., 1962: Brain stem dysfunction with supratentorial mass lesions. Arch. Neurol. *7*, 10 – 32.

68. Mendelow, A. D., Karmi, M. Z., Paul, K. S., Fuller, G. A. G., Gillingham, F. J., 1979: Extradural hematoma: effect of delayed treatment. Brit. Med. J. *1*, 1240 – 1242.

69. Meyer, A., 1920: Herniation of the brain. Arch. Neurol. Psychiatry *4*, 387 – 400.

70. Miller, D., Adams, H., 1972: Physiopathology and management of increased intracranial pressure. In: Critchley, M., O'Leary, J. L., Jennett, B. (eds.), Scientific Foundation of Neurology, pp. 215 – 230. London: William Heinemann Ltd.

71. Miller, J. D., 1975: Volume and pressure in the craniospinal axis. Clin. Neurosurg. *22*, 76 – 105.

72. Miller, J. D., Becker, D. P., 1982: Principles and pathophysiology of head injury. In: Youmans, J. R. (ed.), Neurological Surgery, Vol. 4, pp. 1896 – 1937. Philadelphia: W. B. Saunders Co.

73. Miller, J. D., Becker, D. P., Ward, J. D., Sullivan, H. G., Adams, W. E., Rosner, M. J., 1977: Significance of intracranial hypertension in severe head injury. J. Neurosurg. *47*, 503 – 516.

74. Moiel, R. H., Caram, P. E., 1967: Acute subdural hematomas: A review of eightyfour cases—a six year evaluation. J. Trauma *7*, 660 – 666.

75. Moore, M. T., Stern, K., 1938: Vascular lesions of the brain stem and occipital lobe occurring in association with brain tumors. Brain *61*, 70 – 81.

76. Osborn, A. G., 1977: Diagnosis of transtentorial herniation by cranial computed tomography. Radiology *123*, 93 – 96.

77. Pagni, C. A., 1973: The prognosis of head-injured patients in a state of coma with decerebrated posture. J. Neurosurg. Sci. *17*, 289 – 296.

78. Pasztor, E., Pasztor, A., Bodo, M., Bosch, S., 1975: The role of spinal arachnoid space in compensation of intracranial hypertension. In: Lundberg, N., Ponten, U., Brock, M. (eds.), Intracranial Pressure II, pp. 82 – 85. Berlin-Heidelberg-New York: Springer.

79. Pazzaglia, P., Frank, F., *et al.,* 1979: Clinical course and prognosis of acute post-traumatic coma. J. Neurol. Neurosurg. Psychiatry *38*, 149 – 154.

80. Price, D. J., Knill-Jones, R., 1979: The prediction of outcome of patients admitted following head injury in coma with bilateral fixed pupils. Acta Neurochir. (Wien) *28*, (Suppl.), 179 – 182.

81. Ransohoff, J., Benjamin, M. V., Gage, E. L., Jr., Epstein, F., 1971: Hemicraniectomy in the management of acute subdural hematoma. J. Neurosurg. *34*, 70 – 76.

82. Reid, W. I., Cone, W. V., 1939: The mechanisms of fixed dilation of the pupil resulting from ipsilateral cerebral compression. JAMA *112*, 2030 – 2034.

83. Reilly, P. L., Graham, D. I., Adams, J. H., *et al.,* 1975: Patients with head injury who talk and die. Lancet *2*, 375 – 377.

84. Richards, T., Hoff, J., 1974: Factors affecting survival from acute subdural hematoma. Surgery 75, 253 – 258.

85. Rose, J., Valtonen, S., Jennett, B., 1977: Avoidable factors contributing to death after head injury. Brit. Med. J. 2, 615 – 618.

86. Rosenbluth, P. R., Arias, B., Quartetti, E. V., Carney, A. L., 1962: Current management of subdural hematoma: Analysis of 100 consecutive cases. JAMA 179, 759 – 762.

87. Rossanda, M., Selenati, A., Villa, C., et al., 1973: Role of automatic ventilation in treatment of severe head injuries. J. Neurol. Sci. 17, 265 – 270.

88. Seelig, J. M., Becker, D. P., Miller, J. D., Greenberg, R. P., Ward, J. D., Choi, S. C., 1981: Traumatic acute subdural hematoma: major mortality reduction in comatose patients treated within four hours. N. Engl. J. Med. 304, 1511 – 1518.

90. Shapiro, H. M., Langfitt, T. W., Weinstein, J. D., 1966: Compression of cerebral vessels by intracranial hypertension. II. Morphological evidence for collapse of vessels. Acta Neurochir. (Wien) 15, 223 – 233.

91. Shigemori, M., Syojima, K., Nakayama, K., Kojima, T., Watanabe, M., Kuramoto, S., 1979: Outcome of acute subdural hematoma following decompressive hemicraniectomy. Acta Neurochir. (Wien) 28, (Suppl.), 195 – 198.

92. Sunderland, S., 1958: The tentorial notch and complications produced by herniation through that aperture. Brit. J. Surg. 45, 422 – 438.

93. Sweet, R. C., Miller, J. D., Lipper, M., Kishore, P., Becker, D. P., 1978: The significance of bilateral abnormalities on the CT scan in patients with severe head injury. Neurosurgery 3, 16 – 21.

94. Talalla, A., Morin, M. A., 1971: Acute traumatic subdural hematoma: a review of one hundred consecutive cases. J. Trauma 11, 771 – 777.

95. Troupp, H., Heiskanen, O., 1963: Cerebral angiography in cases of extremely high intracranial pressure. Acta Neurol. Scand. 39, 213 – 223.

96. Vincent, C., David, M., Thiebaud, F., 1936: Le cône de pression temporal dans les tumeurs des hemisphéres cérébraux. Sa symtomatologie; sa gravité; les traitements quil convient de lui opposer. Rev. Neurol. (Paris) 65, 536 – 545.

97. Ward, J. D., Becker, D. P., 1983: Neurosurgery of head injury. In: Ransohoff, J. (ed.), Modern Technics in Surgery. New York: Futura Publishing Co.

98. Ward, J. D., Becker, D. P., Marmarou, A., Choi, S. C., Miller, J. D., Wood, C., Newlon, P. G., Keenan, R., 1984: Failure of propyhlactic barbiturate coma in the treatment of severe head injury. J. Neurosurg. (Submitted).

99. Whaley, N., 1948: Acute subdural hematoma amenable to surgical treatment. Lancet 1, 213 – 214.

# Chronic Subdural Hematoma

J. BRIHAYE

Free University of Brussels (Belgium)

With 16 Figures

## Contents

## 1. Introduction

In spite of a great number of works dedicated to chronic subdural hematoma, the understanding of its physiopathogenesis still remains debatable. The discussions which concerned Virchow's concept of pachymeningitis hemorrhagica interna [29, 40, 153, 183, 186] are nearly forgotten and every neurosurgeon nowadays agrees upon the bold outline written by Cushing (1925) in the preface to Doctor Putnam's dissertation: "In the majority of cases, and perhaps in all, they follow on a trauma so insignificant as to be commonly forgotten by the patient or overlooked in the anamnesis; that the diagnosis should always be considered in a history of mild trauma followed after a latent interval, often of surprising length, by severe headaches associated with psychoses; that, a correct diagnosis being made, the indications for operation are as definite as those for the well recognized extradural hemorrhages associated with fracture of the skull; that perfect recovery is to be expected on evacuation of the clot; that continuance or recurrence of the bleeding is unusual, and, finally, that one's ideas of so-called pachymeningitis hemorrhagica interna with its supposed spontaneous and successive bleedings may possibly have to be entirely recast."

However the important potential of reactivity of the dura mater to any kind of agression must be kept in mind when one considers the etiology of chronic subdural hematoma. The mechanism by which subdural hematoma is growing also remains questionable. If computerized tomography has made the diagnosis of chronic subdural hematoma quite easier, the necessity for surgery to drain the hematoma is at present under discussion.

## 2. Definition and Clinical Features

Subdural hematoma is defined as an accumulation of blood, encysted between the dura mater and the arachnoid membrane (Fig. 1). According to the length of time which separates the onset of clinical manifestations from the known head injury, subdural hematomas are subdivided in acute, subacute and chronic types. A concomitant focal brain injury is another valuable index which could differentiate the acute from the chronic form. McKissock et al. (1960), considering that a temporal classification is imperfect, estimated that the rate of evolution of symptoms most accurately reflected prognosis. Some authors[28, 53, 65, 135, 196] consider the underlying pathology of the membranes found during surgery as a fair index of the age of the hematoma, even though Jamieson and Yelland (1972), have found membranes sometimes well developed within a few days of injury and at other times absent for at least two weeks. For Radcliffe et al. (1972), the shape of the hematoma depends on the age of the patient more than on the date of the hematoma. We have adopted personally the criterion of the existence of membranes, estimating that a well-formed outer wall better indicates the chronic character of the lesion, so imprecise is sometimes the measure of the latent period. In fact, the boundaries between these three forms, acute, subacute and chronic, have to remain flexible[115]. The length of the interval period is differently appreciated but it is frequently considered

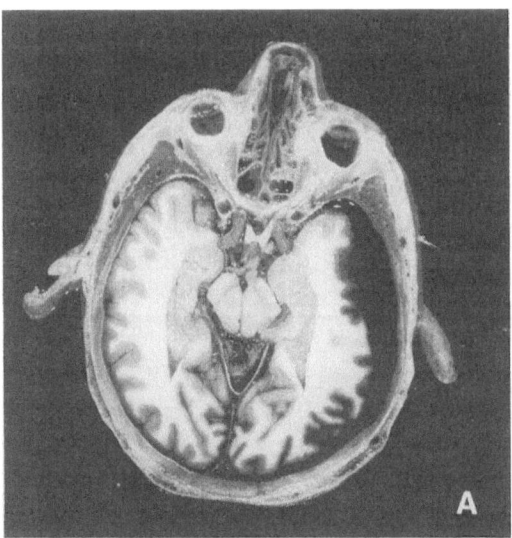

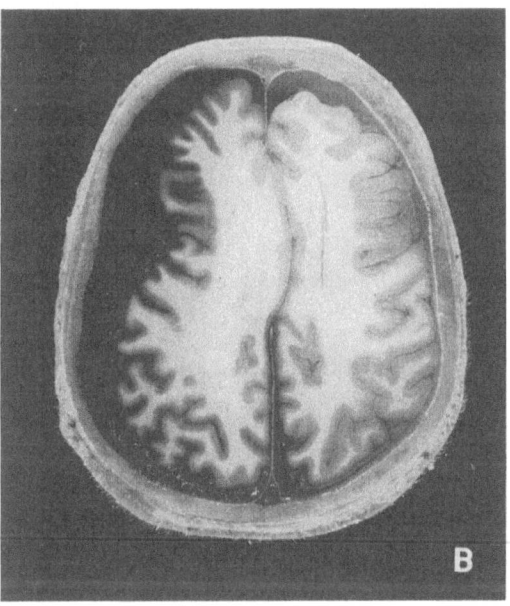

Fig. 1. Anatomic section of the head with a subdural hematoma fixed in situ. Irregular curve of the inner border of the hematic cavity. (Slides due to the courtesy of Doctor Johannes Lang, Professor of anatomy at the University of Würzburg, Federal Republic of Germany)

that an interval of 14 days is a satisfactory measure. Cases in which no history of trauma is reminded are not infrequent; for these, the length of the latent interval cannot be precised.

Very few records regarding the incidence of chronic subdural hematoma in a population are at our disposal. Weber (1969) has observed during the year 1968 in the neurosurgical department in Zurich, 38 cases of chronic subdural hematoma; considering that the clinic takes care of a population of

*Table 1*

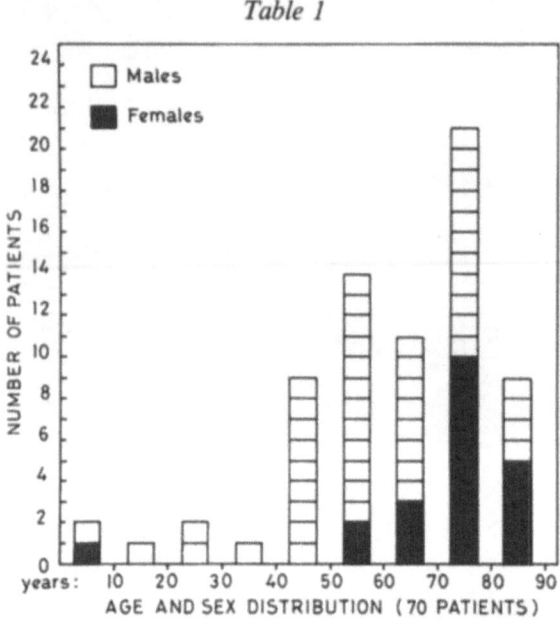

AGE AND SEX DISTRIBUTION (70 PATIENTS)

2.5–3 millions, he roughly estimates that one out of 50,000–100,000 people suffers a chronic subdural hematoma. Fogelholm and Waltimo (1975) in a more systematized study in Helsinki, observed an incidence of 1.72 CSH/1,000,000 people/year in whole Finnish population; however this figure does not represent all of the cases.

The frequency of chronic subdural hematoma among head injuries is better documented. Klug *et al.* (1961), had 3 patients of chronic subdural hematoma under care among 3,742 cases of closed brain injuries, hospitalized in a hospital for miners, having a neurosurgical department; this corresponds to a frequency of 0.05%. Echlin *et al.* (1956) have observed 300 surgically verified cases of subdural hematoma in a series of 30,000 head injuries admitted in a large emergency service in New York; from among the 300 cases, 75 were of the chronic type, that means 0.25% out of the whole group and 25% out of the group of subdural hematomas. El Gindi *et al.* (1979) observed 78 chronic subdural hematomas among 2,000 head injuries (3.9%), partly hospitalized in a military department, partly including war casualties. McKissock *et al.* (1960) count 216 chronic subdural hematomas out of 389 cases of proven subdural hematomas, that means 55% when Munro (1942) only observed 45 cases out of 310 verified subdural hematomas (14.5%). These series are simply indicative of the variables which alter the figures of frequency. In addition, an unknow number of undiagnosed chronic subdural hematomas has to be taken into account.

Age- and sex-incidences are well-known clinical features. Among 70 personal patients under care during the last 15 years, the greater proportion of males and the role of age appear clearly (Table 1); we must specify that hematomas in new-born and young children hospitalized in the department of pediatry have not been considered.

Bilateral chronic subdural hematoma are frequently observed [93]. In our series, 9 patients exhibited a bilateral effusion (12.8%). 12 out of 114 cases (10.5%) for Cameron (1978); 8/108 (7%) for Fogelholm *et al.* (1975); 9.2% for Loew and Kivelitz (1976). As the last authors point out, the percentage of bilateral chronic subdural hematoma varies considerably if children are or not included in the series [98].

Chronic subdural hematoma rarely occurs in the posterior fossa and at the base of the skull; the greatest number develops over the convexity of the cerebral hemisphere; occasionally, it appears in other localizations than the usual fronto-temporo-parietal region: subtemporal, polar, interhemispheric [1, 20, 32, 60, 69, 142, 151, 162, 168].

## 3. Etiopathogenesis

In an attempt at understanding the origin of subdural neo-membranes Schachenmayr and Friede (1978) return to a careful study of the histological features of the hematoma and its membranes. According to the classical concept of the anatomy of meninges, there exists a virtual space between dura and arachnoid; subdural hematomas would result from the effusion of blood in this subdural space. In fact, after fixation in situ, electron microscopic examination of meninges has demonstrated that such a subdural space does not exist. There would be a complex but distinct interface composed of the innermost border of the dura mater (the dura border layer) and the outermost border of the arachnoid (its barrier layer); these two membranes are tightly attached to each other, forming an interface layer of densely packed cells, free of collagen fibers and blood vessels.

Therefore, the subdural space has to be considered as tissue torn artifactually during postmortem procedures or during pathological events. The absence of collagen fibrils and the existence of large extracellular vesicles greatly facilitate a cleavage between dura and arachnoid, due to a lack of coherence [59].

Previously to this anatomical study, Friede (1971) had been struck by the frequent findings of membranous reaction of dura mater. He found indeed in 46 out of 1,044 consecutive necropses, membranous or membranous hemorrhagic lesions of the dura, clinically asymptomatic, for which no causes local or general could be detected. 22 of these membranous lesions were unilateral, 20 bilateral and 27 were located in the falx. Friede distinguished four types of lesions according to their age and thickness. The first type is characterized by thin, densely vascularized neomembranes without hemorrhage or with only a few petechiae; the fourth type is constituted by dense fibrotic lesions with or without encapsulated hematoma or hygroma. Between these two types, there are intermediate forms, incidentally characterized by encapsulated subdural hematomas. In fact, these necropsy findings could be an image of the natural history, at least of some chronic subdural hematomas. The last type could correspond to the spontaneous healing of chronic subdural hematoma, replaced by fibrotic thickening of dura mater.

Friede (1971) concluded his study "with the assumption that neomembrane formation may begin as a primary, probably age-related degenerative process at the inner surface of the dura mater". In a subsequent paper, Friede and Schachenmayr (1978) discovered incidentally neomembranes in 4 patients who died of malignant diseases, cardiac failure, acute pancreatitis and sepsis. They demonstrated that neomembranes derived from proliferation of cells of the dural border layer; there is sprouting of capillaries from the inner dural face into the layers of proliferated dural border cells; there is a tendency within the neomembranes to undergo repetitive multifocal bleeding. Finally, the gradual increase of collagen reinforces the neomembrane, reduces its fragility and terminates in fibrotic healing of the lesion.

Kawano and Suzuki (1981) have even found in organizing hematomas in humans, fibroblasts, collagen and spindle-shaped cells identified as smooth muscle cells by electron microscopy. This could indicate the great potential of cells within the neomembranes.

The arachnoid membrane has also the capacity to react against agression (2.62). Hammes (1944) for example has observed that the meningeal reaction to blood is evident within two hours of the subarachnoid hemorrhage and begins as an outpouring of polymorphonuclear leucocytes, followed by the appearance of lymphocytes and large mononuclear phagocytes derived from the mesothelial lining cells of the arachnoid.

In many cases, chronic subdural hematoma in humans does not terminate spontaneously in a fibrotic scar. On the contrary, it tends to enlarge progressively, providing a silent clinical period before the appearance of symptoms. The mechanism by which the hematoma grows still remains questionable.

Gardner (1932) did not retain the hypothesis of repeated hemorrhage, to explain the progressive enlargement of the hematoma. After having experienced in dogs semipermeable membranes separating blood from cerebro-spinal fluid, he prompted to an osmotic hypothesis: the arachnoid membrane is semipermeable and the cerebro-spinal fluid is drawn into the hemorrhagic cyst by the osmotic tension of the blood proteins contained into the cyst.

Zollinger and Gross (1934), in a patient with a bilateral chronic subdural hematoma, determined the total protein value in the hematoma and in the normal whole blood; they found an important difference in favour of the whole blood that they explain by dilution of the hematoma fluid due to the ingress of cerebro-spinal fluid through the hematoma membrane. They also used the sac of one of the hematoma after surgical removal as an experimental mean, emptying the sac of its content and refilling it with whole blood; a manometer was tied into one end of the sac which was immersed in a beaker containing 0.9% sodium chloride and 0.1% sodium oxalate. After hours, there was a rise in the manometer while fluid of the beaker remained free of proteins. The conclusion drawn by Zollinger and Gross was that the neomembranes do not allow egress of proteins but do allow ingress of water and salts. The progressive breakdown of red cells with liberation of hemoglobin over a long period of time accounts for a differential osmotic tension between the content of the hematoma on one hand, the neighbouring cerebro-spinal fluid and the vessels of the membranes on the other hand. Munro and Merrit (1936) reached the same conclusion after determination of the protein content of the hematoma fluid.

This osmotic theory was largely accepted till 1971 when Weir re-examined the question. Using the freezing point depression method, he determined the osmolality of the subdural hematoma fluid, venous blood and cerebro-spinal fluid in patients and in a control group. He found no significant difference between the samples whatever the age of the hematoma. His conclusion was: "It may be that the late onset of symptoms is due to a dynamic decompensation of cerebral tissue adjacent to the hematoma, possibly without any change in the size of the hematoma." In a subsequent paper, Weir (1980) measured the oncotic pressure of hematoma fluid and venous blood in 20 patients; he did not find a significant difference between them. The same measurement was made by Gjerris and Sorensen (1980) who found the oncotic pressure in hematoma variable, either higher or lower than in plasma, the mean value being slightly higher in hematoma than in plasma; but the difference was not statistically significant. Rabe *et al.* (1972) showed in two children that subdurally instilled labelled serum albumin exchanges with plasma albumin. Gitlin (1955) studying the subdural fluid in children found that the albumin/globulin ratios and albumin/total proteins ratios in the subdural fluid were considerably higher than the same ratios in the corresponding serum samples. This difference would be mainly due to an effusion through the irritated or damaged capillary walls.

It appears from these various contributions that the osmotic theory is unable by itself alone to explain the progressive enlargement of the hematoma.

It was thought for a long time that repetitive hemorrhage could be the mechanism by which the hematoma grows. Fragility of the neocapillaries would be the main cause of this rebleeding. Suzuki and Komatsu (1977) found in their patients with chronic subdural hematoma a high value of estrogen in urine; consequently, they rose the question of the role played by the hormone on the rebleeding phenomenon. Such an unusual finding of course deserves further investigation, but it may be stated that determination of estrogen in urines has not the same value that determination in blood; in addition, we would expect thrombosis rather than bleeding.

Several authors have also demonstrated that there existed a fibrinolytic activity of the neomembranes. Labadie and Glover (1975) undertook a study of hemostatic-fibrinolytic mechanisms in subdural fluid, aspirated at different times in two patients. It appeared probable that subdural effusions possessed factors activating hemostatic mechanisms; there was an accelerated clot formation although the clot formed with subdural fluid was structurally defective. They found also an enhanced fibrinolytic activity of the fluid by the presence of a plasminogen activator; consequently the ineffective clot was rapidly lysing. Ito et al. (1976) investigated the fluid of chronic subdural hematoma in 16 patients. They used $^{51}$Cr-labeled red cells to demonstrate a daily hemorrhage within the hematoma. In addition, no fibrinogen was detected in the subdural fluid, but high levels of fibrinogen degradation products, acting as an anticoagulant, were present. The outer membrane contains a tissue activator, responsible of local hyperfibrinolysis which may well give rise to hemorrhage from the membrane layer. They concluded that "excessive local activation of fibrinolysis plays an important role in the etiology of chronic subdural hematoma". In 1978, Ito et al. carried on their research and found tissue activator in large amount in the outer membrane, so that plasminogen would be consumed by diffusion of the activator and transformed in plasmin which is an active fibrinolytic enzyme. No tissue plasminogen activator was found in the inner membrane. Weir and Gordon (1983) also found in 25 cases of chronic subdural hematoma that subdural fluid contained low fibrinogen and high fibrin degradation product concentrations. These last products have an anticoagulant effect and could inhibit platelet aggregation.

## 4. Experimental Production of Chronic Subdural Hematoma

Experimental production of chronic subdural hematoma have also been attempted in order to check the development of the lesion. Very early experiments are quoted in the paper of Putman and Cushing (1925): Kremiansky 1868, Sperling 1872, van Vleuten 1898, Huegenin 1877. Goodell and Mealey (1963) thought that the early failures to produce experimental hematomas[29, 63, 152, 153] could be due to the small amount of blood, injected into the subdural space of animals; absorption of the clot was indeed the final result of these experiments and no fluid-filled cavities between the membranes were ever observed. Therefore, they injected a greater amount of blood, hypothetizing that fibroplastic proliferation would then occur only at the periphery of the hematoma, allowing the persistence of a cavity into the membranes. Experiments were performed on dogs; influences of variables, as production of intracranial hypotension, hypothermia, attempts to modify the inflammatory response to blood injection were studied. Goodell and Mealy (1971) finally succeeded to produce subdural hematomas, sometimes very large, which ressembled closely the subdural hematoma in humans. But invariably these experimental subdural hematomas organized and regressed. The variables used during the experiments did not modify the resolution of hematomas.

These experiments also demonstrated the natural evolution of liquid blood or clot injected into the subdural space: within 15 hours, a single layer of cells had already migrated to its external surface adjacent to the dura. At 7 days, active phagocytosis of red blood cells and fibroplasia were prominent in the most superficial layer of the hematoma; at that time, an outer membrane was well developed; an inner membrane, one-cell thick, was also present; a sac, enclosing the hematoma, was existing.

In 1972, Watanabe *et al.* modified the experimental protocol of their predecessors, in mixing liquid blood with CSF and in incubating the mixture, before its injection in the subdural space of dogs and monkeys. The clot so prepared was coated with delicate fibrin fibers network. When injected in the subdural space, the clot grew gradually, forming an encapsulated hematoma which did not differ histologically from the human chronic subdural hematoma. The same composed clot injected subcutaneously also produces a chronic encapsulated hematoma. From these findings, the authors concluded that the fibrin membrane of the clot is essential to induce the capsule formation. These experimental hematomas closely resembled the human chronic subdural hematoma in morphological appearance, neurological symptoms and manner of clot.

In 1974, Appelbaum *et al.* repeated similar experiments in the cat and did not find that cerebro-spinal fluid was necessary to produce a special type of clot. The important for the hemorrhage is to be in contact with the inner layer of dura which reacts and cooperates to the formation of the outer membrane. Appelbaum *et al.* found also that the osmolarity of subdural fluid is the same as that of plasma. They observed rebleeding from the sinusoidal neovascular channels within the outer layer of membranes. They were of the opinion that the prime volume of the hematoma is very important and that the intracranial hypotension is also critical. In 1976, Labadie and Glover confirmed the findings of Appelbaum *et al.* that cerebro-spinal fluid has no discernible effect on the behaviour of the implant. They agreed upon the fact that the volume of the implant was an important variable and that the inflammatory reaction constituted an additional stimulus for growth. They demonstrated, as confirmation of this later assumption, that dexamethasone prevented membrane formation.

In conclusion, from this clinical and experimental research, it clearly appears that a multifactorial mechanism proceeds to the formation and development of chronic subdural hematoma. In animals, till now, the provoked subdural hematoma invariably tends to its spontaneous resorption and healing. In humans, the clinical experience demonstrated in a small number of cases spontaneous resorption of the hematoma; but in the majority of patients, chronic subdural hematoma tends to enlarge. Considering the importance of the implant size in the animal experiments, one realizes at once the great role of the surgical drainage which reduces drastically the size of the hematoma.

Keeping in mind these fundamental data disclosed by experimental and clinical research, we will analyze the clinical features of chronic subdural hematoma in humans.

## 5. Clinical Manifestations

The clinical manifestations are manifold and might mimic other pathological processes [10, 50, 109, 188]; they are depending on the size of the hematoma, its localization, rapidity of growing, uni- or bilateral type, on the age and condition of the patient [9, 53].

The classical picture of a posttraumatic chronic subdural hematoma is composed of an evolution in two phases: in the first place, the well-known traumatic event; after its dissipation and a silent period of variable length, the onset of clinical manifestations which usually consists in headaches, mental disorders and motor deficits.

The cause of chronic subdural hematoma is a head injury as far as we consider the slightest sudden displacement of the brain within the cranial cavity (to cough for instance) as a head injury. The trauma is frequently of moderate severity; as emphasized by Loew (1976, 1982) chronic subdural hematoma almost never develops after severe head injury because of the raised intracranial pressure during the initial stage which does not allow distension of the subdural space. The traumatic event can be trivial and so insignificant that the patient and its family have lost its memory and that it is also overlooked by the doctor. Occasionally, it could not have existed; in such cases, the development of the disease appears progressive in one piece[136]. In our series the causative factor remains unknown in 12 cases out of 70, and not mentioned in 3 cases; 15 times, the hematoma followed a road accident of mean severity; in 35 patients the trauma consisted in a fall, often from a step while the patient was drunk.

Subdural hematomas occasionally occur after arterial rupture[14, 26, 31, 41, 42, 159, 199] but then its course is acute or subacute. The usual mechanism of production of the chronic type consists of avulsion of cerebral veins while traversing the subdural space[29, 183]: it is not frequent to find, directly associated with chronic subdural hematoma, a brain cortical lesion with torn vessels (Yance, quoted by Yamashima and Friede 1984). Electron microscopic investigations in humans[200] have demonstrated greater fragility of the bridging veins in their subdural passage than in their other portions; in addition, they are more exposed to traction in the elderly patients by cerebral atrophy. Displacement of the brain produced by head injury or by abrupt raised intracranial pressure, would easily tear the bridging veins[183]. Many other pathological conditions could encourage vessels to bleed, among which disorders of blood coagulation and low spinal fluid pressure syndromes are the most frequently encountered[8, 15, 19, 24, 37, 49, 51, 72, 100, 104, 105, 130, 177, 197]. In our series we observed alcoholism in 14 patients, arterial hypertension and diabetes in 6, anticoagulant drugs in 4, cancer chimiotherapy with fall of platelets in one; 5 times, the hematoma was a complication of cerebro-spinal fluid drainage after shunting procedures which are an important promoting factor of chronic subdural hematoma. In children, subdural effusions are frequently associated with sepsis[154].

The symptom-free period which separates the initial trauma from the first clinical sign is of variable length; it usually ranges from 2 to 8 weeks but could extend to several months. It happens that this latent interval is not entirely free of symptoms: headache or some memory defect can be experienced by the patient along the whole interval. In agreement with our findings, Fogelholm et al. (1975) observed that the time interval from trauma to operation was longer in the older groups; in their series, the medians of the intervals were 5 weeks, 7.5 weeks and 10 weeks in the age groups 20 to 29, 40 to 59, and 60 to 79 years respectively; they also underline the fact that the weight of the brain decreases about 200 g and the space between the brain and skull increases from 6% to 11% of the total intracranial space between the age interval of 50–80[9, 145].

Headaches and mental disturbances are the most frequent and prominent symptoms. In our series psychic disorders were the first manifestations for 30 patients (50%) and headaches for 11 (15.7%); but after a very short time, headaches and mental disorders existed jointly. 90% of the patients reviewed by Svien and Gelety (1964) were suffering of headaches. Feld (1947) has well emphasized the characteristics of headaches in chronic subdural hematoma: they are severe, constant but with variations in intensity, mainly located over the hematoma region for which local tenderness on palpation and percussion may be observed. Mental disorders, in the beginning, are made of slow cerebration with mental confusion and retention memory defect. Thereafter, in absence of adequate treatment, mental disturbances progressively turn to dementia[4,38]; Allen et al. (1940), among 3,100 consecutive autopsies of psychotic patients dead in mental hospitals, found 245 cases of undiagnosed subdural hematomas (7.9%); they expressed the view, according to their experience and a survey of the literature that the subdural bleeding is a commoner post-mortem finding among psychotic patients than it is among general hospital patients. Sphincter incontinence occasionally occurs in parallel with the development of mental impairment, as well as disturbances of the walking balance.

Motor deficit is frequent and was observed early in 14 patients in our series, in conjunction with the onset of headaches and mental disorders. In six cases only the hemiparesis was homolateral to the side of the hematoma; this low figure contrast with what is sometimes reported in the literature[27].

The ophthalmologic disorders are frequent[109]. Mitsumoto et al. (1977) reported anisocoria in 24% of their cases, homonymous hemianopsia in 22%, papilledema in 12%, lesion of the third nerve in 5%, of the sixth in 3%; these figures have to be compared with the findings of the same disorders observed in acute subdural hematomas in which they are respectively 56, 66, 4, 33, and 11%; the prevalence of anisocoria thus appears highest in patients with acute subdural hematoma, the lesion being ipsilateral to the side of the dilated pupil in 81% of all cases (acute and chronic) and contralateral in 19%. In our series, anisocoria was only recorded in two patients and was homolateral to the hematoma in these two cases. As quoted by Jamieson and Yelland, abnormality of one pupil is mainly seen in patients with acute lesions. These clinical manifestations, homolateral to the side of the hematoma, are due to the lateral translation of the brain stem of which the controlateral half is pressed and contused against the edge of the tentorium cerebelli.

Epilepsy, focal or generalized, can happen before or after drainage of chronic subdural hematoma[109]. In our series, Bravais-Jacksonian epilepsy occured three times preoperatively and 2 times postoperatively; generalized seizures 4 times before and twice after surgery. In 5 patients, epileptic seizure was the first clinical manifestation to appear, quickly followed by other disorders; for 3 patients, the seizure was of the Bravais Jacksonian type and occurred after a latent interval of one week, 6 weeks and 6 months respectively; for 2 patients the generalized seizure occurred 2 weeks after the head injury. Out of 50 cases of chronic subdural hematoma reported by Cole and Spatz (1961), a great number (21 patients) suffered epileptic seizures. According to Cambria *et al.* (1966), homolateral Bravais Jacksonian epilepsy could be caused by compression of the opposite hemisphere on the vault.

This broad outline of the clinical picture is modified to some extent according to the volume and location of the hematoma, as well as to the age of the patient. Aronson and Okazaki (1963) found a positive correlation between the size of the hematoma and the percentage of patients showing neurological symptoms; there was also some correlation between the volume of bleeding and the percentage of fatality, attributable largely to the hematoma, as well as with the incidence of secondary brain stem damage. The seriousness of clinical manifestations and the velocity of evolution were markedly less pronounced in patients beyond the age of 75; this makes difficult in old patients the differential diagnosis between chronic subdural hematoma and diffuse cerebral vascular insufficiency. Because of the diminution of brain volume with age, autopsy findings in these elderly patients did not often indicate secondary lesions such as cerebral encephalomalacia or brain-stem hemorrhage.

Stress has been laid upon the impairment of cerebral blood flow due to the brain compression by the hematoma and local edema underneath[9, 25, 67, 138]. Once more, distorsion and compression of the hemisphere on the side of the hematoma are significantly more frequent in patients younger than 65, resulting in raised intracranial pressure. Gjerris and Sorensen (1980) have observed in their patients that the clinical signs disappeared within the first 24 hours following surgery while radiological signs of intracranial pressure still remained obvious.

The location of the hematoma also modifies the clinical picture. Chronic subdural hematoma at the base of the brain or in the posterior fossa is exceptional[1, 90, 151] while it has been reported many times in the interhemispheric fissure[20, 32, 60, 69, 142, 162, 168]: in these cases, paresis of the lower limb is markedly more pronounced than paresis of the upper limb; when the hematoma is bilateral, it happens that the clinical picture made of paraparesis, or quadriparesis, with sphincter disturbances is mimicking a spinal cord compression syndrome[10, 20, 166] (one personal case). Shields *et al.* (1980) estimate that the most likely mechanism of paraparesis could be congestion and kinking of the superior rolandic veins compromising venous drainage and causing localized decreased cortical function.

The clinical evolution is sometimes characterized by transient remission of symptoms. Three patients in our series experienced such a remission: in one case, the first symptom was an epileptic seizure followed by hemiparesis which disappeared after 48 hours; 15 days later mental disorders developed. In another case of chronic subdural hematoma caused by anticoagulant therapy, the first complaint was a sudden headache with drowsiness followed after 2 days by obvious but transient improvement. A third patient had a transitory hemiparesis. Remission of clinical signs would be in relation with modifications in the parenchymatous edema underlying the hematoma[9, 10, 116, 144]. Unfrequently, chronic subdural hematoma could be associated with other posttraumatic complications, as contralateral acute subdural hematoma[171] or for example inappropriate antidiuretic hormone secretion[125].

## 6. Diagnostic Procedures

Chronic subdural hematoma is sometimes clearly demonstrated on *plain X-rays of the skull*, owing to calcification and/or ossification of the membranes (Fig. 2); these hematomas are of very long duration, up to 35 years in the case reported by Debois and Lombard (1980) and usually happen in children and young adults. In general there are no signs of intracranial hypertension; mental disorders and epileptic seizures are the main clinical features[3, 11, 12, 22, 30, 39, 74, 110, 117, 120, 121, 133, 146, 180, 189, 190]. From clinical observation and animal experiments, A. Danis (1973, 1974) has demonstrated that ossification, widespread finding in clinical pathology, is the result of an induction phenomenon on connective tissue, depending on the presence of migrating bone marrow cells locally fixed while calcification seems related to local hypoxic conditions.

*EEG* often indicates the hemisphere over which the hematoma is developing, although it may be normal, mainly in patients with a very low evoluating subdural hematoma. The electrical disturbances have no specific character and they have to be interpreted, taking into account all the other clinical data[76, 89, 109]. Cambria *et al.* (1966) rightly emphasize the signification of "electric silence" which is either marked or indicating by comparison with the other side; electric silence, made of waves with small amplitude and low frequency, suggests the existence of a subdural hematoma and determines the side of its development.

*Echography* may demonstrate displacement of midline structures and suggests the presence of an hemispheric lesion, providing that the lesion is unilateral[109].

The value of *brain scintigraphy* in diagnosis of subdural collection is well known[109]. However its accuracy is far to be absolute; for instance, in 6 patients with verified chronic subdural hematoma and investigated by 99 technetium pertechnetate scanning, Weir (1971) had two negative results while angiography was diagnostic in all cases; Amendola and Ostrum (1977) had the same experience. On the contrary Hurwitz *et al.* (1974) found brain scanning accurate in predicting hematomas in 93% of their 18 cases while echoencephalography only was positive in 44%; they insisted upon the value of delayed scanning; rapid sequential imaging of the radioactive

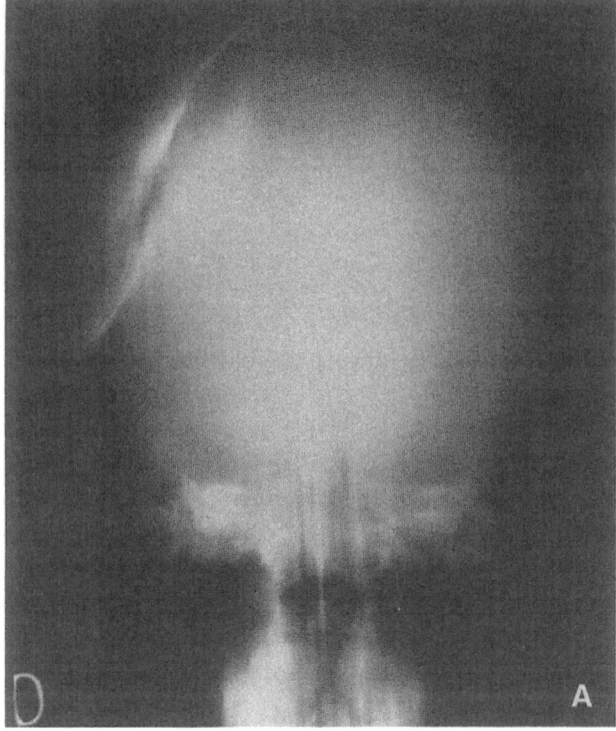

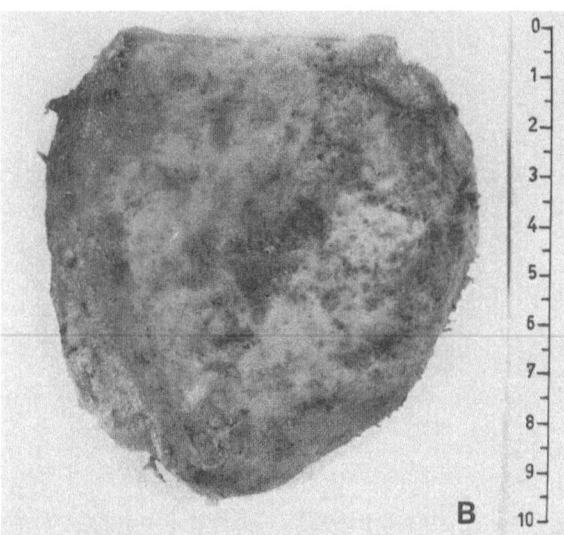

Fig. 2. Ossified subdural hematoma in a boy shunted for hydrocephalus, 9 years previously. A) A. P. radiographic view of the lesion, B) surgically en bloc piece removed

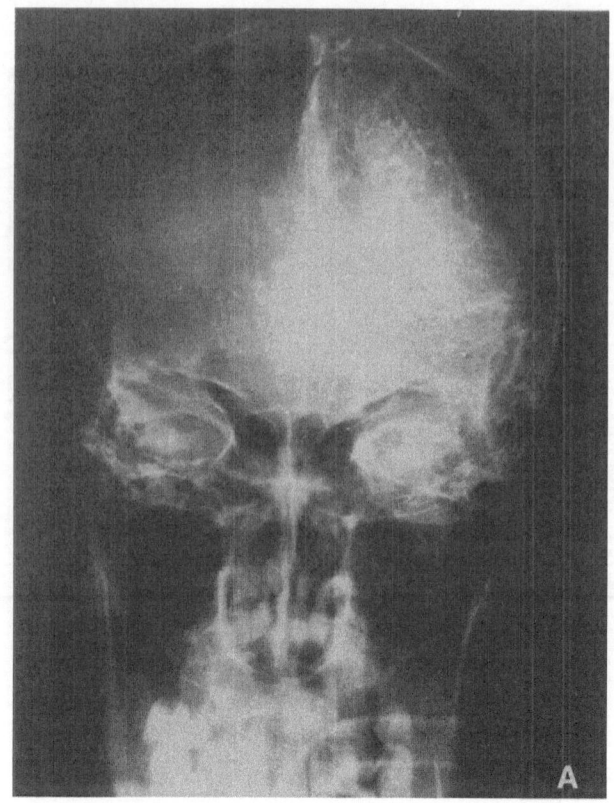

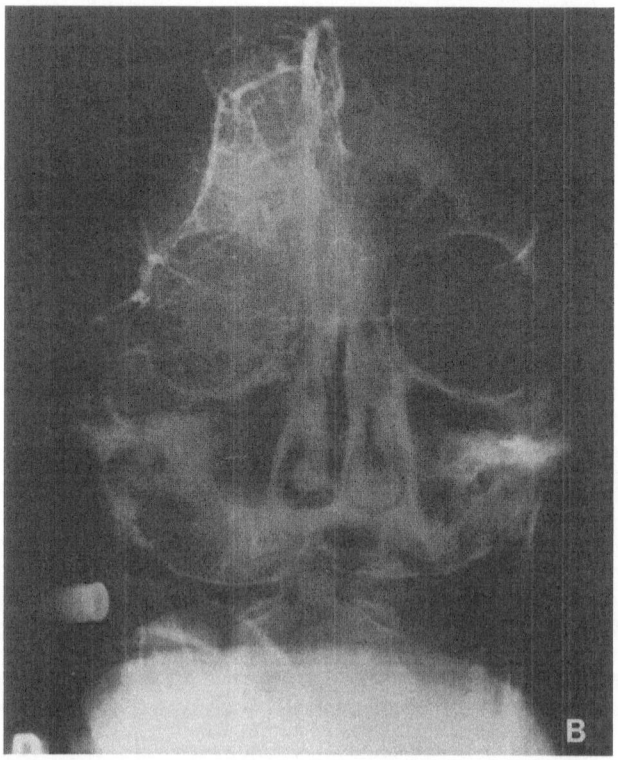

Fig. 3. Two cases (A and B) of chronic subdural hematoma demonstrated by angiography. The classical biconvex or lenticular shape is well seen

bolus may also demonstrate a decreased perfusion in the region of the hematoma. Other results have been obtained by Lombroso *et al.* (1970) in a group of 23 subdural hematomas; in their experience, the two dimensional ultrasound scanning gave better positive indications than the 99-technetium scanning and EEG.

Kjellin and Steiner (1974), thanks to *spectrophotometric examinations of cerebrospinal fluid* in subdural hematomas, found a spectrophotometric xanthochromia of hemorragic origin in all cases examined while, at sight, the cerebrospinal fluid appeared colourless in 52% of the cases. They concluded that "cerebrospinal fluid spectrophotometry is a simple, fast and extremely sensitive method which should be used routinely in the diagnosis of suspected subdural hematoma, if lumbar puncture is not contraindicated".

*The angiographic appearances* of subdural hematoma, acute and chronic, have been well documented at the time when no computerized scanner was available[157, 195, 203]. Even nowadays, arteriography aids the diagnosis in particular situations[104] and in case of isodense bilateral subdural hematoma[123].

Norman (1956) has given a well illustrative diagram of subdural hematomas according to the age of the bleeding: in the acute form, the lesion appears in the AP view as a crescentic image; in the chronic form, the biconvex, lentiform shape is very demonstrative (Fig. 3).

However, we are of the opinion of Radcliffe *et al.* (1972) that this schematic distinction is not always in agreement with the clinical findings; there are real chronic subdural hematoma which keep the crescent shape during their evolution. It is mainly in the capillary and venous phases of the angiogram that the subdural hematoma is the best differenciated (Fig. 3). Gilday *et al.* (1974) have described a transitional form between the acute and chronic hematomas which would be characterized by an irregular contour of the inner membrane; this transitional form does not appear convincing to us, in consideration of our clinical experience. The biconvex shape of the lesion is also proper to the extradural hematoma, but in this case, the lentiform shape appears immediately after the head injury.

Nelson and Freimanis (1963) have emphasized the role played by the position of the anterior cerebral artery and the midline structures in the differential diagnosis of unilateral and bilateral subdural hematomas; however they noticed that a slight displacement of the anterior cerebral artery to the contralateral side (less than 50% of the width of homolateral hematoma) is not sufficiently indicative of an unilateral lesion; therefore they recommend to perform an angiography of the contralateral side.

McLaurin (1965) has also analysed the angiographic appearances in subdural hematomas, taking into account the associated brain lesions, particularly the brain swelling beneath the hematoma; he noted that there was no close correlation between the value of brain compression by the hematoma and the importance of the shift of the anterior cerebral artery; these two angiographic features besides this, behave independently after drainage of the hematoma.

It is worthwhile to know that some pathological conditions could have angiographic appearances of the chronic subdural hematoma; it was the

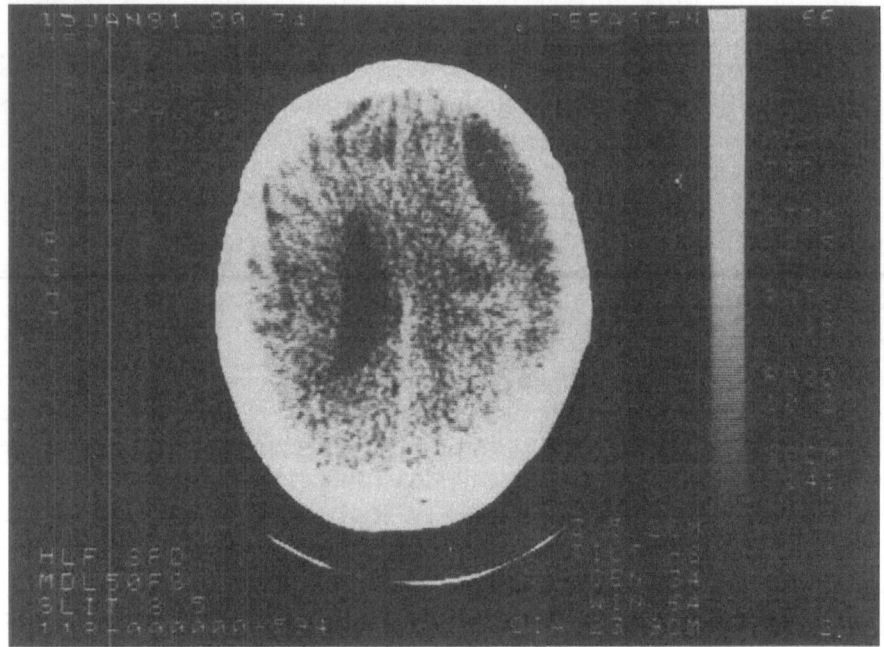

Fig. 4. Chronic subdural hematoma in a patient 82 years old. CT scan 2.5 months after a fall. Biconvex shape of the hematoma with a low attenuation coefficient

case for subdural hydroma, cerebral atrophy and subdural empyema among other disease processes[52, 132].

As soon as it was available, *computerized tomography* has quickly taken the place of other radiological techniques in head injuries.

The characteristic appearance of the avascular zone, crescent-shape in acute subdural hematomas and lenticular or biconvex in chronic forms, well demonstrated by angiography, best judged in the capillary and venous phases, is also perfectly delineated on CT scans (Fig. 4). In addition repeated CT scans allow the follow-up of the hematoma through the various stages of its natural history[75]. At the time of its production, the subdural hematoma is made of fresh blood which appears on the scan as a wide band traced on the cortex surface of the hemisphere; it has a high attenuation

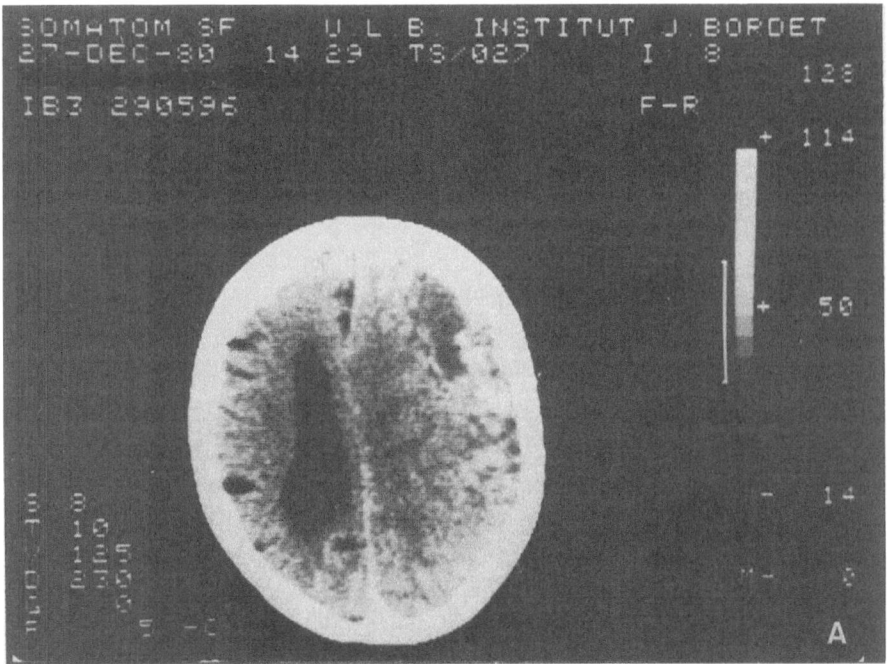

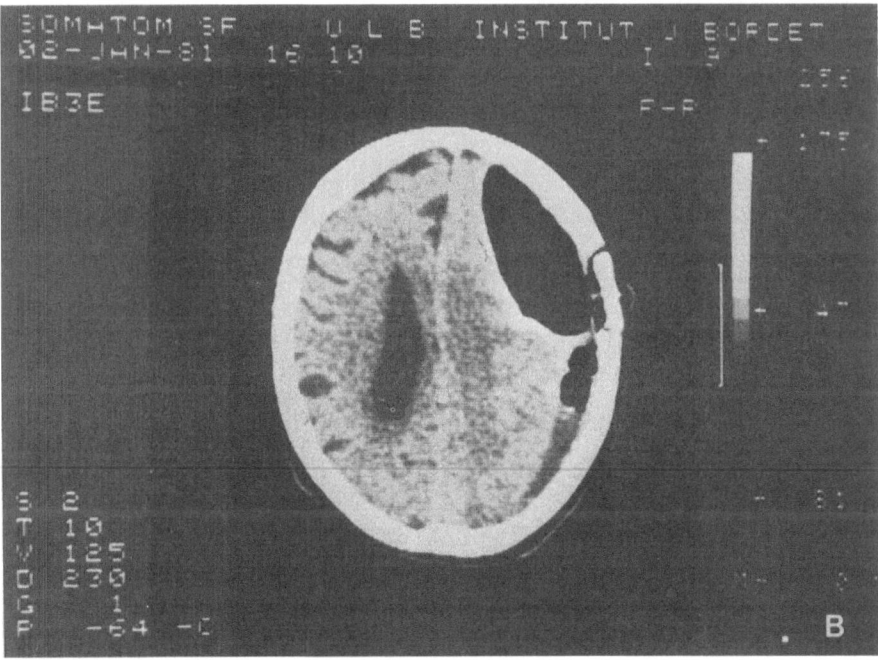

Fig. 5. A) Subdural hematoma with still a high attenuation value, 10 days after fall in a patient 84 years old. The limits of the lesion are poorly defined. B) After surgical evacuation (trephine opening), air fills the cavity in which adherence between the membranes is clearly seen at one point

value (Fig. 5) and a concave margin. As it ages during the following weeks
the hematoma is processing from dense to a progressively less dense and
finally lucent appearance. There is in the literature some disagreement
regarding the rapidity with which this transformation takes place and
therefore with regard to the age of the hematoma[6, 17, 55, 56, 126, 165]. In our

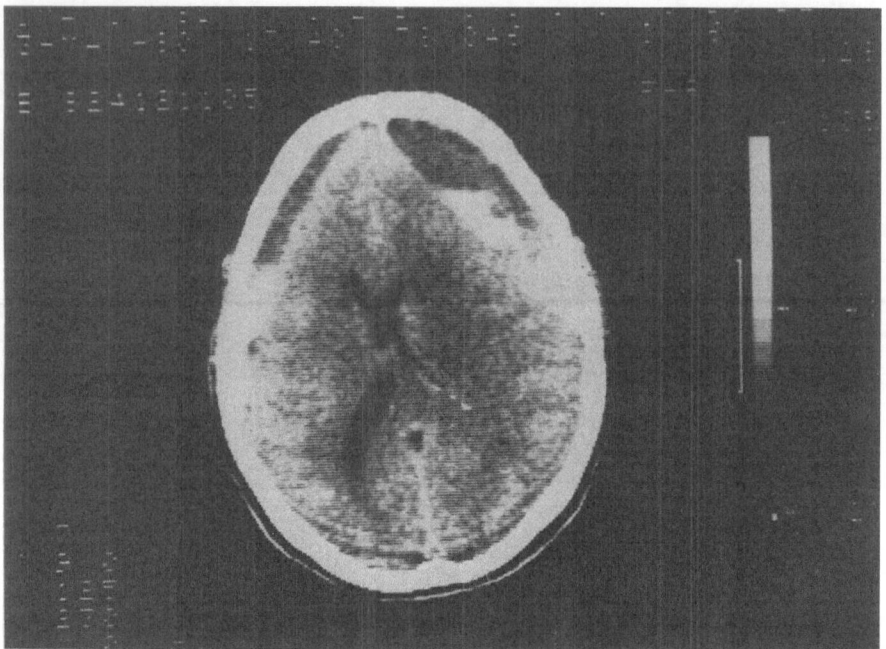

Fig. 6. Unequal bilateral hematoma in a patient 75 years old, 10 days after mild
trauma. There is layering of the cavities, the anterior part having a lesser density
than the adjacent brain and the posterior part still a blood density

experience, there exists no sharp dividing line between the three main
categories: high absorption coefficient, isodense value, low density (Fig. 6).
On an average the hematoma keeps a greater density than the surrounding
brain tissue during the first week; afterwards, for some time, the hematoma
fluid tends to approach the density of the brain tissue and becomes isodense;
for French and Dublin (1977), this period is comprised between 2 and 6
weeks while for Bergström et al. (1977), the isodense phenomenon is reached
after 4 to 9 days and for Kim et al. (1978), after 2 to 3 weeks. After
that, the hematoma tends to be progressively hypodense and lucent (Fig. 7).
As stated by Messina and Chernik (1975), a hematoma might change its
appearance as it ages, but these variations do not signify resorption and
therefore volumetric changes.

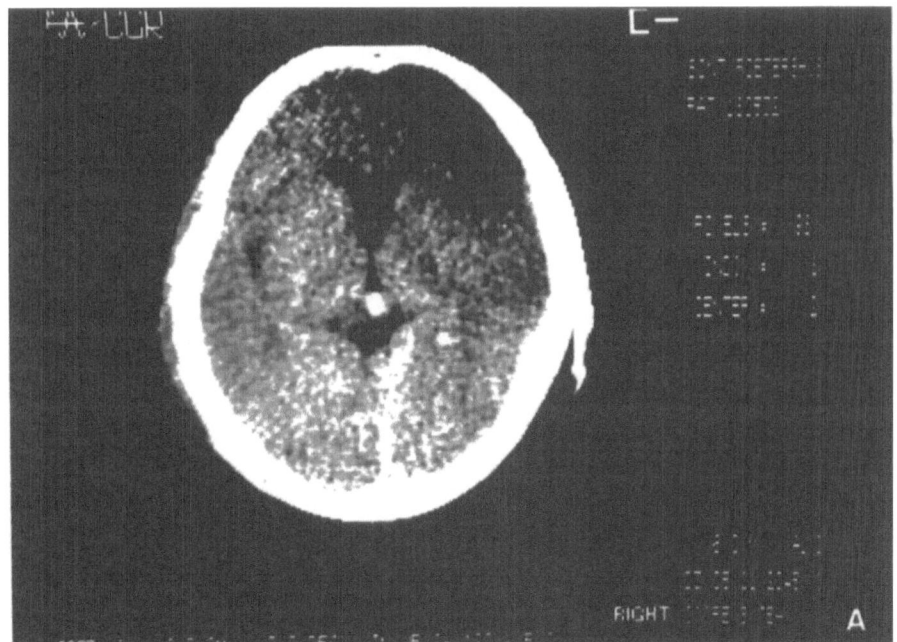

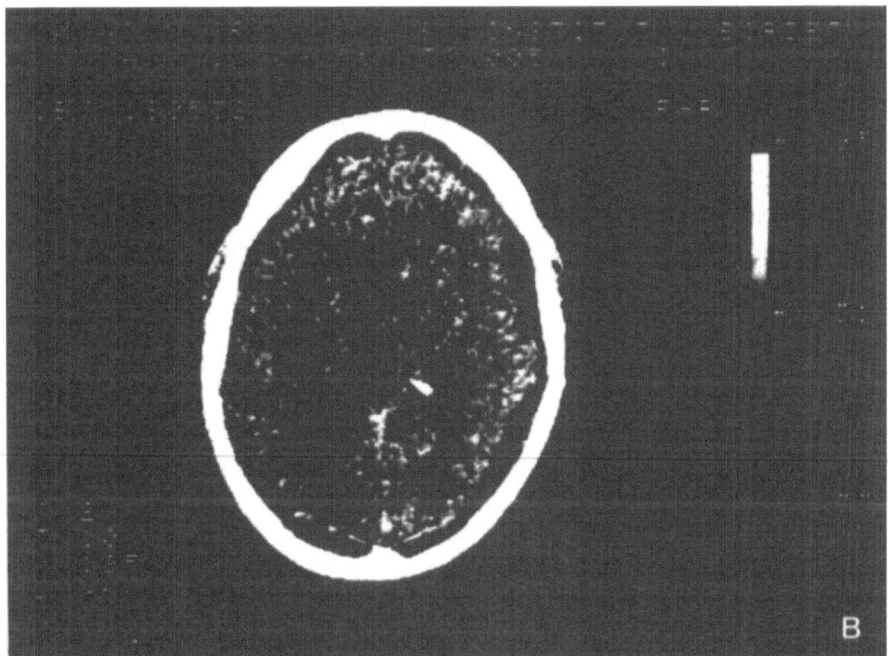

Fig. 7. A) 15 days after trauma in a patient 50 years old. Latent interval of 2 weeks. Isodense subdural hematoma. B) a second CT scan 20 days after the first one demonstrates a crescent-shaped hematoma with low attenuation coefficient. C) 6 months after surgical evacuation, normal appearance of the subdural space on CT scan

In clinical practice, isodense subdural hematoma represents a number of cases: 7 isoattenuating cases out of 69 patients (French and Dublin 1977), 7 out of 43 (Kim *et al.* 1978), 17/87 (Moller and Ericson 1979), 32/195 (Tsai *et al.* 1979).

This description is somewhat theoretical because rebleeding in the subdural cavity is not taken into consideration (Fig. 8); in fact, the absorption

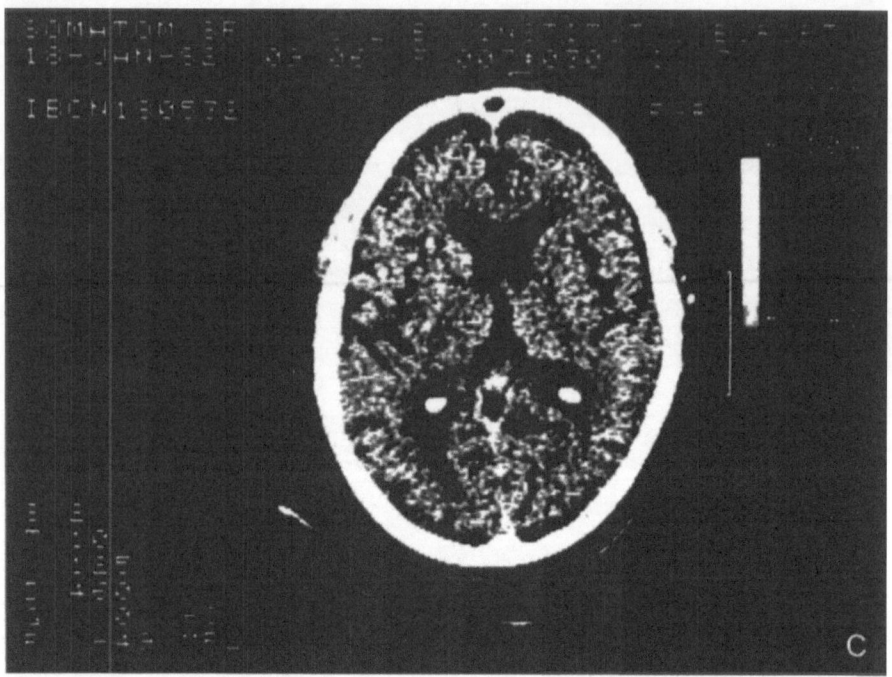

Fig. 7 C

value which appears on CT scan, does not only depend on the length of time from the onset of the lesion. The decreasing density of the hematoma fluid is a multifactorial phenomenon, not yet well understood and which is beyond the scope of this study; it is mainly related to the breakdown of hemoglobin proteins and may be also to ingress and egress of ions and water. The isodense stage represents a limitation in the diagnosis of subdural hematoma since the outline of the lesion is merged into the brain parenchyma. However when the subdural hematoma is unilateral, it can be immediately suspected thanks to the obliteration of the cerebral sulci in the zone of the hematoma and to the shift of the midline structures with mass effect on the ventricles. Nevertheless, as emphasized by Tomaszek *et al.* (1983), in some cases, the volumetric effect of hematoma may be balanced by preexisting brain atrophy which prevents midline shift. In addition to

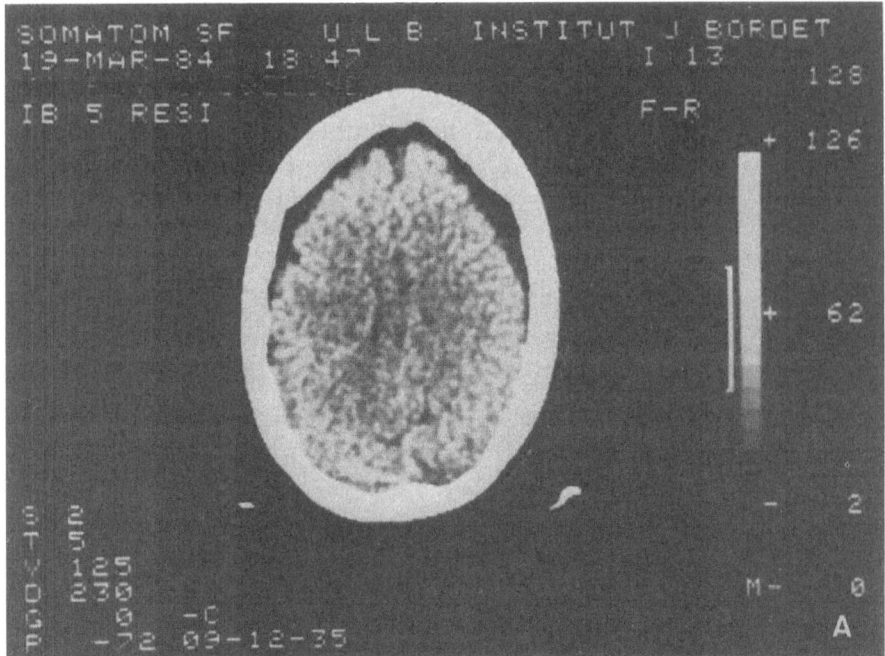

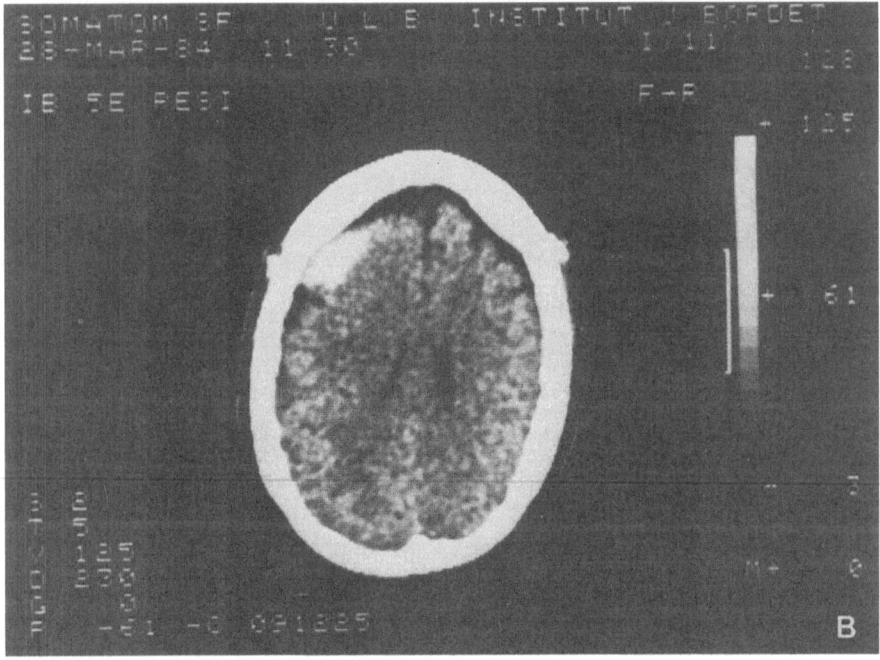

Fig. 8. Recent case of a female 49 years old, not included in the present series. A) CT scan 10 days after a serious traffic accident. Bilateral subdural collection. Trial of medical treatment (bedrest plus dexamethasone) during 9 days without improvement. Drainage through burr holes at the end of the trial of both subdural hematoma. B) CT scan 6 days after drainage. Recurrence of bleeding within the left subdural space which is enlarged

these indicative factors, contrast material injection may enhance the medial border of the hematoma, indicating the separation between hematoma and brain tissue (Fig. 9). When the subdural hematoma is bilateral and isodense the diagnosis may be very difficult. The effacement of cortical sulci and the small size of ventricles are useful clues for the diagnosis (Fig. 10).

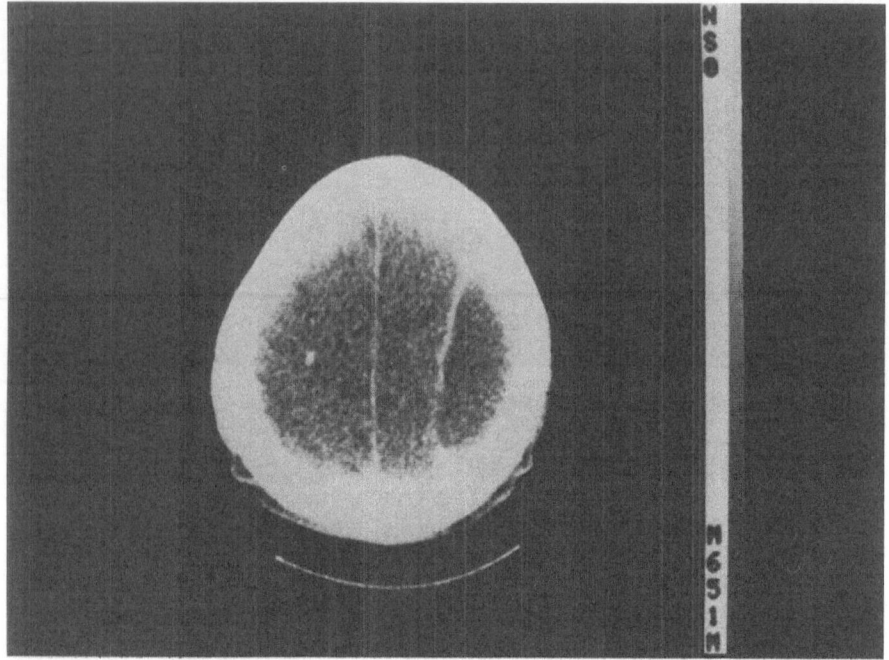

Fig. 9. Chronic subdural hematoma in a patient 61 years old. The contrast-enhanced scan displays a well defined rim on the inner border of the cavity

Greenhouse and Barr (1979) added an overlooked sign which is an abnormally decreased bicaudate cerebroventricular index. Marcu and Becker (1977) have also described a putting together of the anterior ventricular horns which appear sharply pointed; they called this ventricular modification the "hare's ear sign". Jacobson and Farmer (1979) have created the suggestive denomination of "hypernormal" CT scan in dementia. Enhancement of the hematoma could better demonstrate the hematomas, mainly if retarded scan, 4–6 hours after contrast infusion are performed[6, 55, 166]. Messina (1976) has observed uptake of contrast material in hematomas 6 hours after infusion. Amendola and Ostrum (1977) have reported 3 out of 7 cases which were demonstrated after contrast enhancement.

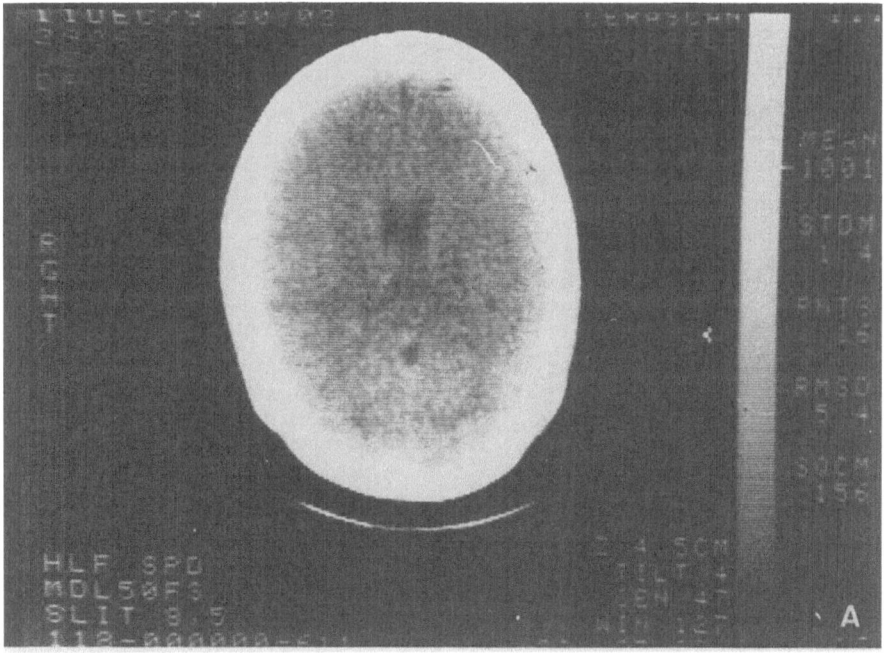

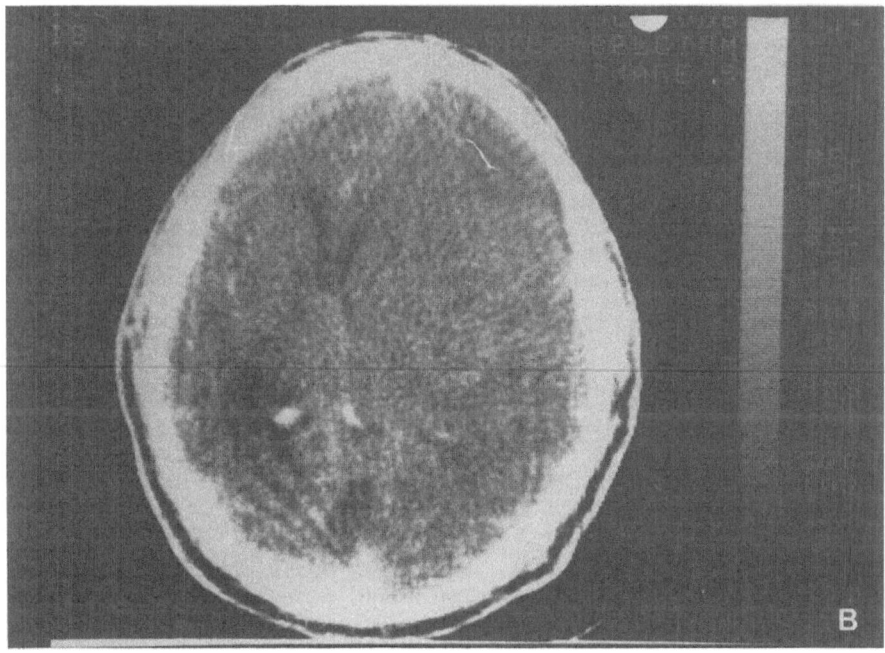

Fig. 10. Isodense bilateral subdural hematoma in 2 cases. A) No ventricular shift
one month after trauma. B) Unequal volume of hematomas 13 days after trauma

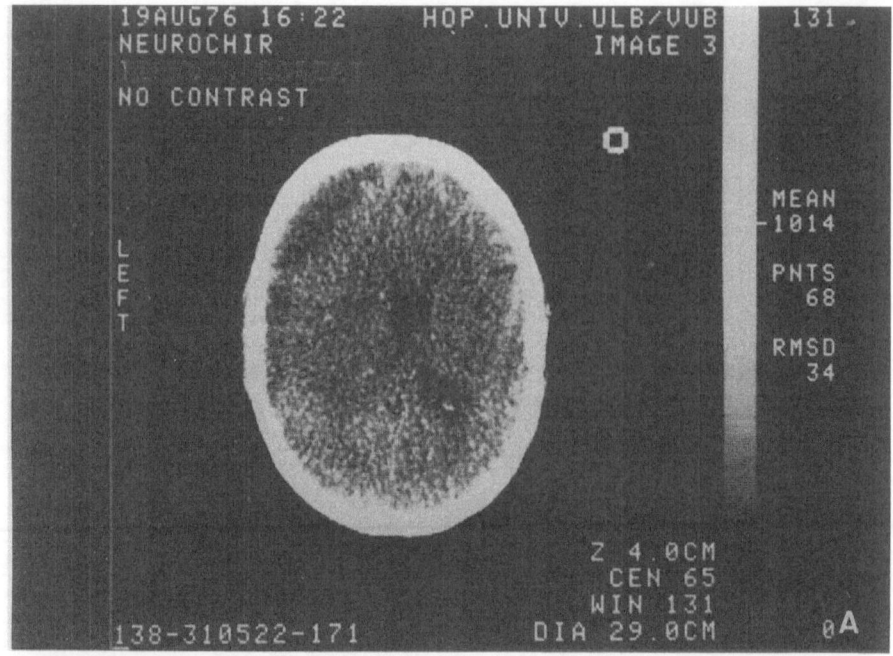

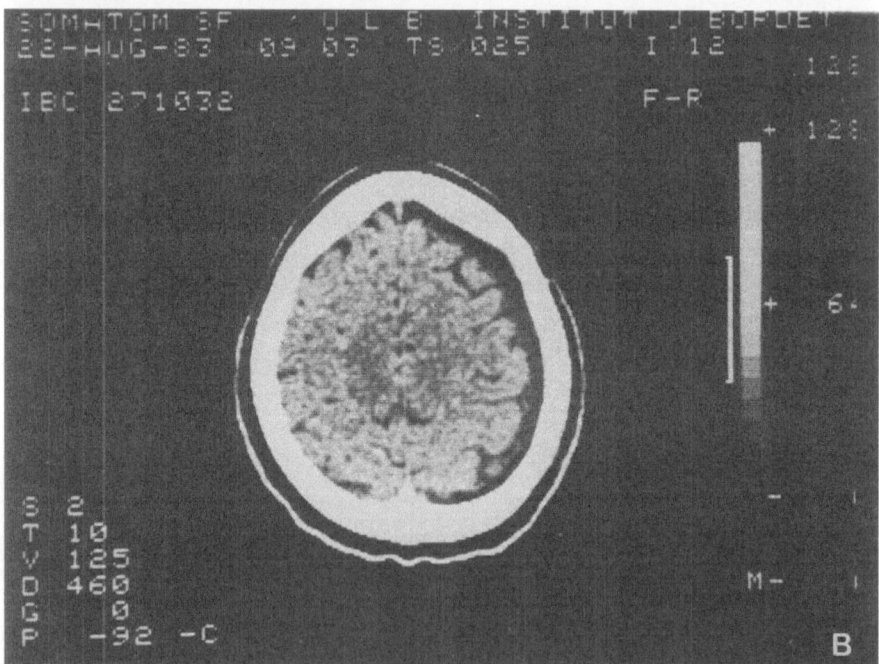

Fig. 11. A) Crescent-shaped chronic subdural hematoma 20 days after trauma. The cortical sulci are obliterated by the brain edema. B) Crescent-shaped hygroma, 5 weeks after trauma. The sulci are not obliterated and the effusion extends on the whole hemisphere

Moller and Ericson (1979) have observed 17 iso-attenuating hematomas in a series of 87 patients; among the bilateral hematomas, 2 were isodense bilaterally and one was isodense on one side only.

The calculation of volume of subdural hematomas has been approached by Sachs J. and Sachs E. (1977) who made use of the formula for the volume of an ellipsoid. Rabe *et al.* (1964) have suggested the isotope dilution method in determining the size of the subdural effusion. Another but rough method consists of filling the cavity during surgery with a measured amount of fluid. French and Dublin (1977) rightly point out that a subdural collection that appears to be thin on CT scan is usually one centimeter or more in its thickest portion at the time of the operation.

When the subdural hematoma appears as a lucent, crescentic-shaped collection, it is not always easy to differentiate it from a subdural hydroma [56, 171]. In our experience, the cortical sulci are better preserved in case of hygroma and its outline is not so markedly defined as it is for subdural hematoma; besides, the hygroma preserves the crescentic shape during all the time of its evolution and extends more often than the chronic subdural hematoma on the whole cerebral convexity (Fig. 11).

In spite of its inestimated value, there are still limitations to computerized tomography [43, 57, 188]; resort to complementary diagnostic procedures must remain in use when CT scan is not in line with the clinical data.

## 7. Surgical Treatment

In spite of a so long time during which chronic subdural hematoma was considered by neurosurgeons, its treatment is still matter for discussion. However, nowadays, it seems accepted by everyone that, when surgery is required, the more simple and the more smooth procedure will be the best for the patient. Whatever the kind of treatment, the aim to achieve is to drain sufficiently the hematoma fluid and to collapse the hematoma cavity in order to encourage resorption of hematoma membranes.

Considering that a number of patients with chronic subdural hematoma are rather old, local anesthesia will be better supported by the patient than general anesthesia.

The more simple management and probably the oldest one is the *subdural tapping,* repeated if necessary. It has been largely used for subdural effusion in infancy since the consistency of the calvarium allows easy puncture.

McLaurin *et al.* (1971) have given an excellent rational of the method, demonstrating that the goal is not to drain completely the hematoma cavity but to empty it sufficiently to stop the process of intracranial hypertension and so doing to promote reversal of the chain of events which keeps the hematoma growing. Tapping is repeated until the decompression is definitely acquired. Such a therapeutical concept presupposes that hematoma membranes are not able to restrict brain growth or brain reexpansion. This concept, which does no more appear debatable to us, has to be taken into account when the other therapeutical procedures will be considered. Tapping can also be achieved in adults through one burr hole drilled at a declivitous point of the cavity; this technique has been largely used for diagnostic as well as therapeutic purposes. However, in order to avoid infection, we remain reluctant to repeat punctures through a wound.

*The burr-hole technique for external drainage* is probably the surgical approach which was the most often performed by the neurosurgeons; it consists of drilling two burr holes over the convexity of the hematoma, one of the burr hole being placed at the inferior part of the lesion. When the hematoma fluid is drained, the cavity is gently irrigated with warm physiologic saline solution, then a draining catheter is introduced in the hematoma and is left in place open in the dressing during one to several days. This simple and effective technique may be carried out everywhere, by every surgeon, under local anesthesia, even in patients in poor condition.

It is recommended when the dura mater over the hematoma is incised, to avoid a sudden and rapid evacuation of the fluid in order to prevent abrupt translation of the brain stem. In a first step, the dura can be punctured and the fluid slowly aspirated; afterwards the dura is incised. All manipulations (irrigation, introduction of the drain) have to be made with caution, in order to avoid rebleeding from the outer membrane. In case of bilateral subdural hematoma, it is recommended to proceed to the simultaneous evacuation of the fluid for the same reason of distorsion of the midline structures (Kaste *et al.* 1979, Tabaddor and Shulman 1977).

Weir and Gordon (1983) have suggested serial measurements in the hematoma fluid "of plasmin and alpha$_2$-antiplasmine complexes as an index of ongoing fibrinolytic activation in vivo, since it raises the possibility of assays of chronic subdural fluid being helpful in predicting which patients might be at greater risk from reaccumulation of hematoma. In such cases, longer periods of external drainage might be indicated and/or the use of fibrinolytic inhibitor drugs".

*A trephination* from 2 to 5 cm in diameter can be used as unique perforation of the calvarium. Through the opening, inspection of the hematoma cavity is facilitated. A piece of the outer membrane can be cutted out for histology. The bone ring is nicked to give passage to the draining tube (Fig. 12). However the temptation could be great to strip off the membranes and this has to be avoided because, even with a 5 cm opening, it will be difficult to take off the whole membranes and to handle the rebleeding or the surface oozing caused by the procedure, with security.

*Craniotomy* with removal of membranes is less and less advocated, though some authors still have recourse to it[158, 185]. Its rational was the

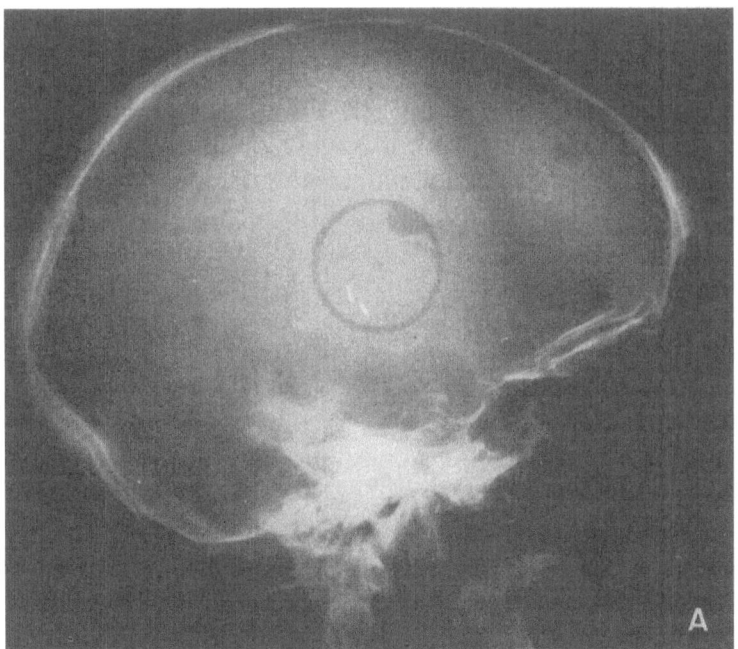

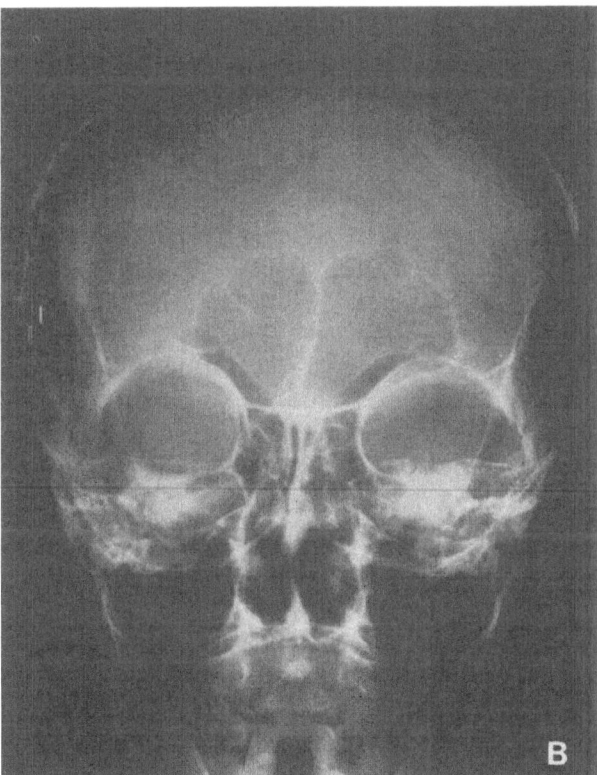

Fig. 12. 2 metal clips, used as markers, are left affixed, one to the dura, the other to the cortex, in order to monitor reexpansion of the hemisphere. The bone ring of the trephination is nicked for passing the catheter outside the skull

removal of the membranes, source of bleeding and cause of constriction of the cerebral hemisphere; but these reasons rapidly lost their evidence[118, 167, 175]. In fact, the focal cerebral swelling often appears more important than the thickness of the membranes and compression by the hematoma[34, 175]. In spite of the fact that the membranes are usually easily peeled from the dura-mater and the arachnoid, membranectomy may be the cause of rebleeding and reaccumulation of fluid.

To our knowledge, indication for an osteoplastic flap and removal of membranes remains when symptomatic continuous reaccumulation of hematoma fluid persists in spite of a correct and long enough drainage.

*Craniectomy* is still advocated by Tyson *et al.* (1980) in rare cases of insufficient improvement after craniotomy and membranectomy and in presence of extensive cerebral swelling; however such a technique must remain exceptional since it is known from clinical experience that long-lasting closed-system drainage of the hematoma may overcome the persistence of an expanded subdural space due to re-accumulation of fluid.

*Calcified or ossified subdural hematoma* deserves consideration with regard to the indication of its surgical excision. The majority of the cases reported in the literature have been surgically removed en bloc. The general opinion of those neurosurgeons who have a personal experience is that surgery did not affect in any way the clinical manifestations, mainly epileptic seizures and mental impairment. The inefficacity of the removal of the lesion is explained by the fact that the hematoma is no more evoluating, the clinical signs being due to permanent cerebral lesions, mainly brain atrophy. However, we must admit that there are particular cases where the calcified or ossified hematoma is still playing a role in the occurrence of clinical manifestations. The patient of Mansuy *et al.* (1964) had a shift of the anterior cerebral artery on angiography; after excision of the lesion, a regression of behaviour disorders and a better medical control of epileptic seizures were observed. In the non-excised case of Debois and Lombaert (1980) there exists also a displacement of the midline structures on CT scans and angiograms. In the first case reported by Afra (1961) there were rapid signs of recovery from the left hemiplegia after surgery; the same observations was made by Perroudon *et al.* (1972). Boyd and Merrell (1943) wrote that the removal of the calcified hematoma may diminish the convulsive attacks and ameliorate the focal neurological manifestations but will probably not improve the symptoms due to intellectual disturbances or deficiencies of cerebral development; Mosberg and Smith (1952) were expressing the same opinion. Our personal case also demonstrated a better medical control of the epileptic seizures (Fig. 2). Therefore from several reports in the literature, it can be said that each case of calcified or ossified hematoma has to be considered carefully, that there is no reason to refuse systematically the surgical removal of the lesion when there exist clinical data which incite to operation.

With regard to surgical techniques, we still have to quote two original operative procedures for which we have no personal experience and which fundamentally consisted of *reduction of the cranial dimensions in infancy* in case of bilateral chronic subdural hematoma. In 1973, Faulhauer, Herrmann and Loew reported an operative technique aiming at eliminating the abnormal subdural space by reducing the size of the dura mater and the cranium: through a large craniotomy, outer and inner membranes are excised and dura, stripped away from the outer membrane, is cut off; thereafter the remaining dura is sutured. The same procedure is repeated on the other side of the cranium. The third step consists of partial resection of the bone bridge over the sagittal sinus, the extremities being drawn together with wire sutures. Finally the two bone flat reajusted are replaced. Skin has also to be often partially resected. Among 14 children operated on, long-term follow-up studies were obtained in 11; apart 2 already brain damaged before surgery, 9 developed into normal infants.

In 1979, Gutierrez, McLone and Raimondi developed a surgical technique quite similar to the procedure proposed by Faulhauer *et al.,* but proceeding from another pathophysiological hypothesis. To quote them, they postulate that "one possible mechanism is the progressive stretching and narrowing of the cortical veins, bridging the subarachnoid and subdural spaces to enter the superior sagittal sinus. This process ultimately leads to thrombosis of these hanging veins. Narrowing and angulation of these veins could result in elevated back pressure favoring the formation of a transudate. 16 children who had progressive and persistent collections of xanthochromic fluid in the subdural spaces secondary to trauma or infection who were treated previously either with subdural tap, burr holes, subdural peritoneal shunt, craniotomy, stripping of membranes and/or a combination of these, were treated by lowering and advancing the superior sagittal sinus with its overlying sagittal suture and performing a duraplasty. This new surgical technique is directed to improve venous drainage from the superior anastomotic vein into the superior sagittal sinus. Angiographic follow-up showed that only 2 patients still had evidence of fluid collection: the rest of the patients showed normal arterial phases, the medullary system was minimally filled and all of these showed remarkable improvement of the venous drainage throughout the superficial cortical veins with no evidence of hanging veins. Intellectual development of these children following lowering of the superior sagittal sinus showed that 8 patients (50%) were normal or above normal; 5 patients (31.2%) were retarded and 3 patients (18.7%) were borderline". This last technique based on a new interpretation of clinical data, indicates that the subdural effusions observed in infancy are not comparable in all their aspects to the chronic subdural hematoma seen in adults.

*Complications* are common to all these surgical techniques but with a variable frequency according to the type of surgery.

*Focal edema,* underlying chronic subdural hematoma is an habitual finding well demonstrated on CT scans; it often extends to the whole hemisphere on the side of the hematoma. It may directly result from compression by the hematoma, interfering with the cortical venous circulation[181]. It may be also provoked or aggravated by the surgical procedure, chiefly when removal of membranes is carried out. Focal edema could justify early treatment with corticoids.

*Delayed reexpansion of the hemisphere* is frequent and an avascular space regularly persists after surgery for a rather long time (from a few days, to 3 or more weeks); it is well seen on repeated CT scans and expresses the fact that the cerebral hemisphere does not expand immediately in spite of an effective evacuation of the hematoma content. When the scanner is not available or disposable, others means allowing follow-up may be used: as Parkinson and Chochinov (1960) did, we often affixe a metal clip on the inner membrane and another one on the dura-mater, through a trephine opening (Fig. 14); thanks to this trick, it was easy on repeated plain X-rays of the skull, to monitor reexpansion of the hemisphere. Vieth *et al.* (1966) used tantalum dust placed on the pia-arachnoid and tantalum clips applied to the dura for measuring the distance between the outer and inner membranes. Still, CT scanner besides the imaging of the subdural space, permits the definition of the remaining or recurrent fluid and the diagnostic of rebleeding within the cavity (Figs. 8 and 13).

Parkinson and Chochinov (1960) have observed delayed reexpansion up to 60 days. The persistance of a residual subdural space after hematoma drainage sometimes contrasts with the rapid improvement of patient's condition. The lack of reexpansion could be find in elderly patients in acquired brain atrophy which prevents rapid and complete reexpansion of the hemisphere; the same situation is also encountered in children whose ultimate prognosis largely depends on preexisting cortical damage[167]. To encourage the hemisphere to come up to the dura mater, were proposed saline injection by lumbar or ventricular puncture, air insufflation within the ventricles, intravenous injection of distilled water[28, 46, 188]. These attempts to swell up again the brain are diversely appreciated; as far as we are concerned, we avoid moving the brain too suddenly.

The development of *epileptic seizures* after surgery is not uncommon. This event does not seem to be in relation with the retained membranes; unfortunately it happened that epilepsy occurred after intraoperative laceration of brain with the catheter or while inner membranes were removed.

One of our patients developed manifestation of *normal pressure hydrocephalus* weeks after drainage of the hematoma. Three of 52 cases

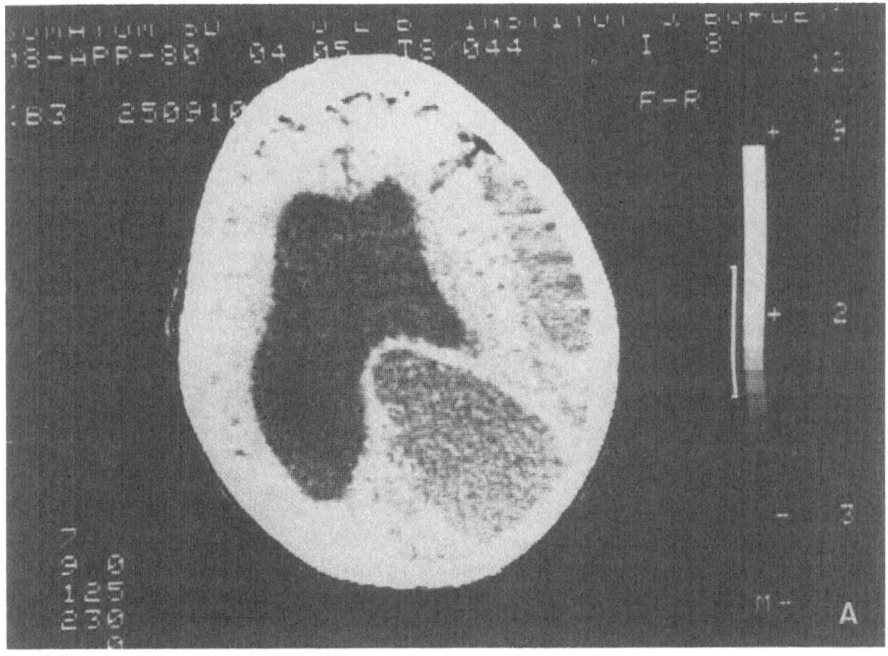

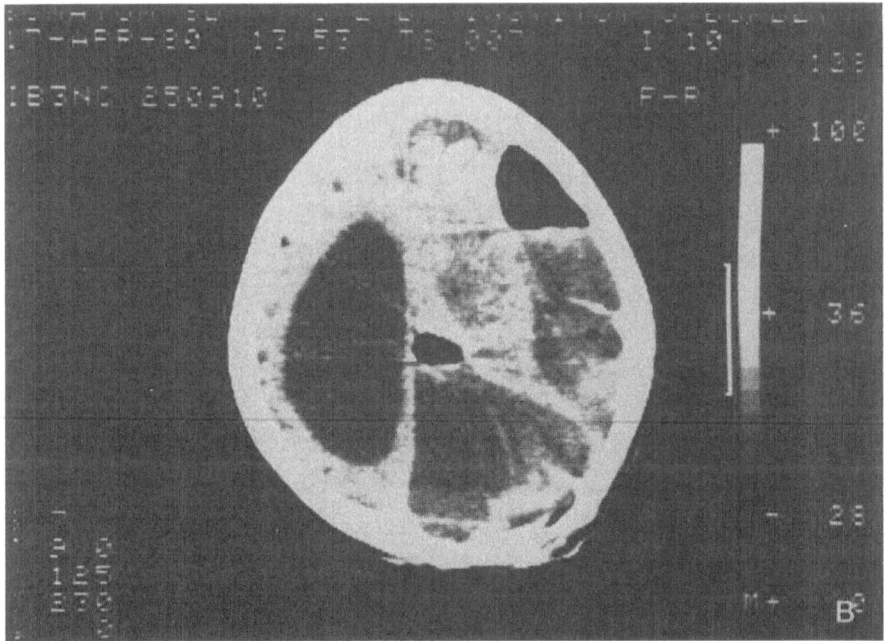

Fig. 13. Patient 70 years old. Latent period probably of several months. A) Enhanced CT scan demonstrating two cavities or a lobulated subdural hematoma. B) 10 days after evacuation of the two hematic sacs. Rebleeding exists with air in the cavities. Reoperation was required

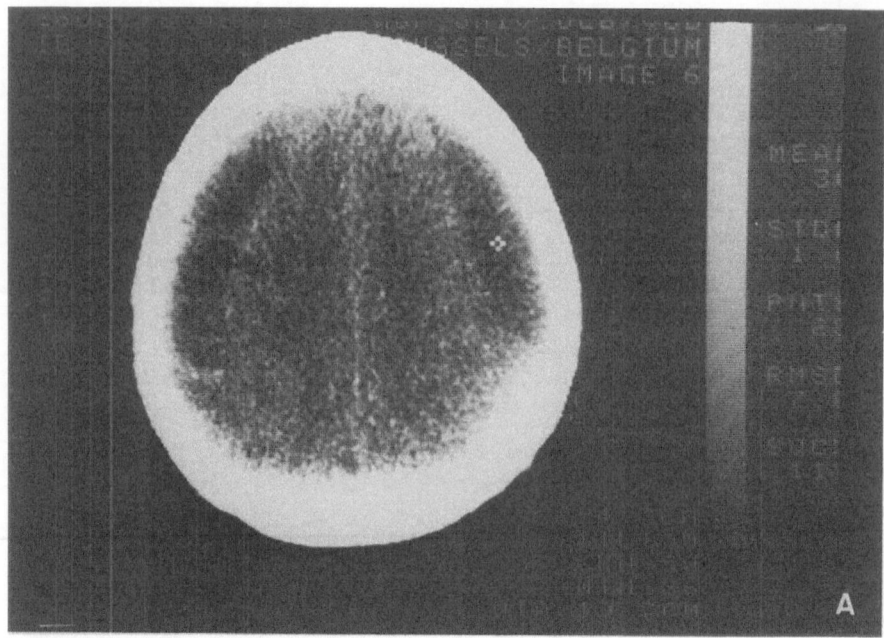

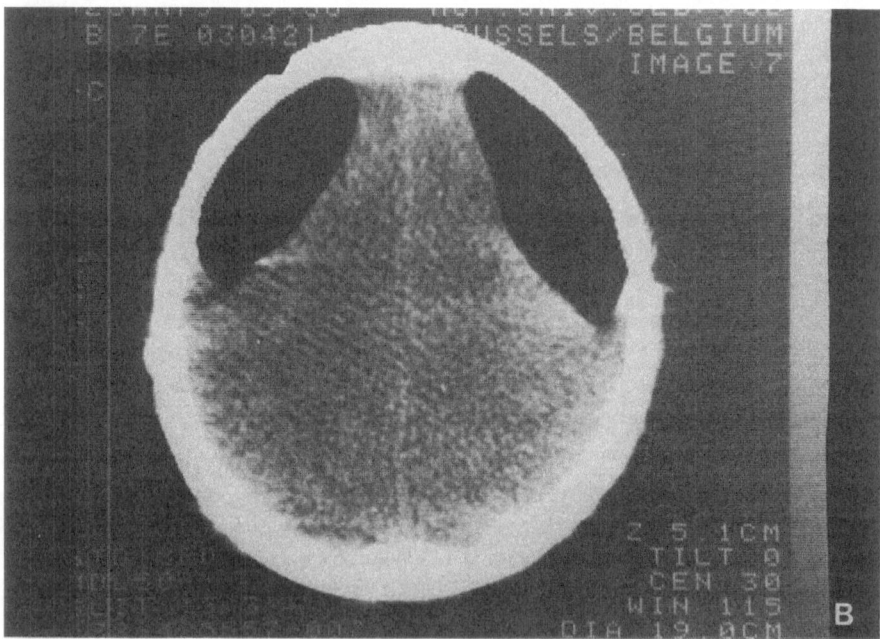

Fig. 14. A) Chronic bilateral subdural hematoma in a patient 75 years old. B) Air entrapped in the cavities, 2 days after drainage. C) 3 days later, the volume of air is markedly and spontaneously reduced

reported by Raskind *et al.* (1972) developed postoperative normal pressure hydrocephalus, explaining clinical deterioration after initial improvement; all three were shunted and improved again.

*Infection* is of rare occurence and is to be feared when repeated tapping is made. In one patient in our series, a subdural empyema developed after burr hole and evacuation of the hematoma; cure was obtained by large drainage of the cavity.

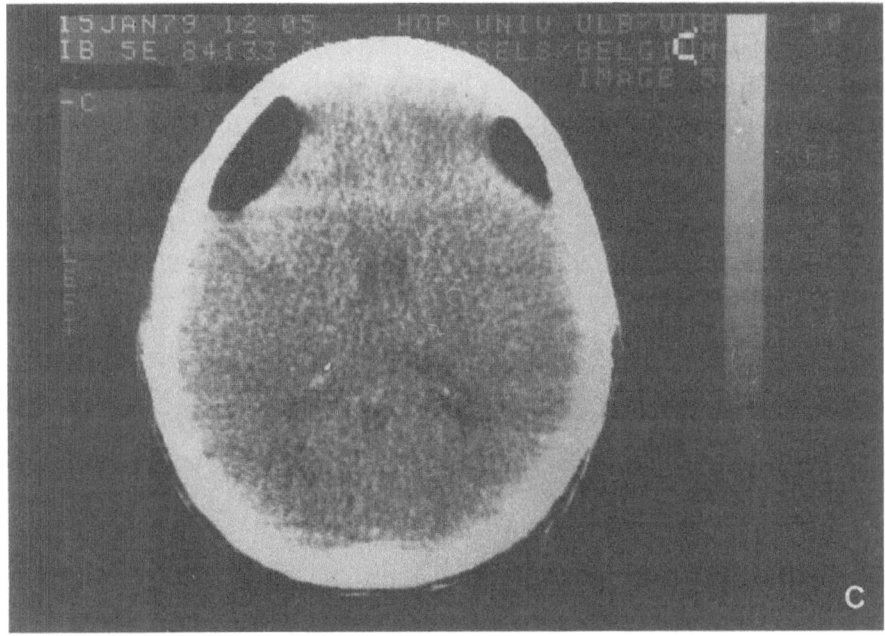

Fig. 14 C

*Bleeding* at the time of tapping may be due to rupture of a cortical vessel by the needle[181]. Late rebleeding (Figs. 8 and 13) from the outer neovascularized membrane is explained by mechanical strain on the membrane or by local alterations of hemostatic-fibrinolytic mechanisms[86, 87, 102, 194]. An exceptional case of probable erythropoiesis or hematopoiesis originated in a subdural hematoma has been reported by Slater (1966) in a child 4 months old.

*Subdural tension pneumocephalus* is realized by postoperative entrapment of air within the subdural space. This trapping is encouraged by the absence of reexpansion of the brain; it could be kept by a valve-like mechanism made of obliteration of the burr hole by membranous cuff. This phenomena is very close to the tension pneumocephalus described in the literature in various pathological conditions[18, 23, 79, 83, 107, 112, 119, 143, 150, 172, 198].

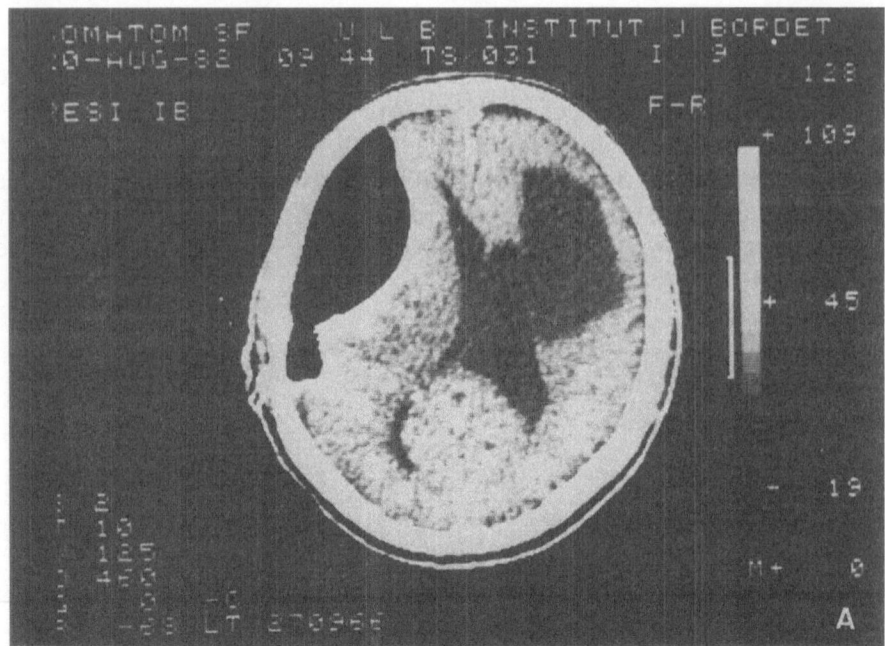

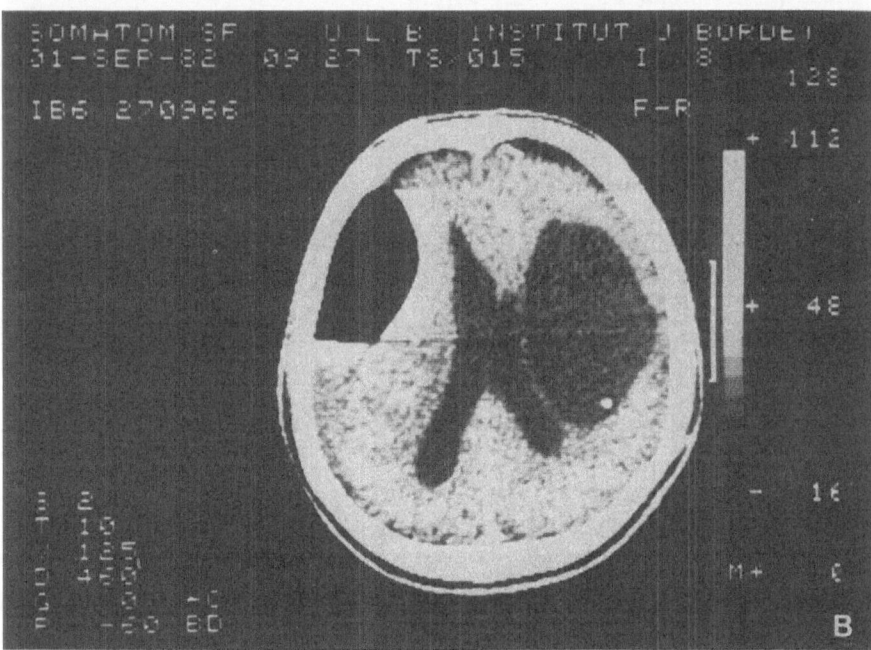

Fig. 15. Patient presenting since birth a huge intracerebral symptomatic cyst, shunted when he was one year old. Revision of the shunt when he was 16 years old because relapse of clinical signs. Chronic subdural hematoma contralateral to the side operated. A) Entrapment of air after surgical drainage. B) 20 days later, persistence of air. The drainage tube of the shunting system is temporarily clipped. C) Two months after, return to normal appearance

Since the patient usually remains in a supine position and because gas in the subdural space is moving with changing head position, the air accumulates anteriorly over both frontal lobes; sometimes it outlines the falx in its anterior part (Fig. 14). Presence of subdural air is not uncommon on CT scan; it was observed eleven times among our 70 patients. Usually it exists without clinical repercussion; sometimes air is under pressure and in great

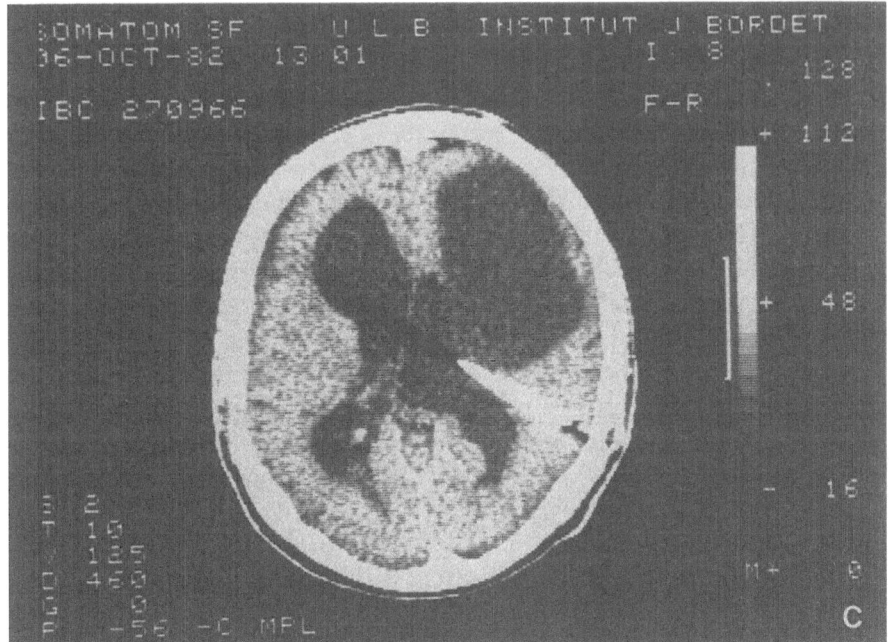

Fig. 15 C

volume, compressing the brain (Fig. 15): tapping the subdural space provokes its egress under pressure through the needle; then it could be responsible of delayed improvement or deterioration of the patient's state. Ectors (1962) thought that air trapped into the hematoma cavity was dilating while warming up from room to body temperature, and consequently was compressing the brain. Raggio (1979), discussing the presentation of Black *et al.* (1979), estimates that this dilatation of the gas is negligible, about 4% depending on the compliance of the parenchyma. Hirsh (1980) reported 2 cases and Bremer and Nguyen (1982) 3 cases (out of 19 cases, 16%) who developed postoperative subdural tension pneumocephalus, causing delayed improvement. Air trapped was also symptomatic in three cases out of the eleven that we observed and it required subsequent drainage; in one other case of subdural hematoma complicating a shunting procedure, the peritoneal tube was firstly clamped and afterwards the valve was changed from medium to a high pressure aperture (Fig. 15).

Subdural tension pneumocephalus therefore should be considered in the differential diagnosis when improvement does not occur after drainage.

Among the 70 cases of our series, 3 were not operated on, 2 underwent craniotomy with removal of membranes and 65 were treated with a closed system drainage, the hematoma content being collected in a sterile urine bag maintained below the level of the patient head. The result of treatment was: 25 patients were classified as excellent or good; 22 as fair and 10 as poor. The too small number of craniotomies does not allow a comparison between the two main surgical techniques. Ten patients presented recurrence of hemorrhage and underwent a second procedure; one developed a subdural empyema and another one a normal pressure hydrocephalus. Eight patients died; 3 were over 80, 4 over 70 and 1 was 62 years old; 3 were comatous and 1 decerebrated at the time of surgery; sepsis and brain stem damage, verified at post-mortem examination in 3 cases, were the main causes of death.

Three patients did not undergo operation: one refused to be drained and was lost to follow-up; in two patients the subdural hematoma was lightly symptomatic and of small volume; they were successfully treated by bed rest.

## 8. Nonsurgical Treatment of Chronic Subdural Hematoma

Bender and Christoff (1974)[16, 113] had the merit to investigate methodically on a fair number of patients the possibilities of medical treatment of subdural hematoma. As they reminded it, once the subdural hematoma was demonstrated, trephination was the usual treatment often without regard to the size of the hematoma or the clinical state of the patient. Meanwhile it was known by autopsy or incidental clinical observation that unsuspected subdural hematoma has regressed spontaneously. Bender and Christoff based the selection of patients for medical treatment on the clinical condition: the more the clinical manifestations are serious or rapidly evolving, the more often the patients are referred to neurosurgery. At the beginning, treatment only consisted of bed rest for a rather long period, thereafter corticosteroids allowed notable reduction of time reserved for bed rest and hospitalization. Only 3 patients received mannitol in addition to corticosteroids.

Among 75 patients exclusively treated with this regimen, no dead occured, 2 poor results were recorded and 3 had recurrences of symptoms. The other patients had a complete recovery.

As a conclusion to their clinical trial, Bender and Christoff (1974) stated: "our policy is to begin with corticosteroid therapy as soon as the diagnosis is suspected. If there is no clinical response to treatment within 24 to 28 hours, mannitol is added intravenously, 200 to 300 gm in 24 hours. Should this combined therapy fail to achieve improvement or should there be any progression, surgery is recommended."

At the same period, Suzuki and Takaku (1970) had postulated, as McLaurin (1971) thought it also, "that the reduction of the internal pressure of a hematoma will cure it, and that therefore the problem may be solved non-surgically if the internal pressure of a subdural hematoma can be reduced by any method, not necessarily craniotomy". Founding their conviction upon the osmotic theory according to which the enlargement of the hematoma provokes strain and hemorrhage in the membranes, they treated their patients with intravenous infusion of 20% mannitol during an average time of 41 days; the average total dosage of 20% mannitol was about 30,000 ml. Therapeutic success, even in severe cases, was obtained in 22 out of 23 patients; one severely ill older patient did not respond to treatment.

Their conviction was backed up by ultrastructural study of membranes taken off from chronic subdural hematomas, some treated with osmotherapy, others only drained surgically[163]. They observed in the wall of capillaries, after osmotherapy, the disappearance of open gaps between adjacent endothelial cells and of degenerating clear endothelial cells; in addition, formation of collagen fibrils within the membrane seemed to be promoted by osmotherapy.

In conclusion, Suzuki and Takaku stated: "If 3 or 4 days of treatment do not effectively reduce the severe symptoms, surgery should be adopted immediately, especially for aged people with severe neurological deficits."

Other reports of therapeutic success with medical treatment appeared[5, 61, 101, 158]. For all that, and stimulated by the publication of Suzuki and Takaku (1970), Gjerris and Schmidt (1974) entered upon a controlled study of patients treated either by craniotomy or by osmotic perfusions. This controlled trial had to be stopped because of repeated failures with mannitol therapy. Therefore Gjerris and Schmidt concluded that mannitol therapy should not be considered as a replacement for surgery in treatment of chronic subdural hematoma.

Medical treatment still remains in dispute. May we state that the first and main point is the selection of patients; those who are in a severe state or with evidence of rapid clinical evolution have to be rapidly referred to neurosurgery; those patients with mild and/or slowly progressing clinical manifestations may undergo trial of medical treatment. The second requirement is to be in a position to closely follow the response to treatment and to be ready at any time to change from medical to surgical management.

## 9. Conclusions

Chronic subdural hematoma is a "posttraumatic" lesion recognized for a very long time[80] and more frequent than it was suspected. Encountered at all ages, it predominates in infancy and in elderly patients, although chronic subdural collections in children are in many cases different from chronic subdural hematomas in adults. Mainly in infancy and old age, the lesion may be bilateral.

The mechanism of the early development and growing of chronic subdural hematoma is not yet fully understood, the thing being that a multifactorial mechanism is very often implied. With few exceptions rupture of bridging veins in their crossing the subdural space from cortex to the sagittal sinus is at the origin of the lesion. Histopathological research has emphasized the great potential of reaction that dura mater and arachnoid exhibit in contact with blood. Exchanges through the hematoma membranes between the content of the hematoma and the neighbouring cerebrospinal fluid and blood normally must occur; osmotic phenomenon is working to a certain extent but does not seem sufficient to explain by itself the enlargement of hematoma. Fragility of neocapillaries which rapidly appear within the outer membrane has to be taken into account. Fibrinolytic substances into the cellular component of the outer membrane seem also to play a role. The general condition of the patient and his regular behaviour (chronic alcoholism, diabetes, arterial hypertension, anticoagulant and chimiotherapy) are frequently reported. All these factors cooperate to the development and growing of the hematoma.

Clinical manifestations are depending on the compressive effect by the lesion and on the slowing of the regional cerebral blood flow by the brain edema underneath the hematoma. Symptomatology is evocative of chronic subdural hematoma when the causative head injury in known and when, after a not too long latent interval, appear headaches and behaviour and memory disorders, often associated with progressive hemiparesis. Symptomatology can be misleading when the causative event is unknown or forgotten and when the latent interval, free of clinical signs, is from several weeks to several months long. The association of progressive mental disorders, even with some complaints of headache and some disturbances of gait, too easily evokes presenility; the figure of 245 cases of subdural hematoma among 3,100 consecutive autopsies of psychotic patients is eloquent[4]. The association of mental disorders with sphincter incontinence and gait disturbances is of common occurence in chronic subdural hematoma, normal (intermittent) pressure hydrocephalus and meningioma arising from the midline of anterior skull base.

Therefore clinical diagnosis is sometimes difficult. So we strongly recommend to ask for complementary investigations for every patient suffering progressive mental disorders associated, or not, with headaches and/or motor deficits. EEG combined with brain scintigraphy remains a valuable detecting procedure. Computerized tomography has replaced cerebral angiography and is the best means of investigation. Even in bilateral isodense lesion, obliteration of circonvolutional sulci and small ventricles incite the radiologist to suspect the hematoma. Complementary investigations are thus mandatory everytime. the clinical diagnosis is uncertain.

Experimental production of chronic subdural hematoma in animals has given importance to two factors with regard to the development of the lesion. The first one is the volume of bleeding in the subdural space: an injection of a too small amount of blood invariably results in rapid resorption of the implant. The second factor is found in the environment of the hematoma: brain atrophy in the elderly procures room for the development of bleeding; elasticity of the skull in infants allows the bleeding to extend. On the contrary, local edema frequently associated with bleeding[85] exerts a pressure on the meninges, being opposed to the hematoma. A local inflammatory reaction of dura mater, provoking appearance of fibrin fibrils, is also a promoting factor for the development of hematoma. Consequently treatment of chronic subdural hematoma in humans must be defined after these experimental variables: the hematoma volume has to be reduced adequately and at the same time patient reequilibration must be secured.

Spontaneous regression of chronic subdural hematoma might occur when the fluid volume and membranes thickness are not too large. Asymptomatic, not resolving chronic subdural hematoma has been seen in old patients providing that brain atrophy leaves room enough for the lesion. Symptomatic, evolving chronic subdural hematoma has to be treated.

Nonoperative management was advocated for chronic subdural hematoma with rather small size and slow clinical evolution. The treatment consists of bed rest and adequate care in order to prevent the slightest brain shock as coughing or constipation. In addition to restraining the formation of membranes and to reducing the pressure within the hematoma cavity, corticosteroids and intravenous mannitol infusion may be given. However such a medical treatment cannot be proposed systematically if the patient is not hospitalized in a neurosurgical department in which, if necessary, management can be rapidly shifted from medical to surgical procedure. Better controlled clinical experience is still required before drawing any firm conclusion regarding the merits of this regimen.

Surgical treatment is based upon a large clinical experience. The necessity of removing membranes is no more accepted, with the exception of very few cases. On the contrary, we are of the opinion that more simple is the technique of drainage, the best it is for the patient. Our rule consists of evacuation of the hematoma fluid under local anesthesia through one or two burr holes, the first one being drilled at a declivitous area of the cavity. It is important to slowly evacuate the hematoma content, above all when there is a high pressure into the cavity; a finger placed in the burr hole makes evacuation smooth. The cavity is gently rinsed, without force, with warm physiologic saline solution. Afterwards a catheter is left and secured in place; it is connected to a sterile urine bag for at least 24 hours. There is no determined limit of time to let the catheter in place; we personally check the volume of fluid daily drained; as soon as we observe a substantial drop in quantity, the drain is taken off. In case of bilateral lesion, the hematomas have to be evacuated simultaneously.

To avoid complications, among which rebleeding and delayed reexpansion of the cerebral hemisphere are the most frequent, it is important to keep these patients, as it is stated for those treated medically, in a good biological balance.

The outcome of chronic subdural hematoma does not depend entirely on the technique of treatment but also on the preexisting brain state of the patient. Still, as stated by Raskin et al.[158], poor results are almost entirely caused by delay in diagnosis and treatment, and thus are largely preventable. Jamieson[91] put a special accent on prevention, reminding us that "the major responsibility for planning organization and conduct of care of patients with head injury rests squarely on our speciality". We need prospective studies for removing the uncertainties which still persist.

## 10. "How to Do It..."

We have discussed in the preceding pages the management of chronic subdural hematoma for patients admitted in a department of neurosurgery or in a general hospital in which a neurosurgeon can be called for. But there exist situations where a non-experienced surgeon has to take care of a patient with chronic subdural hematoma.

Let us recall that chronic subdural hematoma results from a rather slow accumulation of blood into the subdural space, forming a pouch which compresses and hampers the underlying brain.

Chronic subdural hematoma is generally situated in the temporal region of the convexity, extending in part towards the frontal or parietal regions.

Its clinical picture includes disorder of memory, slow cerebration and some mental confusion. Frequently a mild hemiparesis can be observed. In old patients, mainly when no traumatic anamnesis is recorded, the clinical diagnosis may be difficult. Therefore, before making a diagnosis of senile or presenile dementia, it is highly recommended that one proceeds to all diagnostic means available: the shift of a calcified pineal on standard X-rays or the shift of an echo from the midline indicate the presence of a space-occupying lesion. The electroencephalogram sometimes demonstrates a lower voltage above the hematoma. Of course other more sophisticated radiological investigations are indicated if they are available. Lumbar puncture must always be avoided; not only is it not useful but above all it could be very dangerous, provoking entrapment of the temporal lobe with compression of the brain stem.

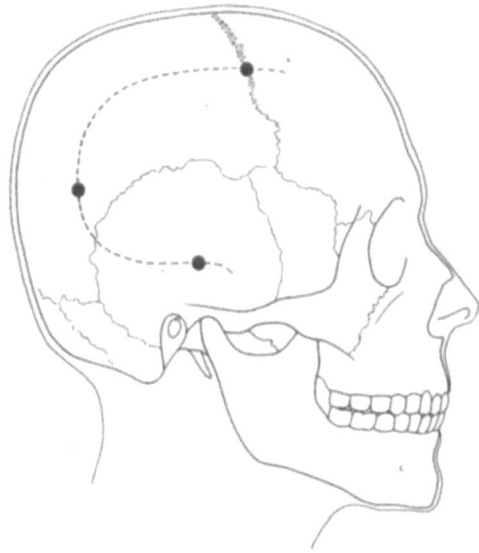

Fig. 16. Design of a possible skin flap (dotted line) with the lower branch curving and descending straightly in front of the ear (not crossing the temporal region). Skin incisions must be made on this line. The temporal burr hole is first drilled 3 cm above the external auditory meatus in order to drain the lower part of the hematoma.
A second burr hole may be made either in the frontal region (4 to 5 cm apart from the mid-sagittal line of the skull) or in the parietal region for gently washing the cavity of the hematoma

When clinical manifestations require a prompt diagnosis, resorting to an exploratory burr hole remains advisable, especially since this burr hole represents at the same time the correct management of the lesion. Tapping the hematoma has indeed to be sometimes undertaken as quickly as possible in order to reduce the shift of brain structures and the compression of the brain stem provoked by the expanding hematoma.

The procedure might be carried out under local anesthesia if the patient is neither comatose nor agitated. Local infiltration of the scalp with a solution of 1% procain and adrenaline is adequate. But general anesthesia with endotracheal tube is in general recommended since it facilitates the surgical procedure and the control of vital functions; when the patient is agitated, general anesthesia is required since restlessness often indicates brain hypoxia.

The patient is placed in a supine position with the temporal region, well in sight, because the main bulk of hematoma tends to lie within this area.

The whole tapping operation can simply be performed without suction and/or diathermy.

The skin incision, 4 cm long, is placed in such a position that it can be used later for turning a skin and bone flaps if it is required (Fig. 16).

A self-retaining retractor draws aside the lips of the incision and usually makes hemostasis of the skin layers.

A burr hole is drilled in the temporal region, 3 cm above and 1 cm forwards to the external auditory meatus, at the dependent part of the hematoma (Fig. 16).

Duramater over the hematoma appears blue in color; it is opened by a stellate incision. The outer membrane of the hematoma, often thick, is incised with the dura allowing the bloodstained fluid to briskly gush out. It is strongly recommended not to let the fluid drain too freely in order to prevent sudden displacement of the brain stem; to achieve this, the simplest way it to put the finger on the dural incision.

When the hematoma appears well drained and the brain is expanding quickly, the dura is left open and the skin and temporal muscle are drawn together with interrupted sutures.

Everytime it is feasible, we recommended to drill a second burr hole placed higher than the first one, in the frontal area, at the level of the coronal suture, 4 to 5 cm from the midline of the vault; if the hematoma is not encountered in this location, a third burr hole has to be made in the parietal area (Fig. 16). The second burr hole is useful for better draining the hematoma: a rubber catheter is introduced within the subdural cavity through the frontal aperture and sterile warm saline solution is very gently injected for washing the cavity from blood clots and stagnant fluid in the most dependent part of the hematoma.

At the end of the washing, if the underlying brain does not expand up to the inner surface of the dura, the catheter introduced through the lowest burr hole might be left in place for 2 or 3 days; our practice is to have the catheter emerging through a separate small stab wound 2 or 3 cm from the skin incision. As usual, the skin incision is sutured in two layers, the pericranium being carefully closed.

When the cavity is not drained with a catheter and if there is reaccumulation of fluid within the subdural space, the cavity may be tapped daily during the following week to evacuate the reformed collection. A blunt needle has to be used for tapping; aspiration is not recommended. the fluid escaping freely. The quantity of fluid usually diminishes progressively after each tapping, the cavity being often dry after 5 or 6 days.

It sometimes happens that air enters into the subdural space through the needle or the catheter but this event usually does not interfere with the postoperative clinical evolution. However, we advise connection of the catheter to a closed bottle everytime it is feasible.

When there are no localizing clinical signs and in the absence of an imaging diagnostic procedure, it is wise to drill a burr hole in the temporal region of the contralateral side in order to make sure that a bilateral subdural hematoma does not exist. In fact, approximately 9% of bilateral chronic subdural hematomas are reported in published series so that contralateral exploration could be life saving.

In conclusion, the surgical procedure for draining chronic subdural hematoma is rather simple, easily and quickly made. The difficulty concerns above all the correct diagnosis of the lesion when there is no anamnesis of trauma and when clinical disorders are slowly developing, the picture mimicking brain tumor, senile dementia or intermittent pressure hydrocephalus.

### Acknowledgement

The author is indebted to Doctor Louis Jeanmart, Professor of radiology at the Free University of Brussels, for assistance in the analysis of radiological documenta.

### References

1. Achslogh, J., 1952: Hématome sous-dural chronique de la fosse cérébrale postérieure. Acta neurol. belg. *52*, 790 – 794.
2. Adams, J. E., Prawirohardjo, S., 1959: Fate of red blood cells injected into cerebrospinal fluid pathways. Neurology *9*, 561 – 564.
3. Afra, D., 1961: Ossification of subdural hematoma. Report of two cases. J. Neurosurg. *18*, 393 – 397.
4. Allen, A. M., Moore, M., Daly, B. B., 1940: Subdural hemorrhage in patients with mental disease. New Engl. J. Med. *223*, 324 – 329.
5. Ambrosetto, C., 1962: Post-traumatic subdural hematoma. Further observations on nonsurgical treatment. Arch. Neurol. (Chic.) *6*, 287 – 292.
6. Amendola, M. A., Ostrum, B. J., 1977: Diagnosis of isodense subdural hematomas by computed tomography. J. Roentgenol. *129*, 693 – 697.
7. Apferbaum, R. J., Guth-Kelch, A. N., Shulman, K., 1974: Experimental production of subdural hematomas. J. Neurosurg. *40*, 336 – 346.
8. Arieff, A. J., Wetzel, N., 1964: Subdural hematoma following epileptic convulsion. Neurology *14*, 731 – 732.
9. Aronson, S. M., Okazaki, H., 1963: A study of some factors modifying response of cerebral tissue to subdural hematoma. J. Neurosurg. *20*, 89 – 93.

10. Arseni, C., Stanciu, M., 1969: Particular clinical aspects of chronic subdural haematoma in adults. Europ. Neurol. *2*, 109 – 122.
11. Arseni, C., Iacob, M., 1970: Calcified intracranial haematoma associated with chronic subdural hygroma. J. Neurol. Neurosurg. Psychiat. *33*, 205 – 207.
12. Bahadir, A. R., Marx, P., 1967: Zur Kasuistik verkalkter und ossifizierter subduraler Hämatome. Neurochirurgia (Stuttgart) *10*, 224 – 228.
13. Bakay, R. A. E., Ward, A. A., 1983: Enzymatic changes in serum and cerebrospinal fluid in neurological injury. J. Neurosurg. *58*, 27 – 37.
14. Bassett, R. C., Lemmen, L. J., 1952: Subdural hematoma associated with bleeding intracranial aneurysm. J. Neurosurg. *9*, 443 – 450.
15. Bell, W. E., Joynt, R. J., Sahs, A. L., 1960: Low spinal fluid pressure syndromes. Neurology *10*, 512 – 521.
16. Bender, M. B., Christoff, N., 1974: Nonsurgical treatment of subdural hematomas. Arch. Neurol. (Chic.) *31*, 73 – 79.
17. Bergström, M., Ericson, K., Levander, B., Svendsen, P., Larsson, S., 1977: Variation with time of the attenuation values of intracranial hematomas. J. Comp. Ass. Tomogr. *1*, 57 – 63.
18. Black, P. McL., Davis, J. M., Kjellberg, R. N., Davis, K. R., 1979: Tension pneumocephalus of the cranial subdural space: a case report. Neurosurgery *5*, 368 – 370.
19. Boop, W. C., Chou, S. N., French, L. A., 1961: Ruptured intracranial aneurysm complicated by subdural hematoma. J. Neurosurg. *18*, 834 – 836.
20. Bortnick, R. J., Murphy, J. P., 1963: Paraparesis with incontinence of bowel and bladder—a syndrom of bilateral subdural hematomas. J. Neurosurg. *20*, 352 – 353.
21. Borzone, M., Capuzzo, T., Perria, C., Rivano, C., Tercero, E., 1983: Traumatic subdural hygromas: a report of 70 surgically treated cases. J. Neurosurg. Sciences *27*, 161 – 166.
22. Boyd, D. A., Merrell, P., 1943: Calcified subdural hematoma. J. nerv. ment. Dis. *98*, 609 – 617.
23. Bremer, A. M., Nguyen, T. Q., 1982: Tension pneumocephalus after surgical treatment of chronic subdural hematoma: report of three cases. Neurosurgery *11*, 284 – 287.
24. Bret, P., Lecuire, J., Lapras, C., Deruty, R., Desgeorges, N., Prudhon, J. L., 1976: Hématome sous-dural et thérapeutique anticoagulante. Neuro-chirurgie (Paris) *22*, 603 – 620.
25. Bordersen, P., Gjerris, F., 1975: Regional cerebral blood flow in patients with chronic subdural hematomas. Acta neurol. Scand. *51*, 233 – 239.
26. Byun, H. S., Patel, P. P., 1979: Spontaneous subdural hematoma of arterial origin: report of two cases. Neurosurgery *5*, 611 – 613.
27. Cambria, S., Daum, S., le Beau, J., 1966: Les hématomes sous-duraux intracrâniens à symptomatologie pyramidale homolatérale. Neuro-chirurgie (Paris) *12*, 473 – 490.
28. Cameron, M. M., 1978: Chronic subdural haematoma: a review of 114 cases. J. Neurol. Neurosurg. Psychiat. *41*, 834 – 839.

29. Christensen, E., 1944: Studies on chronic subdural hematomas. Acta psychiat. Scand. *19*, 69 – 148.

30. Chusid, J. G., de Gutierrez-Mahoney, C. G., 1953: Ossifying subdural hematoma. J. Neurosurg. *10*, 430 – 434.

31. Clarke, E., Walton, J. N., 1953: Subdural haematoma complicating intracranial aneurysm and angioma. Brain *76*, 378 – 404.

32. Clein, L. J., Bolton, C. F., 1969: Interhemispheric subdural haematoma: a case report. J. Neurol. Neurosurg. Psychiat. *32*, 389 – 392.

33. Cole, M., Spatz, E., 1961: Seizures in chronic subdural hematoma. New Engl. J. Med. *265*, 628.

34. Cook, A. W., Browder, E. J., Carter, W. B., 1962: Cerebral swelling and ventricular alterations following evacuation of intracranial extracerebral hematoma. J. Neurosurg. *19*, 419 – 423.

35. Danis, A., 1973: De l'origine des ossifications ectopiques dans le système nerveux central. J. Belg. radiol. *56*, 297 – 302.

36. Danis, A., 1974: Le rôle de la moelle osseuse dans l'ostéogenèse réparatrice. Bull. Acad. Med. Belg. *129*, 173 – 198.

37. Davidoff, L. M., Feiring, E. H., 1953: Subdural hematoma occurring in surgically treated hydrocephalic children. J. Neurosurg. *10*, 557 – 563.

38. Davies, F. L., 1960: Mental abnormalities following subdural hematoma. The Lancet, June *25*, 1369 – 1370.

39. Debois, V., Lombaert, A., 1980: Calcified chronic subdural hematoma. Surg. Neurol. *14*, 455 – 459.

40. De Morsier, G., 1937: Les hématomes de la dure-mère. Diagnostic, pathogénie, traitement. Rev. Neurol. *68*, 665 – 700.

41. Ditullio, M. V., 1977: Epidural hematoma with complete third nerve paralysis in an awake patient. Surg. Neurol. *7*, 193 – 194.

42. Drake, C. G., 1961: Subdural haematoma from arterial rupture. J. Neurosurg. *18*, 597 – 601.

43. Dublin, A. B., Rennick, J. M., Sivalingam, S., 1976: Failure of computerized axial tomography to demonstrate a chronic subdural hematoma. Surg. Neurol. *6*, 23 – 24.

44. Echlin, F. A., Sordillo, S. V. R., Garvey, T. Q., 1956: Acute, subacute and chronic subdural hematoma. J. Amer. Med. Ass. *161*, 1345 – 1350.

45. Ectors, L., 1953: Détails techniques dans le traitement chirurgical de l'hématome sous-dural. Rev. Neurol. *89*, 603 – 604.

46. Ectors, L., 1962: L'hématome sous-dural chronique. Traitement chirurgical. Acta chir. belg. *61*, 570 – 606.

47. El Gindi, S., Salama, M., Tawfik, E., Aboul Nasr, H., El Nadi, F., 1979: A review of 2,000 patients with craniocerebral injuries with regard to intracranial haematomas and other vascular complications. Acta Neurochir. (Wien) *48*, 237 – 244.

48. Faulhauer, K., Herrmann, H. D., Loew, F., 1973: Operative treatment of extremely large bilateral subdural effusions in infancy. Acta Neurochir. (Wien) *28*, 179 – 187.

49. Faulhauer, K., 1982: The overdrained hydrocephalus. Clinical manifestations and management. In: Advances and Technical Standards in Neurosurgery (Krayenbühl, H., *et al.,* eds.), Vol. 9, pp. 3–24. Wien-New York: Springer.

50. Feld, M., 1947: Contribution à l'étude des hématomes sous-duraux spontanés. Rev. Neurol. *79,* 97–108.

51. Ferguson, G. G., Barton, W. B., Drake, C. G., 1968: Subdural hematoma in hemophilia: successful treatment with cryoprecipitate. J. Neurosurg. *29,* 524–528.

52. Ferris, E. J., Lehrer, H., Shapiro, J. H., 1967: Pseudo-subdural hematoma. Radiology *88,* 75–84.

53. Fogelholm, R., Heiskanen, O., Waltimo, O., 1975: Chronic subdural hematoma in adults. Influence of patient's age on symptoms, signs and thickness of hematoma. J. Neurosurg. *42,* 43–46.

54. Fogelholm, R., Waltimo, O., 1975: Epidemiology of chronic subdural haematoma. Acta Neurochir. (Wien) *32,* 247–250.

55. Forbes, G. S., Sheedy, P. F. II, Piepgras, D. G., Houser, O. W., 1978: Computed tomography in the evaluation of subdural hematomas. Radiology *126,* 143–148.

56. French, B. N., Dublin, A. B., 1977: The value of computerized tomography in the management of 1,000 consecutive head injuries. Surg. Neurol. *7,* 171–183.

57. French, B. N., 1978: Limitations and pitfalls of computed tomography in the evaluation of craniocerebral injury. Surg. Neurol. *10,* 395–401.

58. Friede, R. L., 1971: Incidence and distribution of neomembranes of dura mater. J. Neurol. Neurosurg. Psychiat. *34,* 439–446.

59. Friede, R. L., Schachenmayr, W., 1978: The origin of subdural neomembranes. II. Fine structure of neomembranes. Amer. J. Pathol. *92,* 69–78.

60. Gannon, W. E., 1961: Interhemispheric subdural hematoma. J. Neurosurg. *18,* 829–830.

61. Gannon, W. E., Cook, A. W., Browder, E. J., 1962: Resolving subdural collections. J. Neurosurg. *19,* 865–869.

62. Gannon, W. E., 1962: Roentgenologic signs of resolving subdural hematomas. Radiology *79,* 420–424.

63. Gardner, W. J., 1932: Traumatic subdural hematoma with particular reference to the latent interval. Arch. Neurol. Psychiat. (Chic.) *27,* 847–858.

64. Garrel, S., Kramarz, P., 1965: Etude électroencéphalographique de l'hématome sous-dural du nourrisson. A propos de 45 observations. Rev. Neurol. *113,* 271–278.

65. Gilday, D. L., Wortzman, G., Reid, M., 1974: Subdural hematoma: is it or is it not acute? Radiology *110,* 141–145.

66. Gitlin, D., 1955: Pathogenesis of subdural collections of fluid. Pediatrics *16,* 345–351.

67. Gjerris, F., Sorensen, S., 1980: Colloid osmotic and hydrostatic pressures in chronic subdural haematomas. Acta Neurochir. (Wien) *54,* 53–60.

68. Gjerris, F., Schmidt, K., 1974: Chronic subdural hematoma. Surgery or Mannitol treatment. J. Neurosurg. *40,* 639–642.

69. Glista, G. G., Reichman, H., Brumlik, J., Fine, M., 1978: Interhemispheric subdural hematoma. Surg. Neurol. *10*, 119−122.

70. Glover, D. E., Labadie, L., 1976: Physiopathogenesis of subdural hematomas. Part 2: inhibition of growth of experimental hematomas with Dexamethazone. J. Neurosurg. *45*, 393−397.

71. Goodell, Ch. L., Mealey, J., 1963: Pathogenesis of chronic subdural hematoma. Experimental studies. Arch. Neurol. (Chic.) *8*, 429−437.

72. Goodman, J. M., Mealey, J., 1969: Postmeningitis subdural effusions. The syndrome and its management. J. Neurosurg. *30*, 658−663.

73. Greenhouse, A. H., Barr, J. W., 1979: The bilateral isodense subdural hematoma on computerized tomographic scan. Arch. Neurol. (Chic.) *36*, 305−307.

74. Griponissiotis, B., 1955: Ossifying chronic subdural hematoma. Report of a case. J. Neurosurg. *12*, 419−420.

75. Grumme, Th., Lanksch, W., Kazner, E., Aulich, A., Meese, W., Lange, S., Steinhoff, H., Wende, S., 1976: Zur Diagnose des chronischen subduralen Hämatoms im Computer-Tomogramm. Neurochirurgia (Stuttgart) *19*, 95 −103.

76. Gutierrez-Luque, A. G., McCarty, C. S., Klass, D. W., 1966: Head injury with suspected subdural hematoma. Effect on EEG. Arch. Neurol. (Chic.) *15*, 437−443.

77. Gutierrez, F. A., McLone, D. G., Raimondi, A. J., 1979: Physiopathology and a new treatment of chronic subdural hematoma in children. Child's Brain *5*, 216−232.

78. Hammes, E. M., 1944: Reaction of the meninges to blood. Arch. Neurol. Psychiat. (Chic.) *52*, 505−514.

79. Hirsh, L. F., 1980: Intracranial air following subdural hematoma drainage with delayed recovery. Neurochirurgia (Stuttgart) *23*, 55−58.

80. Hoessly, G. F., 1966: Intracranial hemorrhage in the 17th century. A reappraisal of Johann Jacob Wepfer's contribution regarding subdural hematoma. J. Neurosurg. *24*, 493−496.

81. Hubschmann, O. R., 1980: Twist drill craniotomy in the treatment of chronic and subacute subdural hematomas in severely ill and elderly patients. Neurosurgery *6*, 233−236.

82. Hurwitz, S. R., Halpern, S. E., Leopold, G., 1974: Brain scans and echoencephalography in the diagnosis of chronic subdural hematoma. J. Neurosurg. *40*, 347−350.

83. Ikeda, K., Nakano, M., Tani, E., 1978: Tension pneumocephalus complicating ventriculoperitoneal shunt for cerebrospinal fluid rhinorrhoea: case report. J. Neurol. Neurosurg. Psychiat. *41*, 319−322.

84. Isch-Treussard, C., Rohmer, F., Philippides, D., 1965: L'électroencéphalogramme dans les hématomes sous-duraux chroniques du nourrisson. Rev. Neurol. *112*, 298−301.

85. Ishii, S., Hayner, R., Kelly, W. A., Evans, J. P., 1959: Studies of cerebral swelling. II. Experimental cerebral swelling produced by supratentorial extradural compression. J. Neurosurg. *16*, 152−166.

86. Ito, H., Yamamoto, S., Komai, T., Mizukoshi, H., 1976: Role of local hyperfibrinolysis in the etiology of chronic subdural hematoma. J. Neurosurg. *45*, 26–31.

87. Ito, H., Komai, T., Yamamoto, S., 1978: Fibrinolytic enzyme in the lining walls of chronic subdural hematoma. J. Neurosurg. *48*, 197–200.

88. Jacobson, P. L., Farmer, T. W., 1979: The "hypernormal" CT scan in dementia: bilateral isodense subdural hematomas. Neurology *29*, 1522–1523.

89. Jaffe, R., Librot, I. E., Bender, M. B., 1968: Serial EEG studies in unoperated subdural hematoma. Arch. Neurol. (Chic.) *19*, 325–330.

90. Jamieson, K. G., Yelland, J. D. N., 1968: Extradural hematoma. Report of 167 cases. J. Neurosurg. *29*, 13–23.

91. Jamieson, K. G., 1970: Extradural and subdural hematomas. Changing patterns and requirements of treatment in Australia. J. Neurosurg. *33*, 632–635.

92. Jamieson, K. G., Yelland, J. D. N., 1972: Surgically treated traumatic subdural hematomas. J. Neurosurg. *37*, 137–149.

93. Kaste, M., Waltimo, O., Heiskanen, O., 1979: Chronic bilateral subdural heamatoma in adults. Acta Neurochir. (Wien) *48*, 231–236.

94. Kaste, M., Hernesniemi, J., Somer, H., Hillbom, M., Konttinen, A., 1981: Creatine kinase isoenzymes in acute brain injury. J. Neurosurg. *55*, 511–515.

95. Kawano, N., Suzuki, K., 1981: Presence of smooth-muscle cells in the subdural neomembrane. J. Neurosurg. *54*, 646–651.

96. Kim, K. S., Hemmati, M., Weinberg, P. E., 1978: Computed tomography in isodense subdural hematoma. Radiology *128*, 71–74.

97. Kjellin, K. G., Steiner, L., 1974: Spectrophotometry of cerebrospinal fluid in subacute and chronic subdural hematomas. J. Neurol. Neurosurg. Psychiat. *37*, 1121–1127.

98. Klein, R., 1963: L'hématoma sous-dural du nourrisson. Neurochirurgia (Stuttgart) *6*, 152–163.

99. Klug, W., Loew, F., Wustner, S., 1961: Zur Frage der Häufigkeit chronischer subduraler Hämatome nach Schädelverletzungen. Zbl. Neurochir. *21*, 51–56.

100. Kothandaram, P., 1970: Dural liposarcoma associated with subdural hematoma. Case report. J. Neurosurg. *33*, 85–87.

101. Kurti, X., Xhumari, A., Petrela, M., 1982: Bilateral chronic subdural haematomas: surgical or non-surgical treatment. Acta Neurochir. (Wien) *62*, 87–90.

102. Labadie, E. L., Glover, D., 1975: Local alterations of hemostatic-fibrinolytic mechanisms in reforming subdural hematomas. Neurology *25*, 669–675.

103. Labadie, E. L., Glover, D., 1976: Physiopathogenesis of subdural hematomas. Part I: Histological and biochemical comparisons of subcutaneous hematoma in rats with subdural hematoma in man. J. Neurosurg. *45*, 382–392.

104. Lacour, F., Trevor, R., Carey, M., 1978: Arachnoid cyst and associated subdural hematoma. Arch. Neurol. (Chic.) *35*, 84–89.

105. Lepoire, J., Montaut, J., Renard, M., Duplay, J., 1964: Les hématomes sous-duraux spontanés au cours des traitements anticoagulants prolongés. Neurochirurgia (Stuttgart) 7, 184—193.

106. Liedberg, N., 1941: Zur Frage des chronischen subduralen Hämatoms. Acta chir. Scand. 85, 165—179.

107. Little, J. R., MacCarty, C. S., 1976: Tension pneumocephalus after insertion of ventriculoperitoneal shunt for aqueductal stenosis. Case report. J. Neurosurg. 44, 383—385.

108. Loew, F., 1982: Management of chronic subdural haematomas and hygromas. In: Advances and Technical Standards in Neurosurgery (Krayenbühl, H., et al., eds.), Vol. 9, pp. 113—131. Wien-New York: Springer.

109. Loew, F., Kivelitz, R., 1976: Chronic subdural haematomas. In: Handbook of Clinical Neurology (Vinken, P. J., Bruyn, G. W., eds.), Vol. 24, pp. 297—327. Amsterdam: North-Holland Publ. Comp.

110. Lombardi, G., 1973: Les hématomes calcifiés. J. Belg. radiol. 4, 337—339.

111. Lombroso, C. T., Erba, G., Yogo, T., Logowitz, N., St. Hilaire, J., 1970: Two dimensional sonar scanning for detection of intracranial lesions. A comparison with isotope scans, electroencephalograms, and radiological studies in 97 cases. Arch. Neurol. (Chic.) 23, 518—527.

112. Lunsford, L. D., Maroon, J. C., Sheptak, P. E., Albin, M. S., 1979: Subdural tension pneumocephalus. Report of two cases. J. Neurosurg. 50, 525—527.

113. Lusins, J., Jaffe, R., Bender, M. B., 1976: Unoperated subdural hematomas. Long term follow-up study by brain scan and electroencephalography. J. Neurosurg. 44, 601—607.

114. McKissock, W., Richardson, A., Bloom, W. H., 1960: Subdural haematoma. A review of 389 cases. The Lancet 1, 1365—1369.

115. McLaurin, R. L., Tutor, F. T., 1961: Acute subdural hematoma. Review of 90 cases. J. Neurosurg. 18, 61—67.

116. McLaurin, R. L., 1965: Contributions of angiography to the pathophysiology of subdural hematomas. Neurology 15, 866—873.

117. McLaurin, R. L., McLaurin, K. S., 1966: Calcified subdural hematomas in childhood. J. Neurosurg. 24, 648—655.

118. McLaurin, R., Isaacs, E., Lewis, P., 1971: Results of nonoperative treatment in 15 cases of infantile subdural hematoma. J. Neurosurg. 34, 753—759.

119. Magnaes, B., Nornes, H., 1972: Traumatic tension pneumo-hydrocephalus. The intracranial pressure pattern and the pathogenetic factors. Acta Neurochir. (Wien) 27, 17—27.

120. Mansuy, L., Levy, A., Beaujard, M., 1953: Hématome sous-dural calcifié chez un enfant. Rev. Neurol. 89, 585—591.

121. Mansuy, L., Girard, P. F., Boucher, M., Tete, R., 1964: Les hématomes sous-duraux calcifiés (à propos d'une observation d'hématome calcifié pré-frontal bilatéral). Rev. Neurol. 111, 5—16.

122. Marcu, H., Becker, H., 1977: Computed-tomography of bilateral isodense chronic subdural hematomas. Neuroradiology 14, 81—83.

123. Markwalder, T. M., 1981: Chronic subdural hematomas: a review. J. Neurosurg. 54, 637—645.

124. Markwalder, T. M., Steinsiepe, K. F., Rohner, M., Reichenbach, W., Markwalder, H., 1981: The course of chronic subdural hematomas after burr-hole craniostomy and closed-system drainage. J. Neurosurg. *55*, 390 – 396.

125. Maroon, J. C., Campbell, R. L., 1970: Subdural hematoma, with inappropriate antidiuretic hormone secretion. Arch. Neurol. (Chic.) *22*, 234 – 239.

126. Messina, A. V., Chernik, N. L., 1975: Computed tomography: the "resolving" intracerebral hemorrhage. Radiology *118*, 609 – 613.

127. Messina, A. V., 1976: Computed tomography: contrast media within subdural hematomas. A preliminary report. Radiology *119*, 725 – 726.

128. Mitsumoto, H., Conomy, J. P., Regula, G., 1977: Subdural hematoma. Experience in a general hospital. Cleveland Clin. Quart. *44*, 95 – 99.

129. Mitsumoto, H., Conomy, J. P., Regula, G., 1977: Ophthalmologic aspects of subdural hematoma. Cleveland Clin. Quart. *44*, 101 – 106.

130. Miyazaki, S., Fukushima, H., Kamata, K., Ishii, S., 1983: Chronic subdural hematoma after lumbar-subarachnoid analgesia for a cesarean section. Surg. Neurol. *20*, 459 – 460.

131. Moller, A., Ericson, K., 1979: Computed tomography of isoattenuating subdural hematomas. Radiology *130*, 149 – 152.

132. Moritz, R., Szdzuy, D., Moser, E., 1976: Zur Problematik des angiographischen Nachweises von Subduralempyemen im Interhemisphärenspalt. Zbl. Neurochir. *37*, 111 – 118.

133. Mosberg, W. H., Smith, G. W., 1952: Calcified solid subdural hematoma. Review of literature and report of an unusual case. J. Nerv. Ment. Dis. *115*, 163 – 173.

134. Moyes, P. D., Thompson, G. B., Cluff, J. W., 1965: Subdural peritoneal shunts in treatment of subdural effusions in infants. J. Neurosurg. *23*, 584 – 587.

135. Munro, D., Merritt, H. H., 1936: Surgical pathology of subdural hematoma based on a study of one hundred and five cases. Arch. Neurol. Psychiat. *35*, 64 – 78.

136. Munro, D., 1942: Cerebral subdural hematomas. A study of three hundred and ten verified cases. New Engl. J. Med. *227*, 87 – 95.

137. Negron, R. A., Tirado, G., Zapater, C., 1975: Simple bedside technique for evacuating chronic subdural hematomas. Technical note. J. Neurosurg. *42*, 609 – 611.

138. Nelson, S. W., Freimanis, A. K., 1963: Angiographic features of convexity subdural hematomas with emphasis on the differential diagnosis between unilateral and bilateral hematomas. Amer. J. Roentgenol. *90*, 445 – 461.

139. Norman, O., 1956: Angiography differentiation between acute and chronic subdural and extradural haematomas. Acta radiol. *46*, 371 – 378.

140. Nyström, S., Mäkelä, T., 1964: Das akute, subakute und chronische subdurale Hämatom. Bericht über 100 Fälle. Acta Neurochir. (Wien) *11*, 565 – 578.

141. O'Brien, P. K., Norris, J. W., Tator, Ch. H., 1974: Acute subdural hematomas of arterial origin. J. Neurosurg. *41*, 435 – 439.

142. Ogsbury, J. S., Schneck, S. A., Lehman, R. A. W., 1978: Aspects of interhemispheric subdural haematoma, including the falx syndrome. J. Neurol. Neurosurg. Psychiat. *41*, 72 – 75.

143. Osborm, A. G., Daines, J. H., Wing, S. D., Anderson, R. E., 1978: Intracranial air on computerized tomography. J. Neurosurg. *48*, 355—359.
144. Parkinson, D., Chochinov, H., 1960: Subdural hematomas. Some observations on their postoperative course. J. Neurosurg. *17*, 901—904.
145. Perlmutter, I., Gables, C., 1961: Subdural hematoma in older patients. JAMA *176*, 112—114.
146. Perroudon, C., Dumas, R., Bochu, M., Buffard, P., Mansuy, L., Girard, P. F., 1972: Les hématomes sous-duraux calcifiés. A propos d'un cas. Ann. Radiol. *15*, 719—723.
147. Piepsz, A., Bormans, J., Segers, A., Noterman, J., Decostre, P., 1975: Value of brain scanning in pediatric subdural collections. Acta Pediat. Scand. *64*, 2—6.
148. Pierron, D., George, B., Ouahes, O., Riche, M. C., Cophignon, J., 1981: Tomodensitométrie et hématomes intracrâniens post-traumatiques sans manifestation clinique. Neuro-chirurgie (Paris) *27*, 213—216.
149. Pihkanen, T. A., Vauhkonen, M. L., 1967: Haematoma subdurale in the patient material of a neuropsychiatric hospital. Acta Neurol. Scand. *43*, 192—193.
150. Pitts, L. H., Wilson, Ch. B., Dedo, H. H., Weyand, R., 1975: Pneumocephalus following ventriculoperitoneal shunt. Case report. J. Neurosurg. *43*, 631—633.
151. Pourpre, Tournoux, Rebuffat, 1957: Hématome sous-dural de la fosse postérieure. Neuro-chirurgie (Paris) *3*, 200—202.
152. Putman, T. J., Cushing, H., 1925: Chronic subdural hematoma. Its pathology, its relation to pachymeningitis hemorrhagica and its surgical treatment. Arch. Surg. *11*, 329—393.
153. Putman, T. J., Putman, I. K., 1927: The experimental study of pachymeningitis hemorrhagica. J. Nerv. Ment. Dis. *25*, 260—272.
154. Rabe, E. F., Flynn, R. E., Dodge, Ph. R., 1962: A study of subdural effusions in an infant. With particular reference to the mechanisms of their persistence. Neurology *12*, 79—92.
155. Rabe, E. F., Young, G. F., Dodge, Ph. R., 1964: The distribution and fate of subdurally instilled human serum albumin in infants with subdural collections of fluid. Neurology *14*, 1020—1028.
156. Rabe, E. F., Flynn, R. E., Dodge, P. R., 1968: Subdural collections of fluid in infants and children. A study of 62 patients with special reference to factors influencing prognosis and the efficacy of various forms of therapy. Neurology *18*, 559—570.
157. Radcliffe, W. B., Guinto, F. C., Adcock, D. F., Krigman, M. R., 1972: Subdural hematoma shape. A new look at an old concept. Amer. J. Roentgenol. *115*, 72—77.
158. Raskind, R., Glover, M. B., Weiss, S. R., 1972: Chronic subdural hematoma in the elderly: a challenge in diagnosis and treatment. J. Amer. Geriat. *20*, 330—334.
159. Rengachary, S. S., Szymanski, D. C., 1981: Subdural hematomas of arterial origin. Neurosurgery *8*, 166—173.

160. Rosenørn, J., Gjerris, F., 1978: Long-term follow-up review of patients with acute and subacute subdural hematomas. J. Neurosurg. *48*, 345–349.
161. Sachs, J., Sachs, E., 1977: A simple formula for calculating the volume of subdural hematomas. Neurosurgery *1*, 60–61.
162. Samii, M., Schindler, E., Hey, O., 1974: Ein subdurales Hämatom des Interhemisphärenspalts. Acta Neurochir. (Wien) *30*, 319–326.
163. Sato, S., Suzuki, J., 1975: Ultrastructural observations of the capsule of chronic subdural hematoma in various clinical states. J. Neurosurg. *43*, 569–578.
164. Schachenmayr, W., Friede, R. L., 1978: The origin of subdural neomembranes. 1. Fine structure of the dura-arachnoid interface in man. Amer. J. Pathol. *92*, 35–68.
165. Scotti, G., Terbrugge, K., Melancon, D., Belanger, G., 1977: Evaluation of the age of subdural hematomas by computerized tomography. J. Neurosurg. *47*, 311–315.
166. Shields, C. B., Stites, T. B., Garretson, H. D., 1980: Isodense subdural hematoma presenting with paraparesis. Case report. J. Neurosurg. *52*, 712–714.
167. Shulman, K., Ransohoff, J., 1961: Subdural hematoma in children. The fate of children with retained membranes. J. Neurosurg. *18*, 175–181.
168. Sibayan, R. Q., Gurdjian, E. S., Thomas, L. M., 1970: Interhemispheric chronic subdural hematoma: report of a case. Neurology *20*, 1215–1218.
169. Slater, J. P., 1966: Extramedullary hematopoiesis in a subdural hematoma. Case report. J. Neurosurg. *25*, 211–214.
170. Stone, J. L., Lang, R. G. R., Sugar, O., Moody, R. A., 1981: Traumatic subdural hygroma. Neurosurgery *8*, 542–550.
171. Stone, J. L., Rifai, M. H. S., Sugar, O., Lang, R. G. R., Oldershaw, J. B., Moody, R. A., 1983: Subdural hematomas. I. Acute subdural hematoma: progress in definition, clinical pathology, and therapy. Surg. Neurol. *19*, 216–231.
172. Stroobandt, G., Evrard, Ph., 1970: Pneumatocèle intracérébral traumatique à caractère expansif. Acta Neurol. Belg. *70*, 542–550.
173. Suzuki, J., Takaku, A., 1970: Nonsurgical treatment of chronic subdural hematoma. J. Neurosurg. *33*, 548–553.
174. Suzuki, J., Komatsu, S., 1977: Estrogen in patients with chronic subdural hematoma. Surg. Neurol. *8*, 243–247.
175. Svien, H. J., Gelety, J. E., 1964: On the surgical management of encapsulated subdural hematoma. A comparison of the results of membranectomy and simple evacuation. J. Neurosurg. *21*, 172–177.
176. Tabaddor, K., Shulman, K., 1977: Definitive treatment of chronic subdural hematoma by twist-drill craniostomy and closed-system drainage. J. Neurosurg. *46*, 220–226.
177. Talalla, A., Halbrook, H., Barbour, B. H., Kurze, Th., 1970: Subdural hematoma associated with long-term hemodialysis for chronic renal disease. JAMA *212*, 1847–1849.
178. Talalla, A., McKissock, W., 1971: Acute "spontaneous" subdural hemorrhage. Neurology *21*, 19–23.

179. Terbrugge, K., Melancon, D., Belanger, G., 1977: Evaluation of the age of subdural hematomas by computerized tomography. J. Neurosurg. *47*, 311 – 315.

180. Tiberin, P., Beller, A. J., 1963: Observations on so-called brain stones or cerebral calculi. Neurology *13*, 464 – 476.

181. Tindall, G. T., Payne, N. S., O'Brien, M. S., 1976: Complications of surgery for subdural hematoma. Clin. Neurosurg. *23*, 465 – 482. ·

182. Tomaszek, D. E., Tyson, G. W., Mahaley, M. S., 1983: Unilateral subdural hematoma without midline shift. Surg. Neurol. *20*, 71 – 73.

183. Trotter, W., 1914: Chronic subdural haemorrhage of traumatic origin, and its relation to pachymeningitis haemorrhagica interna. Brit. J. Surg. *2*, 271 – 291.

184. Tsai, F. Y., Huprich, J. E., Segall, H. D., Teal, J. S., 1979: The contrast-enhanced CT scan in the diagnosis of isodense subdural hematoma. J. Neurosurg. *50*, 64 – 74.

185. Tyson, G., Strachan, W. E., Newman, P., Winn, H. R., Betler, A., Jane, J., 1980: The role of craniectomy in the treatment of chronic subdural hematomas. J. Neurosurg. *52*, 776 – 781.

186. Van Gehuchten, P., Martin, P., 1932: Les hématomas sous-duraux chroniques. Rev. Neurol. *11*, 178 – 197.

187. Vieth, R. G., Tindall, G. T., Odom, G. L., 1966: The use of Tantalum dust as an adjunct in the postoperative management of subdural hematomas. J. Neurosurg. *24*, 514 – 519.

188. Vigouroux, R. P., Baurand, C., Guillermain, P., Reynier, Y., Gomez, A., Lena, G., Vincentelli, F., Gondim-Oliveira, J., 1982: Traumatismes cranio-encéphaliques. Encyclopédie Med. Chirurg. 17585 A 10, 22 – 24.

189. Waga, S., Sakakura, M., Fujimoto, K., 1979: Calcified subdural hematoma in the elderly. Surg. Neurol. *11*, 51 – 52.

190. Watts, C., 1976: The management of intracranial calcified subdural hematomas. Surg. Neurol. *6*, 247 – 249.

191. Weber, G., 1969: Das chronische Subduralhämatom. Schweiz. med. Wschr. *41*, 1483 – 1488.

192. Weir, B., 1971: The osmolality of subdural hematoma fluid. J. Neurosurg. *34*, 528 – 533.

193. Weir, B., 1980: Oncotic pressure of subdural fluids. J. Neurosurg. *53*, 512 – 515.

194. Weir, B., Gordon, P., 1983: Factors affecting coagulation: fibrinolysis in chronic subdural fluid collections. J. Neurosurg. *58*, 242 – 246.

195. Wickbom, I., 1949: Angiography by post-traumatic intracranial haemorrhages. Acta Radiol. *32*, 249 – 258.

196. Wintzen, A. R., 1980: The clinical course of subdural haematoma. Brain *103*, 855 – 868.

197. Wintzen, A. R., Tijssen, J. G. P., 1982: Subdural hematoma and oral anticoagulant therapy. Arch. Neurol. (Chic.) *39*, 69 – 73.

198. Witcombe, J. B., Torrens, M. J., Gye, R. S., 1976: Intracerebral pneumatocele: an unusual complication following intraventricular drainage in a case of benign intracranial hypertension. Neuroradiology *12*, 161 – 164.

199. Wright, J. R., Slavin, R. E., Wagner, J. A., 1965: Intracranial aneurysm as a cause of subdural hematoma of the posterior fossa. J. Neurosurg. *22*, 86–89.
200. Yamashima, T., Friede, R. L., 1984: Why do bridging veins rupture into the virtual subdural space? J. Neurol. Neurosurg. Psychiat. *47*, 121–127.
201. Yashon, D., Jane, J. A., White, R. J., Sugar, O., 1968: Traumatic subdural hematoma of infancy. Long-term follow-up of 92 patients. Arch. Neurol. (Chic.) *18*, 370–377.
202. Yashon, F., White, R. J., Bryk, J. P., Dakters, J. G., 1971: Simplified supplementary treatment of chronic subdural fluid collections. Neurochirurgia (Stuttgart) *14*, 8–13.
203. Zingesser, L. H., Schechter, M. M., Rayport, M., 1965: Truths and untruths concerning the angiographic findings in extracerebral haematomas. Brit. J. Radiol. *38*, 835–847.
204. Zollinger, R., Gross, R. E., 1934: Traumatic subdural hematoma. An explanation of the late onset of pressure symptoms. JAMA *103*, 245–249.

# Subdural Hydromas

S. MATSUMOTO and N. TAMAKI

Department of Neurosurgery, Kobe University School of Medicine, Kobe (Japan)

With 6 Figures

## Contents

## Terminology and Definition

Subdural hydroma is one of the most confused or controversial pathological conditions because of its vague definition and wrong use of terminology. The term, "subdural hydroma" was first proposed by Dandy (1940). But the terms, subdural hematoma, hygroma, hydroma, effusion and fluid collection have been sometimes confusingly used to indicate the same or different conditions of an abnormal collection of fluid in the subdural space.

Hydroma and hygroma should be considered synonymous to prevent from causing confusion, although Kinley *et al.* (1951) used the term, "hygroma" to indicate a collection of xanthochromic fluid free in the subdural space with a nonencapsulating neomembrane, and "hydroma" to indicate a collection of clear or slightly xanthochromic fluid free in the subdural space with no evidence of a membrane. Subdural hydroma may be differentiated from chronic subdural hematoma by the absence of a neomembrane. But some cases with subdural hydroma may have an associated neomembrane as indicated at surgery and also already reported by Dandy (1940).

The association of a neomembrane appears to be depend on the stage of the lesions. Chronic lesions of both types may have neomembranes. Consequently the abnormal collection of fluid in the subdural space occurring after head injury may be classified into two large categories, hematomas and hydromas.

Subdural hematoma may be defined as the accumulation in the subdural space of abnormally large quantities of blood clot, or fresh reddish or old chocolate brown hematomatous fluid with or without a neomembrane. Subdural hydroma should be standardized for an accumulation in the subdural space of clear, xanthochromic, or sometimes slightly bloodtinged cerebrospinal fluid with or without a neomembrane.

Relatively large bleeding may secondarily follow the preexisting subdural hydroma and may result in formation of the subdural hematoma. Thus the pathological condition, subdural hydroma indicating a subdural collection of the cerebrospinal fluid due to rupture of the arachnoid membrane itself is a definitive and obvious clinical entity and should be differentiated from subdural hematoma, although both conditions may be related as described above.

### Historical Background

Naffziger (1924) first described clinically and in pathophysiological detail the subdural fluid collection following head injury. He assumed that this pathological condition resulted from cerebrospinal fluid escape into the subdural space through a rupture of the arachnoid membrane. This mechanism, in which a tear has occurred in the arachnoid membrane allowing escape of the cerebrospinal fluid into the subdural space, appears to be reasonable, since a subdural hydroma may develop soon after the head injury. He attributed the further accumulation of the fluid to less resistence to flow of cerebrospinal fluid through a rupture of the arachnoid than in the other subarachnoid space over the brain. Dandy (1940) proposed first the term "subdural hydroma" for indicating the collection of CSF in the subdural space, and pointed out the torn arachnoid membrane as a cause of

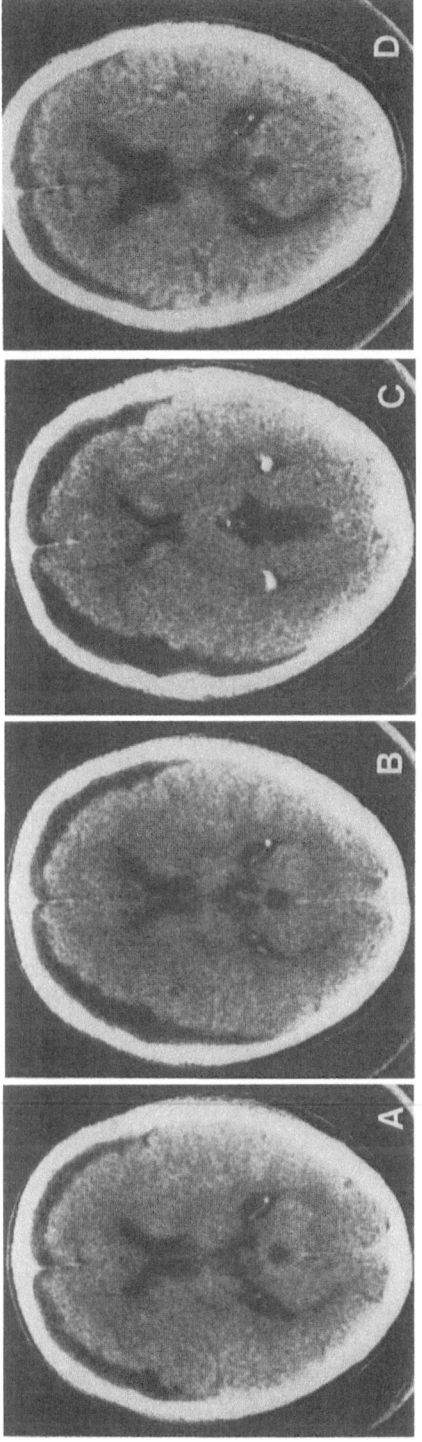

Fig. 1. CT scans of a 77-year-old man, showing that subdural hydroma could be demonstrated 5 hours after mild head injury (A: 5 hours) and it enlarged progressively for a several weeks to result in production of headache, memory disturbance and disorientation (B: 11 days, C: 40 days), which at last needed burr hole aspiration 2 months after head injury. CT scan on last follow-up examination (D) performed 19 months after surgery revealed the remaining of the small amount of subdural hydroma, although marked reduction in size of subdural hydroma was noted in comparison with that seen on the preoperative CT scans and clinical symptom disappeared completely after surgery

subdural collection of CSF. He (1946) also used the term "external hydroencephalus" indicating this pathological condition.

Da Costa and Adson (1941) assumed that blocking the return to the subarachnoid spaces for further CSF circulation and absorption occurred due to the closure of the arachnoid tear by strong compression to the brain surface from the subdural space and/or due to brain edema. Their theory was supported by the fact that the subdural hydroma was found to occur from a few hours to several weeks and subdural hematoma has been present for many months before the diagnosis was confirmed. They demonstrated also the tear in the arachnoid and the escape of CSF in the region of the Silvian fissure.

Since the advent of computed tomography as a diagnostic tool, it is reconfirmed that the fluid accumulated in the subdural space is from the escape of CSF through arachnoid tear, because the subdural hydroma may be found immediately after the head injury, and may enlarge for a few days or weeks as indicated by a review of our cases described later (Fig. 1).

## Pathophysiology

In order to understand the pathophysiology of the subdural hydroma the clinical anatomy of the meninges and their interspaces will be briefly described.

Three membranes are overlying the brain surface. The pia, the innermost membrane, is a relatively tough membrane and firmly adheres to the brain surface, covering the entire brain parenchyma and extending into the fissures and sulci. The arachnoid membrane adheres to the inner smooth surface of the dura, which is firmly attached to the inner surface of the skull by connective tissue.

The subdural space, which is present between the arachnoid and the dura, is considered to contain a small amount of fluid, which is distinct from CSF, as demonstrated by Penfield (1924). There are no structural connections between the arachnoid membrane and the dura mater other than the arachnoid granulations which enter the superior sagittal sinus and lateral lacunes in the dura, and the blood vessels which traverse the subdural space.

The arachnoid membrane is very fragile, and easily torn, through which CSF pours out, as observed at surgery. There is a network of trabecular filaments traversing the subarachnoid space, which acts as a cusion for the brain.

The relative different movement between the skull and brain brought about by head injury may result in the sliding movement between the dura and arachnoid membrane. The arachnoid membrane may be torn by this acceleration or deceleration movement of the brain. The leakage of the CSF into the subdural space may occur through the rupture of the arachnoid membrane. So *et al.* (1975) found evidence of a communication between the subdural and subarachnoid spaces in surgically proven cases of traumatic subdural hydroma by [111]In-DTPA cisternography.

The leakage of CSF from the arachnoid tear may transiently or progressively occur by a pressure gradient between the subarachnoid space and subdural space. If the outflow of the CSF into subdural space does not cease and progressively continues, or bleeding occurs newly into the subdural space, the subdural fluid collection may lead to the clinical symptoms and signs.

Da Costa and Adson (1941) pointed out that the fluid in the subdural space may remain free or may become encapsulated with in a thin membrane. The membrane may become thicker, when the hydroma has been of long duration, although never as thick as the membrane of a subdural hematoma. Oka *et al.* (1972) observed membrane formation in five out of 26 cases of subdural hydroma, in all of which three weeks had elapsed between the time of head injury and operation.

It is not clear why the fluid should collect progressively in the subdural space in some cases, and resolve in other cases. Cohen *et al.* (1927) assumed a valve-like action at the site of the torn arachnoid, so that the CSF can escape into the subdural space but cannot return to the subarachnoid spaces by compressing the arachnoid membrane to the brain. We postulate in addition that the one way direction of the bulk flow of the cerebrospinal fluid plays an important role in the enlargement of the subdural hydroma.

Small hemorrhages also appear to play a role in the increasing size of the subdural hydroma at least in some cases. Gutierez *et al.* (1979) postulated that stretching and narrowing of the cortical veins, traversing the subdural spaces to enter the superior sagittal sinus, could result in disturbance of cerebral hemodynamics, which also might favor further formation and enlargement of collection of fluid in the subdural space.

We sometimes observe a great tendency to reaccumulate after evacuation or removal of the fluid, in comparison with the chronic subdural hematomas, which are cured easily by surgery. The possible causes of a tendency to reaccumulate appear to be the small expansibility of brain due to brain atrophy, which is often seen in elderly patients, and failure of the arachnoid tear to heal and close.

The subdural fluid may contain a little blood and varies in color from pinkish to xanthochromic according to the time interval of the bleeding after head injury. Subdural hydroma may result not only from trauma, but also from meningitis, extradural infections, sinus thrombosis, hydrocephalus, intracranial surgery, and dural metastasis, consequently the nature of the subdural fluid may vary within wide limits. It varies with the etiological factor involved.

From the clinico-pathological standpoint, the following classification is offered:

A. Traumatic,
a) primary cause,
b) secondary cause.
B. Spontaneous (nontraumatic),
a) early stage of hydrocephalus (external hydrocephalus),
b) infection,
c) sinus thrombosis,
d) dural metastatic tumor.
C. Postsurgical,
a) craniotomy,
b) CSF shunt procedures.

In this chapter category A, traumatic subdural hydroma will be mainly described with a brief description of those of other causes.

The chronic subdural hematoma may develop if the bleeding occurs from the neomembrane or from blood vessels such as bridging veins or cortical vessels and may be encapsulated by further formation of the neomembrane (Fig. 2).

Miyazaki et al. (1980), Yamada et al. (1979), and Taguchi et al. (1982), recently demonstrated by serial CT scanning that the existence of the subdural collection of CSF is the most important factor for producing chronic subdural hematoma.

Even the acute subdural hematoma of arterial origin may follow the subdural hydroma, if the small arteries traversing the subdural space rupture (Fig. 3). Thus the subdural hydroma may become causative lesion of all kinds of subdural hematoma, acute, subacute or of the chronic type.

Especially for the formation of chronic subdural hematoma subdural hydroma may be one of the prerequisite pathological conditions. Watanabe et al. (1972) confirmed also experimentally that a mixture of CSF with blood was required for producing the subdural hematoma simulating the symptomatic human chronic subdural hematoma.

## Incidence

As far as the incidence of the subdural hydroma is concerned, Pia (1961) reported 15.4% of all subdural hematomas and hydromas in adults and 61.4% of those in children. According to the recent report described by Stone et al. (1983) subdural hydromas are seen in 10% of 712 surgical cases with closed head injury over 4 years of age. Oka et al. (1972) pointed out that the incidence of traumatic subdural hydroma was about 7% of all patients with traumatic intracranial mass lesions which needed operation. Thus the

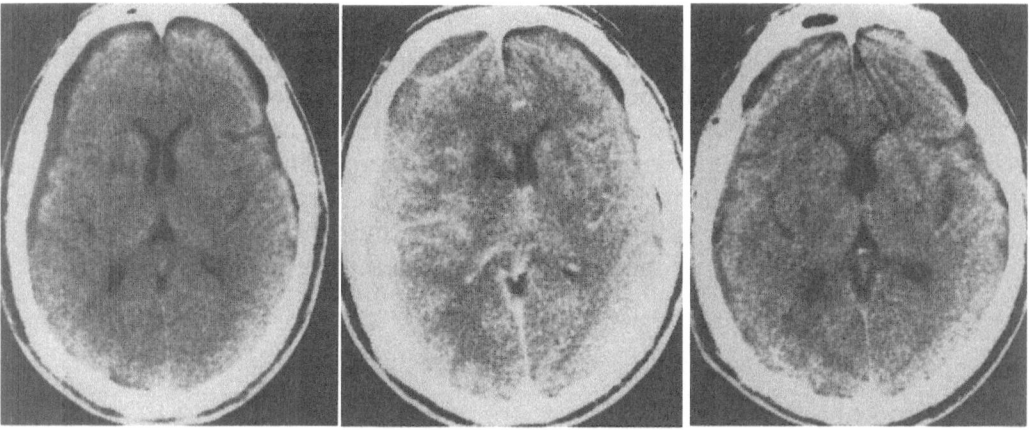

Fig. 2. CT scans of a case with subdural hydroma (left), which transformed into chronic subdural hematoma (center). Burr hole aspiration permitted complete disappearance of subdural lesion (right)

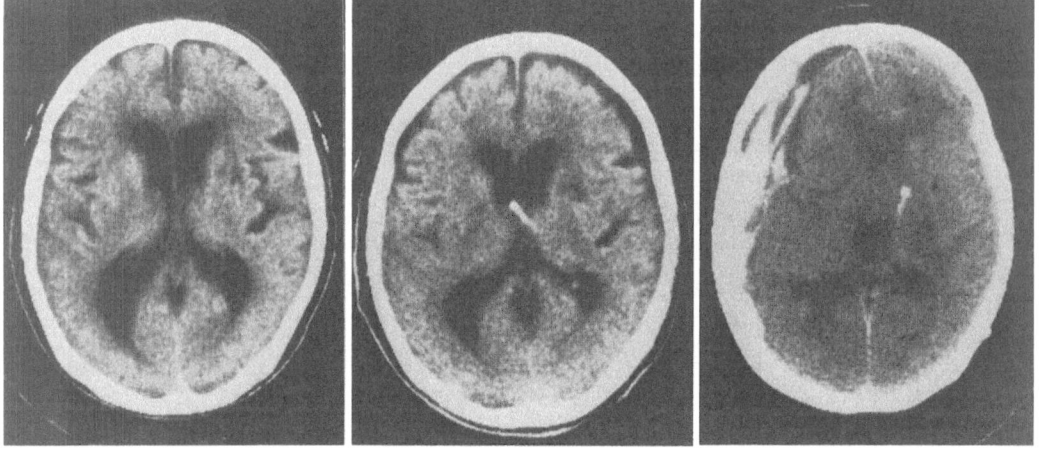

Fig. 3. CT scans of a 74-year-old woman, who underwent a ventriculo-peritoneal shunt for normal pressure hydrocephalus (left), showing bilateral thin subdural hydroma after shunt (center) followed by acute subdural hematoma of arterial origin (right), which was identified at surgery

incidence of subdural hydroma which need operation appears to be estimated from 10 to 20 percent of all head injury operation cases in adult, and much higher incidence is noted in children than in adults. With frequent use of CT as a diagnostic tool the incidence of subdural hydroma appears to be significantly increased than that earlier.

## Sex and Age

The subdural hydroma is much more frequent among men than among women. This is due to the larger incidence of head injury among the former. Review of 18 cases, experienced by us recently after the advent of CT scan, revealed that all patients were male. The patients ranged in age from 26 to 82 years with the median age of 58.

The elderly and the patients of any ages with shunt for hydrocephalus are particularly susceptible to subdural hydroma and subdural hematoma. The

Table 1. *Sex and Age of the Patients with Subdural Hydroma*

| Sex | Number of patients | Age | Number of patients |
|---|---|---|---|
| Male | 18 | –30 | 1 |
| Female | 0 | 31–40 | 2 |
| | | 41–50 | 4 |
| | | 51–60 | 3 |
| | | 61–70 | 3 |
| | | 71–80 | 4 |
| | | 81– | 1 |
| | | mean: 57.8 years | |

reason is that the special intracranial condition, a combination of brain atrophy and low intracranial pressure, which may result in a potential widening of the subdural space and an arachnoid tear, seems to render one more susceptible to the effects of even trivial head injury. The age distribution was similar in 40, 50, 60 and 70 decades (Table 1).

## Location

The subdural hydroma is usually bilateral but may be unilateral, the reason of which appears to result from the anatomical condition that there is free communication between the bilateral subdural spaces and from the fact that the fluid accumulated in the subdural space can move relatively freely to the other side. That the subdural hydroma is at the early stage by no means a nonencapsulating lesion, unlike the chronic subdural hematoma, may be also one explanation. The subdural hydroma may frequently extend upward over the one side of the entire hemisphere from the Sylvian fissure, and it may extend into the other side usually to the lesser extent than the former (Fig. 4). But it may not infrequently extend over both hemispheres to the same extent (Fig. 5).

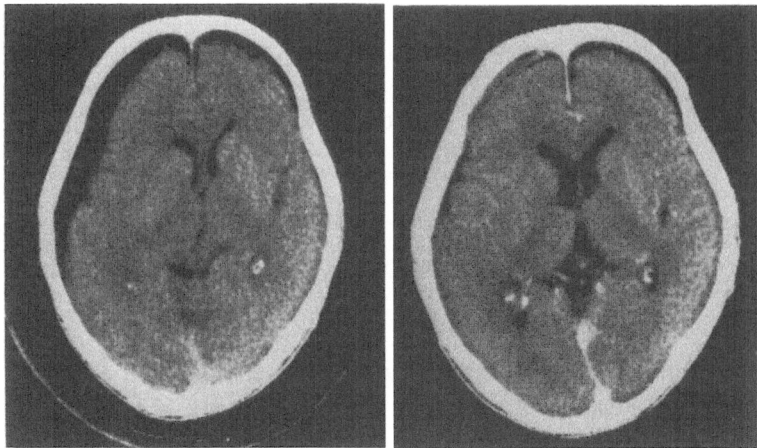

Fig. 4. CT scan showing asymmetrical subdural hydroma, which was most frequently seen. Preoperative CT (left), postoperative CT (right)

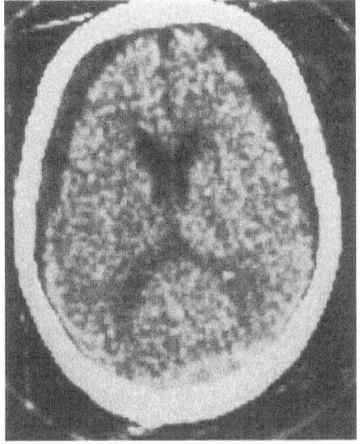

Fig. 5. CT scan showing symmetrical subdural hydroma

Table 2. *Location of Subdural Hydroma*

| Location | Number of patients |
|----------|--------------------|
| Bilateral | 18 |
| Unilateral | 0 (3) |

Figures in parenthesis shows the numbers of chronic subdural hematoma developed following subdural hydroma.

In our series of 18 cases surgically treated, all patients had bilateral lesions, most of which showed asymmetrical accumulation of the fluid on both sides. Three out of 18 cases which developed chronic subdural hematoma following subdural hydroma had a unilateral lesion, when the subdural hematoma was diagnosed (Table 2).

### Severity of Head Injury

There was only one case who had no history of head trauma. The remaining 17 cases had a history of head injury, in ten of which the head injuries were light or trivial without loss of consciousness or with a short time of unconsciousness. The remaining 7 cases had loss of consciousness of longer than 6 hours duration (Table 3).

Table 3. *Severity of Head Injury*

| Duration of unconsciousness | Number of patients |
| --- | --- |
| None | 1 |
| Within 6 hours | 10 |
| Over 6 hours | 7 |

### Interval from Head Injury to CT Diagnosis

The subdural hydroma occur much earlier after head injury than the chronic subdural hematoma does. In our series of 16 cases diagnosed by CT scanning, thirteen out of 16 cases (81%) were found to have developed by 3 weeks after injury. The shortest time from head injury to CT diagnosis was 5 hours (Table 4).

It appears that the arachnoid tear occurs immediately after head injury, but it may take a few days to weeks to form the subdural hydroma presenting with symptoms and signs. The chronic subdural hematoma, however, is generally believed to develop a few months after head trauma. This is one 'of the most different points between subdural hydroma and chronic subdural hematomas.

### Symptoms and Signs

The syndrome of the posttraumatic subdural hydroma is nothing pathognomonic. The symptoms and signs of subdural hydroma may occur in acute, subacute, and chronic types. The signs and symptoms of increased

Table 4. *Interval from Head Injury to CT Diagnosis*

| Period between injury and CT diagnosis | Number of patients |
|---|---|
| –5 | 5 |
| 6–10 | 4 |
| 11–20 | 4 |
| 21– | 3 |
| 130– | (2) |

Figures in parenthesis indicate the numbers of cases followed by chronic subdural hematoma.

intracranial pressure such as headache, nausea, vomiting, disorientation, inactivity, consciousness disturbance, and focal signs such as hemiparesis, aphasia, increased contralateral reflexes, and positive pathological reflexes may develop. The outstanding symptom is headache, which may occasionally occur on the same side of the subdural hydroma. Disorientation and decreased activity and mentation may be present in the elderly patients.

The symptoms may develop immediately after the injury, or they may appear after a free interval of longer or shorter duration varing from a few hours to weeks. Ingebrightson (1969) attributed the postconcussion syndrome such as headache, dizziness and failure in recent memory to accumulation of CSF in the subdural space. "Silent" subdural hydromas of delayed evolution may be seen in a small percent of head injury patients, as pointed out by French *et al.* (1978).

## Diagnosis

Skull X-ray and cerebral angiography have played an important role in making the diagnosis of subdural hydroma prior the era of CT diagnosis. Angiography, however, is recently rarely performed. The CT scanner has improved our ability to diagnose and treat subdural hydroma. Accurate size, location, sequential change in size, the result of the treatment, and the association with hematoma or hydrocephalus can be evaluated with ease.

The differentiation of subdural hydroma from chronic subdural hematoma is usually not difficult when the subdural hematoma demonstrated the high density or isodensity extracerebral marginal lesions on CT scans. It may be sometimes, however, difficult to differentiate subdural hydroma from chronic subdural hematoma showing low density marginal layer on CT scans. Grumme *et al.* (1976) demonstrated low density marginal layers in 37% of the patients with chronic subdural hematoma, and Scotti *et al.*

(1977) pointed out that as high as 76% of the patients with chronic subdural hematoma had the low density lesions on CT scans.

In our series of 18 cases of subdural hydromas diagnosed only by CT scans the subdural shadow on CT revealed a much lower density than the low density seen in chronic subdural hematoma. The subdural shadow on CT scans seen in our cases showed as low as the CSF cavities do.

Masuzawa et al. (1983) also pointed out that clear distinction could be made between a hematoma and hydroma. When compared to the density of the ventricular cavity, all of the low density hematomas were higher in density, while all hydromas appeared CSF dense or lower.

## Treatment

The result of treatment of subdural hydroma was improved by the early use of CT scanning.

Seven cases was followed up without surgical treatment because of minimal symptoms such as light headache and dizziness, three of which showed complete disappearance of subdural fluid collection on CT scans. Decrease in size of subdural hydroma was seen in one case, and there were no changes in size of subdural hydroma in 2 cases at least by one year follow-up. French et al. (1978) also observed that some patients with subdural hydroma have a tendency to resolve spontaneously. These suggest that operation may be unnecessary in those patients who present with no or insignificant symptoms.

In 4 cases unilateral simple burr hole aspiration and irrigation was performed, which resulted in complete disappearance of subdural hydroma in one, decrease in size in one and no change in size in two cases.

Continuous drainage of subdural space was performed in two cases for a few days and two weeks, one of which showed disappearance of subdural hydroma and the other a decrease in size of subdural hydroma on CT scans.

Subdural-peritoneal shunt was undertaken in three cases, two of which showed disappearance and one of which a decreased size of subdural hydroma on serial CT scans.

Combined burr hole aspiration and subsequent ventriculo-peritoneal shunt was performed in one case, and combined burr hole aspiration followed by subdural-peritoneal shunt and ventriculo-peritoneal shunt in the other case because of later development of hydrocephalus following surgery for subdural hydroma, both of which made a satisfactory recovery without evidence of the presence of subdural hydroma on CT scans and with good control of hydrocephalus.

All the patients made satisfactory recoveries without neurological signs and symptoms irrespective of the different methods of the surgical procedures (Table 5).

Table 5. *Results of Treatment*

| Method of treatment | Number of patients | CT findings after treatment | | | Clinical symptoms |
|---|---|---|---|---|---|
| | | No change | Decreased size | Disappearance | |
| Conservative | 7* | 2 | 1 | 3 | all improved or cured |
| Burr hole aspiration | 4 | 2 | 1 | 1 | |
| External drainage | 2 | 0 | 1 | 1 | |
| Subdural-peritoneal shunt | 3 | 0 | 1 | 2 | |
| Burr hole aspiration + ventriculo-peritoneal shunt | 1 | 0 | 0 | 1 | |
| Burr hole aspiration + subdural-peritoneal shunt + ventriculo-peritoneal shunt | 1 | 0 | 0 | 1 | |

* One case was lost for follow up.

Those with a relatively thin subdural hematoma and slight neurological signs can be left untreated and followed by repeated CT scans, or they may be treated with steroid, mannitol and other osmotic drugs.

Conservative treatment using steroid or mannitol, as advocated by Suzuki *et al.* (1970) and Bender *et al.* (1974) as a treatment of subdural hematoma, may be attempted in some cases of subdural hydroma.

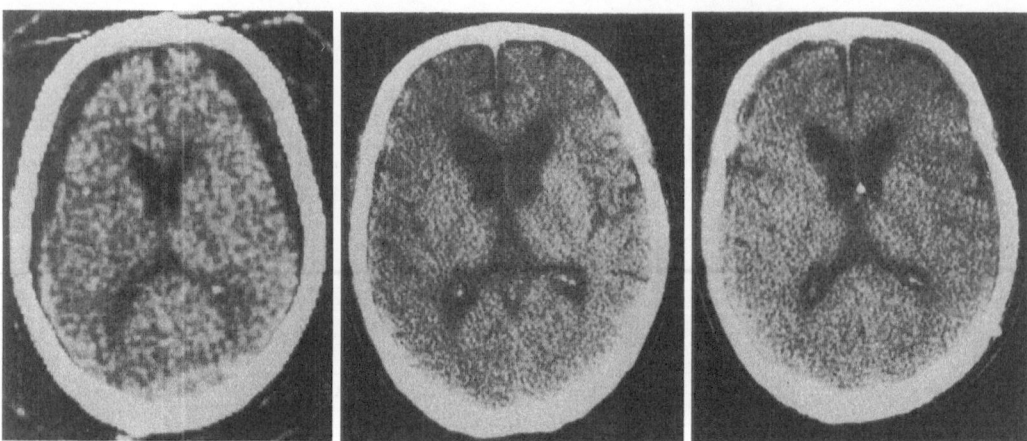

Fig. 6. CT scans of a 82-year-old man who developed bilateral subdural hydroma (left) after mild head injury, which was cleared up by bilateral burr hole aspiration. One year after surgery he complained of progressive inactivity, disorientation, dementia, gait disturbance and urinary incontinence. CT scan at that time (center) showed no evidence of subdural hydroma, but presence of ventriculomegaly and sulcal collapse. CT scan after ventriculo-peritoneal shunt (right) showed reduction in size of lateral ventricles. The patient returned to normal life after ventriculo-peritoneal shunt

The first choice of surgical treatment is generally considered to be burr hole aspiration and irrigation as used in the treatment of chronic subdural hematoma. In urgent cases when there is alteration in consciousness and neurological deficits, burr hole aspiration should be performed promptly.

Another surgical method, closed system suction drainage as suggested by Weir (1983) and Yashon *et al.* (1970) is also selected for the cases resistent to the burr hole method.

Despite these several methods of treatment disappearance of subdural hydroma is not always found after surgery on CT scans, although these procedures led to satisfactory recoveries from the clinical aspects.

The reason why these procedures do not infrequently result in a complete disappearance of subdural hydroma may be explained by the fact that the site of the arachnoid tear does not easily seal and close, and continuous leakage of CSF from the subarachnoid space into the subdural space may persist.

In those patients who have persistent accumulation of the CSF in the subdural space and clinical symptoms, a subdural-peritoneal shunt may be added, which will provide the continuous drainage of the subdural space. A ventriculo-peritoneal shunt is recommended for the patients with subdural hydroma followed by hydrocephalus (Fig. 6). On the basis of the hypothesis that subdural fluid accumulation might be related to a disturbance of CSF circulation, Njiokiktjien *et al.* (1980) recommended the ventriculo-peritoneal shunt for selected children with subdural hydroma.

## References

1. Bender, M. B., Christoff, N., 1974: Non surgical treatment of subdural hematomas. Arch. Neurol. *31*, 73–79.
2. Cohen, I., 1927: Chronic subdural accumulations of the cerebrospinal fluid after cranial trauma. Report of a case. Arch. Neurol. Psychiat. *18*, 709–723.
3. Da Costa, D. G., Adson, A. W., 1941: Subdural hydroma. Arch. Surg. *43*, 559–567.
4. Dandy, W. E., 1940: Chronic subdural hydroma and serious meningitis (Pachimeningitis serosa: Localized external hydrocephalus). In: Lewis, D. (ed.), Practice of Surgery, Vol. 12, pp. 306–310. Hagerstown, Md.: W. F. Prior Company Inc.
5. Dandy, W. E., 1946: Treatment of an unusual subdural hydroma (external hydrocephalus). Arch. Surg. *52*, 421–428.
6. Dickinson, E. H., Pastar, B. H., 1948: Two cases of acute subdural hygroma simulating massive intracranial hemorrhage. J. Neurosurg. *5*, 98–101.
7. French, B. N., Cobb, C. A., Corkill, G., Youmans, J. R., 1978: Delayed evolution of posttraumatic subdural hygroma. Surg. Neurol. *9*, 145–148.
8. Gannon, W. E., Cook, A. W., Browder, E. J., 1963: Resolving subdural collections. J. Neurosurg. 865–869.
9. Grumme, T. H., Lanksch, W., Kagner, E., Anlich, A., Meese, W., Lange, S., Steinhoff, H., Wnede, S., 1976: Zur Diagnose des chronischen subduralen Hämatoms im Computer-Tomogramm. Neurochirurgia *19*, 95–103.
10. Gutierrez, F. A., McLone, D. G., Raimondi, A. J., 1979: Physiopathology and a new treatment of chronic subdural hematoma in children. Child's Brain *5*, 216–232.
11. Ingebrightsen, B., 1969: Arachnoid rupture as cause of the postconcussion syndrome. A new theory of the pathophysiology. Acta Neurol. Scand. *45*, 231 –237.
12. Kinley, G., Riley, H. D., Beck, C. S., 1951: Subdural hematoma, hygroma, and hydroma in infants. J. Pediat. *38*, 667–686.
13. Masuzawa, H., Sato, J., Kamitani, H., Yamashita, M., 1983: The contents of chronic subdural hematoma and its CT density, with special reference to differentiation from subdural hygroma. Neurol. Med. Chir. (Tokyo) *23*, 123–130.

14. Miyazaki, S., Ohmori, H., Kanazawa, Y., Munekata, K., Fukushima, H., Kamata, K., 1980: The pathogenesis of chronic subdural hematoma—Sequential study with computerized tomography. Neurol. Med. Chir. (Tokyo) *20*, 875−881.

15. Munro, D., Merrit, H. H., 1936: Surgical pathology of subdural hematoma, based on a study of one hundred and five cases. Arch. Neurol. Psychiat. *35*, 64−78.

16. Naffziger, H. C., 1924: Subdural fluid accumulations following head injury. J.A.M.A. *82*, 1751−1752.

17. Njiokiktjien, C. J., Valk, H., Ponssen, H., 1980: Subdural hygroma: Results of treatment by ventriculo-abdominal shunt. Child's Brain *2*, 285−302.

18. Oka, H., Motomochi, Y., Suzuki, Y., Ando, K., 1972: Subdural hygroma after head injury. A review of 26 cases. Acta Neurochir. (Wien) *26*, 265−273.

19. Penfield, W. G., 1924: The cranial subdural space (A method of study). Anat. Rec. *28*, 173−175.

20. Pia, H. W., 1961: Das traumatische subdurale Hydrom. Zbl. Neurochir. *21*, 74−84.

21. Portnoy, H. D., Croissant, P. D., 1974: Combined drainage of ventricular and subdural fluid. Surg. Neurol. *2*, 41−42.

22. Robertson, W. C., Gomez, M. R., 1978: External hydrocephalus. Early findings in congenital communicating hydrocephalus. Arch. Neurol. *35*, 541−544.

23. Scotti, G., Terbrugge, K., Melancon, D., 1977: Evaluation of the age of subdural hematoma by computerized tomography. J. Neurosurg. *47*, 311−315.

24. So, S. K., Gerberg, E., Sakimura, I., Wright, W., 1975: Tracer accumulation in a subdural hydroma: case report. J. Nucl. Med. *17*, 119−121.

25. Stone, J. L., Rifai, M. H. S., Sugar, D., Lang, R. G. R., Oldershaw, J. B., Moody, R. A., 1983: Subdural hematomas. I. Acute subdural hematoma: progress in definition, clinical pathology and therapy. Surg. Neurol. *19*, 216−231.

26. Taguchi, Y., Nakamura, N., Sato, J., Hasegawa, Y., 1982: Pathogenesis of chronic subdural hematoma, sequential study with computerized tomography. Neurol. Med. Chir. (Tokyo) *22*, 276−282.

27. Watanabe, S., Shimada, H., Ishii, H., Ishii, S., 1972: Productions of clinical form of chronic subdural hematoma in experimental animals. J. Neurosurg. *37*, 552−561.

28. Winertock, D. P., Spetzler, R. F., Hoff, J. T., 1975: Acute, posttraumatic subdural hygroma. Natural course with angiographic documentations. Radiology *115*, 373−375.

29. Yamada, H., Nihei, H., Watanabe, T., Shibui, S., Murata, S., 1979: Chronic subdural hematoma occuring consequently to the posttraumatic subdural hygroma—on the pathogenesis of the chronic subdural hematoma. Brain & Nerve *31*, 115−121.

30. Yashon, D., White, R. J., Bryk, J. P., Dakters, J. G., 1970: Simplified supplementary treatment of chronic subdural fluid collections. Neurochirurgia *14*, 8−13.

# Extracerebral Hematomas in Children

## M. Choux

Département de Neurochirurgie pédiatrique, Hôpital des Enfants, C.H.U. Timone, Marseille (France)

With 8 Figures

## Contents

Post-traumatic extracerebral hematomas in children represent various types of hemorrhages with a different incidence and especially a different prognosis. Some, the extracranial ones, are frequent and without patholog- ical consequences. Others, the extradural or subdural ones, are more rare but represent severe complications of head injuries. We will describe first the extracranial hematomas which are present in many head trauma in children. We will distinguish subcutaneous, subgaleal and subperiosteum hema- tomas. In a second part we will study the intra-cranial but extracerebral hematomas, in other words, those situated by the dura (extradural and subdural hematomas). We will emphasize, for each, the pediatric character- istics since the general aspects of these hematomas have been described in another chapter.

## I. Extracranial Hematomas

In this section, hemorrhages at three different levels are included: subcutaneous, subgaleal and subperiosteum. There is considerable confu- sion over the anatomy and the terminology of these types of hemorrhage. Any collection of blood over the skull can be etymologically referred to as a cephalhematoma but, it is clearer to restrict cephalhematoma to hemor- rhage between periosteum and skull. Some authors have classified subgaleal hematoma with subcutaneous hematoma (Potter and Craig 1976) or with cephalhematoma (Larroche 1977). Accurate localization of an extracranial hematoma is necessary to avoid clinical confusion and erroneous treatment. Anatomically, one can distinguish at the level of the scalp and the skull four different layers, the skin with the superficial fascia, the galea or epicranial aponeurosis, the periosteum and the bone. Between each level a collection of blood can occur (Table 1).

### A. Subcutaneous Hematoma

A post-traumatic subcutaneous hematoma is quite frequent even in minor injury in an infant. This hematoma appears soon after the trauma and can have a large extension over the skull and sometimes bilaterally. It can remain in place a long time and not rarely it is the skin bulging which is the revealing symptom of a head trauma. A posttraumatic subcutaneous hematoma is much more frequent in children than in older patients. It is particularly common in infants and in our experience a third of hospitalized children under two years old, with head injury, present with a localized or extensive bulging at the level of the scalp even without any erosion or contusion of the skin. We have demonstrated the particular vascular richness of the skin and the superficial fascia, in young children. A mild trauma of the vault may determine a subcutaneous hematoma, sometimes very extensive and associated with signs of anemia.

Table 1. *Extracranial Hematomas Localization*

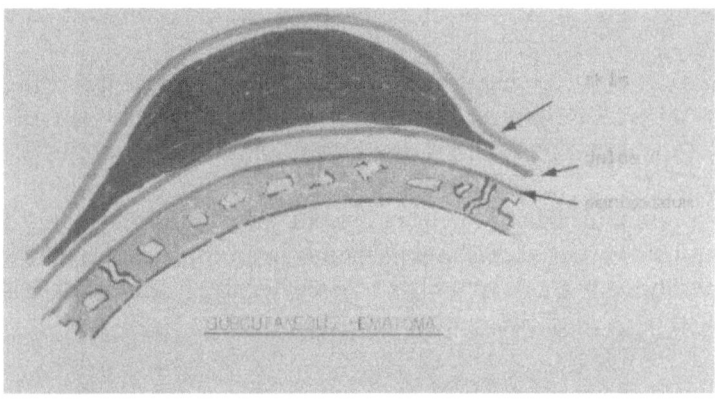

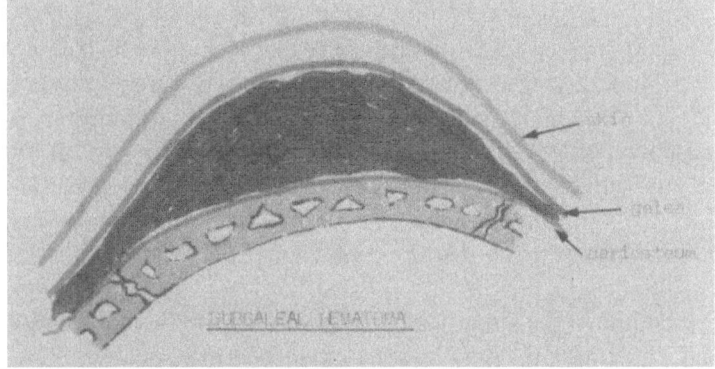

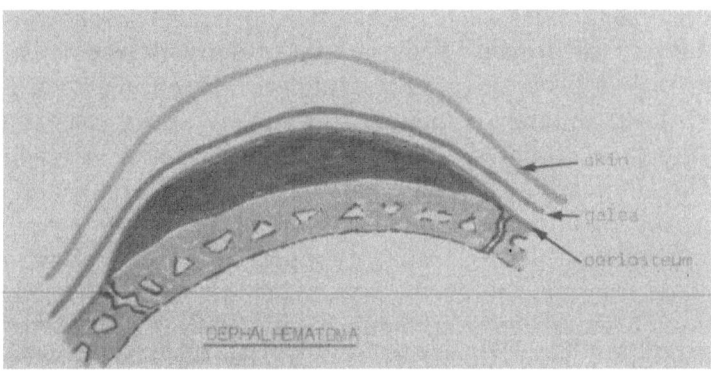

A subcutaneous hematoma can appear in any place on the skull but parietal and frontal localizations are the most frequent. At the level of the orbital region it is of value to establish the time of appearance of such a hematoma. When the orbital hematoma, unilateral or bilateral, develops immediately after an injury the bleeding origin is the subcutaneous deep portion of the superficial fascia. In contrast, in the case of an orbital hematoma appearing a few hours or on the second day after the injury, an underlying skull fracture exists. In many cases a subcutaneous hematoma is the revealing sign of an unsuspicious head trauma without any initial symptoms.

A puncture of these hematomas is not only unnecessary but can be dangerous by facilitating a local infection. Even in the case of a very extensive subcutaneous hematoma, an evacuation by needle is contra-indicated.

When a puncture has been performed the hematoma can rapidly recur. In the majority of the cases a subcutaneous hematoma disappears in a few days or sometimes weeks, but we have seen extensive hematomas disappearing completely in only two months.

### B. Subgaleal Hematoma

A subgaleal hematoma occurs between the galea (or epicranial aponeurosis) and the pericranium. It has been called also subaponevrotic hematoma. The galea is attached laterally to the zygomatic arch, the auricular muscle, anteriorly to the orbital ridges of the frontal bone, and posteriorly to the tissues of the posterior cervical triangle. This large subgaleal space contains connective tissue and small veins, especially emissary veins between the dural sinuses and the superficial veins of the scalp.

A hematoma into the subgaleal space is not limited by adherences to the sutures and consequently may spread over the entire scalp.

Subgaleal hematomas occur most often in neonates following either vaginal delivery or forceps delivery. In obstetrical trauma subgaleal hematoma frequently occurs over the right parietal bone. If we consider that the left occiput anterior is the most frequent appearance, the right hemicranium can be injured against the maternal pelvis. After birth the subgaleal hematoma may spread slowly over the entire scalp and require monitoring for the effects of blood loss.

In infants a subgaleal hematoma can appear after a cranial trauma with or without a fracture. In many cases it is not easy to distinguish a subcutaneous hemorrhage from a subgaleal one. A subcutaneous hematoma is generally more limited because the adherences between the galea and the scalp. A subgaleal hematoma may extend extensively to both sides and elevate large portions of the scalp. Accumulations of blood enlarge for 1 to 15 days and after resolve over 1 to 4 weeks. In the majority of cases the bleeding has a venous origin because very few arteries cross the subgaleal space which explains the slow progression of the hematoma, during the first days.

Subgaleal hematomas in children may occur after many types of trauma. Some authors mention subgaleal hematomas after minor trauma (Scott

1936, Hamlin 1968, Adeloye 1975, Kuban 1983). In some cases a hair pulling mechanism must be considered (Cantu 1971, Faber 1976, Falfo 1981).

Subgaleal hematoma can occur without any skull lesion. Adeloye (1975) reports his experience with 55 subgaleal hematomas in Nigerian patients, 48 were less than 10 years old. 27 of the patients (50%) had no fracture. Kuban (1983) presents 6 cases of subgaleal hematomas in four children and two infants. Not one had a fracture. Hypoprothrombinemia may explain the frequence of subgaleal hemorrhage in African babies who frequently do not receive vitamine K (Robinson 1968).

The mechanism of such a hematoma in the subgaleal space may be multiple but two can be considered. A radial force in the case of hair pulling, can disrupt venous vessels of the subgaleal space. A tangential movement in case of birth trauma or head injury will displace the mobil gallea over the fixed pericranium. As has been mentioned for subcutaneous hematomas, subgaleal hematomas must not be aspirated. The risk of infection is important and reaccumulation of blood following aspiration may need a transfusion. Finally, evacuation of the liquid by needle does not reduce significantly the time of resolution. Subgaleal hematomas rarely calcify and when they do, it is incompletely.


## C. Cephalhematomas

Cephalhematoma is a hemorrhage between the periosteum and the bone. It is most often unilateral and limited locally by the periosteal union at the cranial sutures. Consequently, as a rule, a cephalhematoma does not cross the midline as a subgaleal hematoma can do. It is usually parietal in location but can involve the frontal or the occipital bones (Fig. 1).

Differentiation of cephalhematoma from a subcutaneous hematoma (caput) in a neonate is generally easy. The cephalhematoma look less soft than a subcutaneous mass, it does not cross the suture lines and may increase in size after the birth. More difficult is to determine if the deep mass is a cephalhematoma or a subgaleal hematoma. Both may increase during the first days and may have the same clinical aspects at the beginning.

Asubperiosteal hematoma is found in about 0.50 to 2% of deliveries and more frequently in neonates of primiparous mothers.

*Reported incidence of cephalhematoma:*

Sjovall (1936) 0.41%,
Kendall-Woloshin (1952) 2.49%,
Tan (1970) 0.20%,
Zelson (1974) 1.50%.

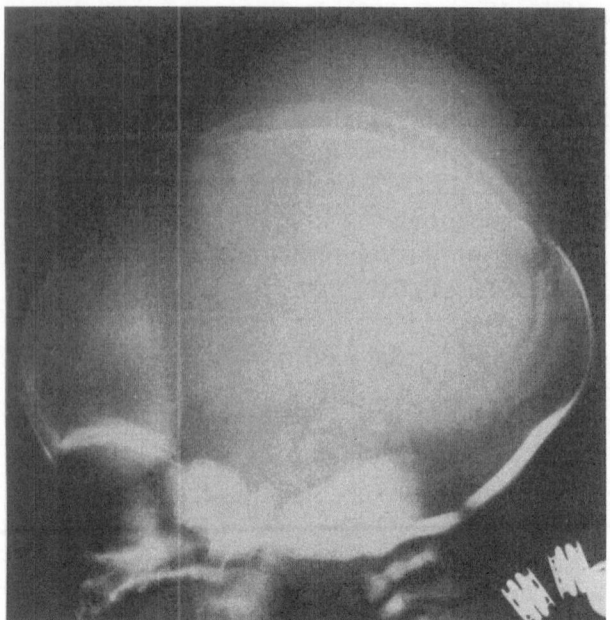
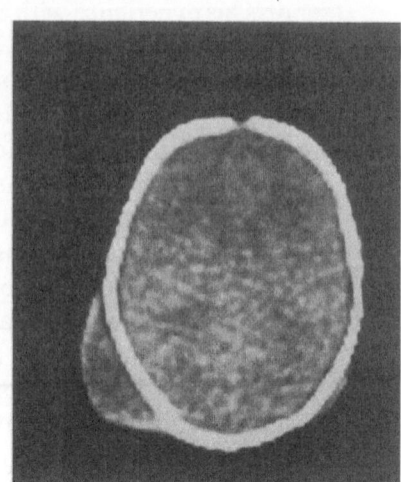

Fig. 1. Cephalhematoma in newborn

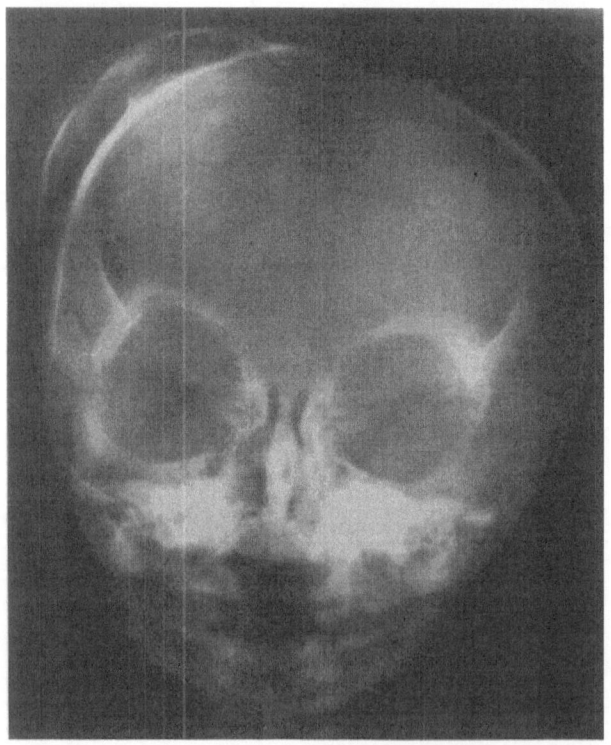
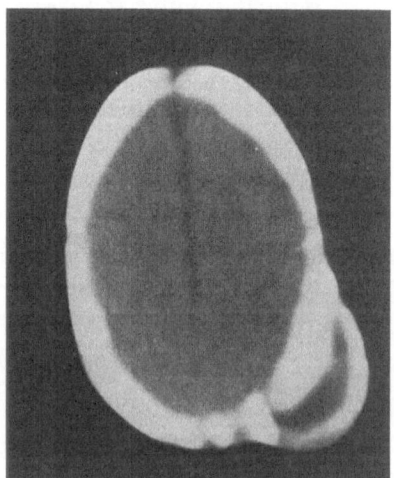

Fig. 2. Calcified cephalhematoma

In the literature cephalhematoma occur more frequently after forceps delivery:

Kendall: 64 of the 69 neonates (93%),

Zelson: 67 of the 111 neonates (60%).

Kendall and Woloshin mention an incidence of 25% of fracture, although Harwood-Nash and Zelson indicates an incidence of 5%. A high incidence of skull fracture exists in newborns with bilateral cephalhematomas (18% for Zelson).

Aspiration of cephalhematoma must be prohibited even if the hematoma takes a long time to resolve. A calcification of the membranes can appear (in approximately 10% of the cases) but only in few cases a marked calcified hematoma needs surgical removal. In the majority of cases the calcified rim is thin enough to be remodelled in a way to obtain a normal head shape. Calcification usually occurs 2 to 5 weeks after birth but in a few cases it occurs early in the first week (Fig. 2).

## II. Intracranial Hematomas

### A. Subdural Hematomas

Subdural hematoma is the most frequent intra-cranial hematoma after head injuries in children. In this chapter we will study only subdural hematomas in children, secondary to a head trauma and with an initial hemorrhagic liquid. Consequently we will not mention other subdural effusions such as subdural hygromas or hydromas which will be considered in another chapter.

Subdural hematoma can be classified depending on the age of the children and the age of the lesion. Considering the age of the children one must distinguish subdural hematomas in the newborn as a result of birth trauma, subdural hematoma in infants and subdural hematoma in older children. Considering now the age of the lesion, subdural hematoma may be classified as acute (the first two days), subacute (3 days to 3 weeks) or chronic (after 3 weeks). This distinction is essential since the majority of authors in their reports on subdural hematomas consider essentially chronic hematomas. In fact many subdural hematomas are diagnosed later when the liquid is xanthochromic or clear. The initial cause of the hematoma remains unknown and consequently one speaks more commonly of subdural effusion. To be clear we discuss more precisely acute and subacute post-traumatic subdural hematomas without ignoring that a chronic subdural hematoma is the logical evolution of an ignored or untreated acute hematoma.

Accurate diagnosis and immediate treatment of acute subdural hematomas can avoid a chronic evolution of the collection of liquid and its major consequence a psychomotor impairment. Previously Ingraham and Matson in 1949, stressed on early diagnosis and surgical treatment of these hematomas in infancy. It is clear that the incidence of classical chronic subdural effusions in infants will diminish significantly at the moment that acute hematoma will be recognized initially and treated adequately.

Acute subdural hematoma in children is a clinical entity, quite different from that seen in adults, where they are three or four times more frequent than in children. If many series of acute subdural hematomas in adults have been reported in the literature, very few can be found in childhood. Until 1965, only single case reports have been published. Suzuki in 1970 with 8 cases; Sparacio in 1971 with 6 cases, Gutierrez in 1975 with 27 cases, Hayakawa in 1984 with 22 cases; Alvarez-Garijo in 1981 with 7 cases are the authors who have published the main series of acute subdural hematomas. The exact incidence of post-traumatic acute or subacute subdural hematomas is difficult to know in the major series of head traumas since there is no distinction between acute or chronic hematomas. Hendrick in a series of 4,465 cases of head trauma mention that a subdural hematoma occurred in 235 children (5.2%). Ingraham and Matson report a higher incidence (12%). In a personal series of 6,700 pediatric head traumas, 288 subdural hematomas were found (4.3%).

Subdural hematomas are mostly frequent in children under two years of age and especially under one year. Hendrick points out that 86% occur in infants and 59.2% in the 0–6 months age group. In our series infants represent 73% and 46% were under 6 months of age. In two pediatric series of acute subdural hematomas the proportion of infants is 88.8% (Gutierrez) and 70% (Hayakawa).

## Anatomical Aspects

The majority of acute subdural hematomas are supratentorially situated (90 to 95%). A posterior fossa hematoma is more common in children than in adults. In fact this latter site is particular to neonates after birth injury.

An acute or subacute subdural hematoma of the supra-tentorial region is generally less extensive than a chronic one. It occupies the fronto-parietal area with a temporal extension. A localized frontal, temporal or occipital hematoma is very uncommon. If chronic hematomas are more often bilateral, acute hematomas are generally unilateral. In children there is a significant incidence of interhemispheric acute subdural hematoma. In the series of Zimmerman acute convexity hematomas in children are as frequent as inter-hemispheric hematomas. In adults, acute convexity hematomas are four times more frequent than in children.

## Causes of Subdural Hemorrhage

Subdural hematoma may originate from an arterial or venous bleeding. In cases of arterial sources, usually from cortical arteries, the subdural hematoma is generally associated with a cerebral contusion and the evolution is acute. When the hematoma has a venous origin we can distinguish three types of injury:

1. tearing of bridging veins extended from the brain to the dural sinuses,
2. lesions or lacerations of dura-mater,
3. lesions of a venous sinus by a fracture or a disjunction of a suture.

The most frequent cause is the first one but considering that in young children the same mechanism can cause different lesions, it is possible to find at the same time a rupture of a bridging vein and a laceration of the dura. The commonest site of tearing of bridging veins is at the level of the sagittal sinus and this explains the frequency of para-sagittal hematomas. It is interesting to stress the difficulty or the impossibility to visualize these interrupted veins either by angiography or during surgery or even during an autopsy. The bleeding from these veins can stop spontaneously or can be intermittent, explaining the reccurrence of some hematomas. If the rupture of the bridging veins remains the main cause of posttraumatic subdural hematoma, we want to stress the importance of the second type of injury in neonates or in infants, the laceration of the dura, even without a skull fracture. The lesions are generally a disruption of the different layers of the dura, more than a complete tearing. These lesions are more often found at the level of dural folds and more frequent near the tentorium. In two recent cases of our series it was possible, during the postmortem examination, to visualize such a lesion. An important clot over the cerebral hemisphere was found and attached to the dura in a localized point. The dura was not ruptured but lacerated in this localized region, close the sagittal sinus. Such a mechanism has been clearly demonstrated in newborn infants presenting with a fetal skull deformity.

## 1. Subdural Hematomas in the Newborn

The first well documented reports of subdural hematomas in neo-natal life after birth trauma were those of Craig in 1938, Schipke in 1954 and Schwartz in 1961. Capon (1922) mentions that in about two percent of all infants born died with a subdural hemorrhage. The relation to a difficult delivery was clear. The improvement of obstetrical methods has changed the incidence of this complication even if it remains important in preterm infants. Larroche in 1977, among 700 necropsies, found 18% of subdural bleeding in term infants and 11% in preterm infants who died.

Breech delivery is a particular cause of brain lesion and especially of subdural hematoma (Sulama). Many authors have mentioned that subdural hemorrhage is more common in primipare than in multipare. In the series of Takagi, posterior fossa subdural hematomas are more frequent in primipare (84%).

The causes of the subdural hematomas in the newborn have been mentioned previously. One cause must be added because it characterizes neonate head trauma and especially the posterior fossa localization. It is the skull lesion at the level of the posterior intra-occipital synchondrosis with the separation of the lateral and the squamous part of the occipital bone.

The cerebral convexity and the parasagittal regions are the commonest site of subdural hematomas after birth trauma but the posterior fossa localization is not rare. Many have been discovered at autopsy. Coblentz in 1940 describes the first case. Since them about 50 cases have been reported in the literature. The most documentated report was those of Takagi in 1982, who presents 25 cases of posterior fossa subdural hemorrhage (2 treated surgically and 23 untreated, found at autopsy) and he reviewed all the literature of this localization.

*Clinical symptoms* vary with the site and the importance of the hematoma. The onset of symptoms after birth is within the first 24 hours but Alvarez-Garijo found in his series of 7 cases a free interval from 16 to 72 hours.

The distress appears with respiratory difficulty, palor, stupor, weak-cry, unequal pupils. The neonate rapidly deteriorates and becomes comatose. When the subdural hematoma is massive the initial sign can be palor and anemia.

Cerebral convexity hematoma may lead to neurological manifestations such as focal seizures, hemiparesis, eye deviation. Retinal hemorrhages are present in 30 to 50% of the cases.

In posterior fossa hematomas the mean time of onset of the symptoms after birth is shorter (8.6 hours for Takagi). This author found a respiratory abnormality in 100% of the cases, a cyanosis in 32% and convulsions in 20%.


*Diagnostic investigations*

skull X-rays show that skull fractures are relatively rare and depressed fractures exceptional. A displacement of the different parts of the occipital bone can be presents,

the diagnosis of subdural hematoma is confirmed by CT scanning. It shows the characteristic aspects of a high density lesion overlying one or both hemispheres. Initially subdural hematomas in the newborn are more often unilateral. A contusion of the underlying brain may be seen as well as an important shift of midline structures. In cases of posterior fossa localization a dilatation of the supra-tentorial ventricular compartment can be discovered early.

*Treatment.* Subdural taps may be both a method of diagnosis and a treatment. Even with the improving results of CT scanning a subdural tap at the beginning, could give useful information on the precise quantity and quality of the fluid and its pressure. In a newborn in very bad condition, evacuation of some quantity of blood could help to pass an initial and critical period. But it is well known that subdural taps at the level of the fontanelle can ignore a hematoma located in the temporal or the parieto-occipital region. Negative subdural taps in cases of subdural hematomas are not exceptional.

In the neonate we recommend, initially, repeated taps to evacuate a liquid hematoma. Sometimes a craniotomy or burr holes are needed in cases of subdural clot. In our experience a complete evacuation of a subdural hematoma is possible by subdural taps only in the majority of cases. These punctures must be repeated daily or sometimes twice a day. In cases of subdural hematomas associated with an important brain contusion and a skull lesion, a craniotomy is needed. The morbidity of these cases remains important and a notable proportion of patients develop a chronic subdural effusion.

## 2. Subdural Hematomas in Infants and Young Children

*Causes.* A number of children have no history of trauma, but without a history of meningitis or severe dehydration it is clear that the great majority of subdural hematomas are traumatic. An important injury is not always necessary and few repeated mild-head traumas, which are considered as "normal" by the family, may determine a subdural hematoma which often is a chronic one at at the moment of diagnosis.

In practice a significant number of cases result from falls: from crib, chair, wrapping tables, or from the arms of the parents. Many are unobserved falls, especially when they are totally asymptomatic. A violent and repeated shaking of a baby without evidence of external trauma may be sufficient to create a subdural hematoma after rupture of bridging veins or repeated acceleration-deceleration of the brain. This relatively new mechanism has been documented by Guthkelch in 1971 and Caffey in 1972 after the experimental work of Ommaya in 1968, studying the effects of sudden deceleration in rhesus monkeys. This mechanism probably explains why a large number of children with subdural hematomas present without significant head impact and without skull fractures (Till, McClelland). Subdural hematomas are not rare in abused children. Caffey in 1946 reported 6 cases of multiple fractures in the long bones of infants presenting with chronic subdural hematomas. Silverman in 1953 defined the syndrome as a traumatic lesion. Kempe and Silverman in 1962 created the term "battered child syndrome". Guthkelch (1971) and Caffey (1972) explain the main manifestations of child abuse as "whiplash, shaken infant syndrome". McClelland (1980) reports 21 cases of cerebral injury in child abuse. 6 of them were admitted with a whiplash shaken infant syndrome and 4 had evidence of acute subdural hematomas. Hahn in 1983 reports 77 cases of child abuse with 126 craniocerebral injuries (average 1.6 percent). 30 presented with subdural hematomas.

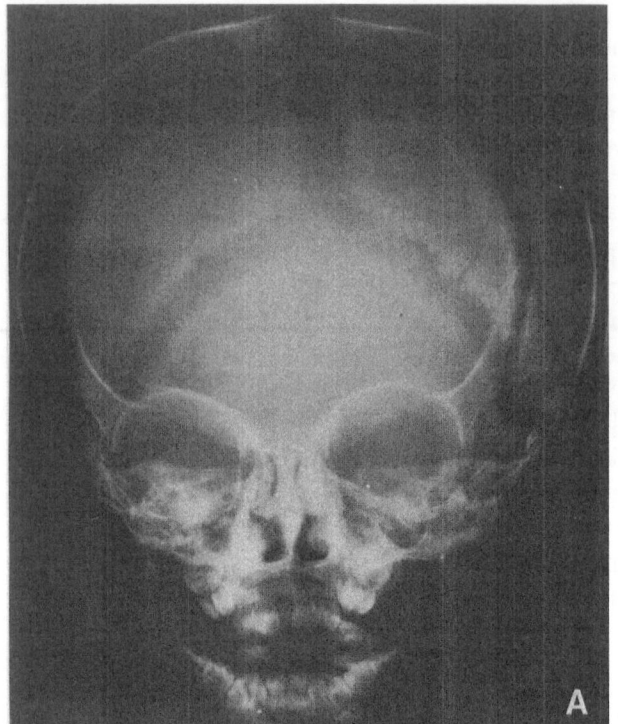
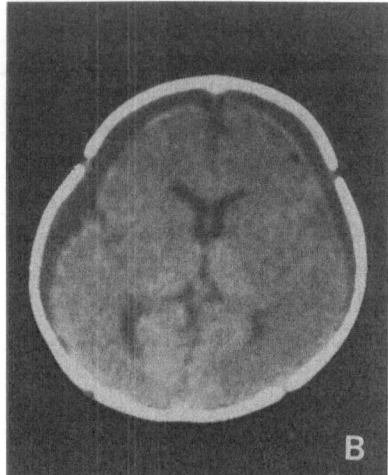

Fig. 3. Eight-month-old bettered child. A) Important disjonction of all the sutures. B) Acute subdural bilateral hematoma

If subdural hematomas are a part of the battered child syndrome, its true incidence is variable in the literature, 28% for McHenry, 29% for Hahn, 20% for our data (Fig. 3).

*Mechanism.* The same mechanisms we have mentioned for newborn injuries can be found in the infant. But at this age the majority of subdural hematomas are of venous origin by rupture of bridging veins. Very few have a true arterial origin, from cortical arteries with contused underlying brain. We must note too that the majority of subdural hematomas in the literature are not explained by a skull lesion.

*Clinical aspect.* In infants, generally, the clinical aspect of acute or subacute subdural hematomas are less dramatic than in a newborn. The

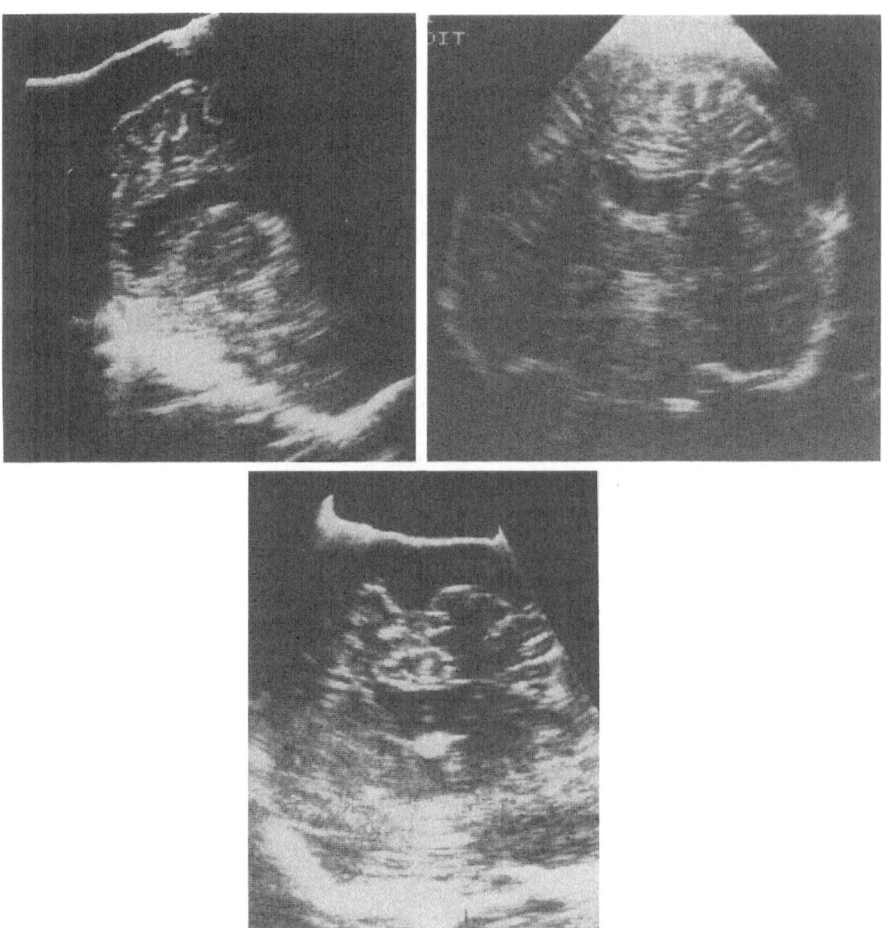

Fig. 4. B-mode ultrasonogram showing three different subdural hematomas

level of consciousness is diminished but a comatous state is rare. The child looks pale, irritable. The anterior fontanelle is tense. Convulsions occur in 50 to 70% of the cases. Focal neurological signs can be found. Unequal pupils may represent. Retinal hemorrhage is present in 63.1% of the cases of Gutierrez and 55% of the cases of Hayakawa. In cases of associated brain damage clinical symptoms and neurological deficits are important. In small children traumatic shock can mask signs of acute intracranial hypertension.

### Diagnostic Investigation

X-ray examinations reveal a fracture of the skull in a variable proportion in the literature since many series do not specify which are acute and which are chronic subdural hematomas. Hendrick reports that only 12% of children under two years of age had a demonstrable fracture. In his series the incidence of fracture increases with age: 7% between 0 to 6 months old and 22% between 6 months to 2 years old. Ingraham and Matson report 11% with fractures. In a series of acute subdural hematomas only the incidence of skull fracture is higher 40.7% for Gutierrez, 59% for Hayakawa. In our personal series the proportion of associated fractures in

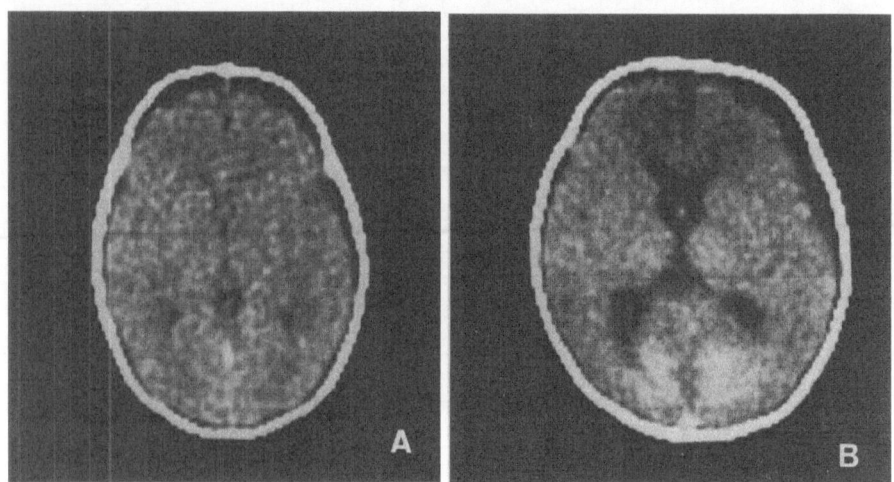

Fig. 5. CT scanning aspects of acute or subacute subdural hematomas. A) Moderate subdural hematoma in a 3-year-old child treated by subdural drainage by burr hole. B) Acute right subdural hematoma in a 14 months old child treated by subdural external drainage

infants is 18% but in cases of pure acute subdural hematomas the incidence rises to 45%. Depressed fractures associated with subdural hematomas are very uncommon. In a personal series of 51 depressed fractures in infants we have found only one subdural hematoma.

B-mode ultrasonography is a well-proved method of determining the presence and the size of a subdural hematoma and to follow the therapeutical evolution (Fig. 4).

CT scanning (Fig. 5) demonstrates the hematoma as a peripheral increased density that covers the cerebral hemisphere. Kaufman has demonstrated that an acute subdural hematoma can be isodense in an anemic patient since the density is indirectly related to the blood hemoglobin level. CT scanning reveals eventually an associated brain lesion which can play a role in the mass effect. The use of cerebral angiography in children has diminished tremendously and indications remain rare.

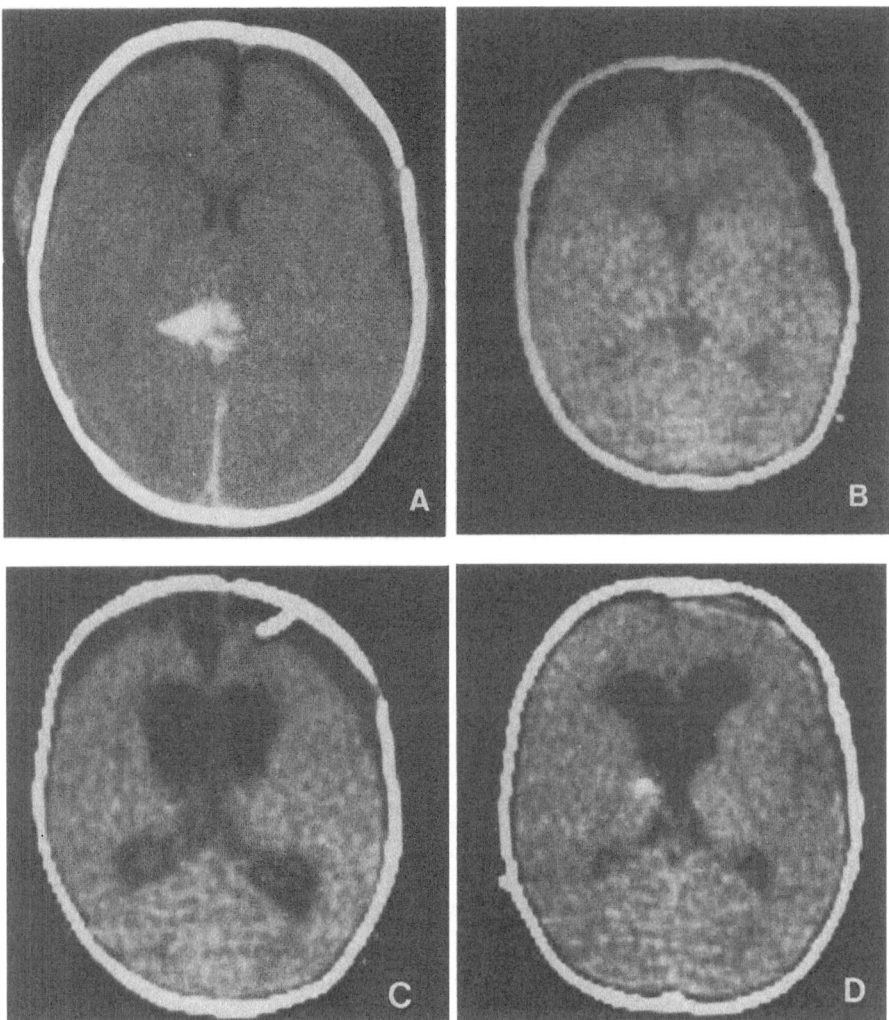

Fig. 6. Evolution of an acute subdural hematoma in a 4-month-old boy after a vehicle accident. A) Novembre 11, 1982: Right acute subdural hematoma by contre coup mechanism. B) Novembre 26, 1982: Bilateral subdural hematoma treated by subduro peritoneal shunt. C) December 16, 1982: Secondary acute hydrocephalus treated by ventriculo peritoneal shunt. D) June 14, 1983: Disappearance of subdural hematoma. Stabilized hydrocephalus. Normal neurological evolution

*Treatment.* Three methods of treatment can be used: subdural taps, burrhole or trepanation opening and craniotomy for evacuation of the clot (Fig. 6),

subdural tapping is recognized to be effective for the diagnosis in urgent cases, but not effective as definite treatment, since some acute subdural hematomas can be coagulated. In this last case negative subdural taps do not exclude the diagnosis of a subdural hematoma,

an opening of the skull by a burr hole or trepanation is the best method to evacuate a liquefied subdural hemorrhage or a clot. A secondary irrigation can be useful,

an osteoplastic bone flap for removal of an extensive subdural hematoma or a solid clot in an infant is the treatment of choice for Gutierrez. In our experience we are convinced that the majority of acute subdural hematomas can be evacuated and drained with a trepanation uni- or bilaterally,

craniotomy can be reserved for cases in which the subdural clot cannot be removed totally through a burr hole or when a persistent extensive hematoma cannot be controlled.

*Results.* The overall mortality of patients with posttraumatic acute or subacute subdural hematomas is always high in the literature.

Rosenvorn in a series of 149 patients of all ages, reports a mortality of 73% for acute and 27% for subacute subdural hematomas in spite of steroids, hyperventilation and decompression to treat edema. In this series the mortality rate in children is 57% for acute hematomas in comparison with 71% in patients between 16–64 years old. Gutierrez mentions a general mortality of 20% in a series of 27 pediatric acute subdural hematomas. For Hayakawa the overall mortality is 13.6%. In our personal experience the mortality is near 17%. These results confirm a more favourable prognosis in children than in adults since most reports of acute subdural hematoma in adults give a mortality of 65 to 90%.

Regarding now the correlations between treatment and mortality, it appears clearly that in the surgical group the mortality is higher in accordance with the fact that it is the group of most injured children. Gutierrez mentions a mortality of 26/6% in the surgical group (3 craniotomies and 1 bilateral burr holes) against 8.3% in the subdural taps group. In our series we have a mortality of 17% in infants treated by burr holes opening or trepanation.

The morbidity depends on the age of the child, the severity of consciousness disturbance in the acute stage and the modality of treatment. The later prognosis is worse in children under one year of age and in patients with a prolonged period of coma. It seems that more patients treated by only subdural taps develop a chronic subdural collection.

In Gutierrez's series it appears that 41.6% of patients treated with repeated subdural taps converted to chronic subdural collection and only 13.3% in the surgical group. In our series only 8% of patients developed a chronic subdural hematoma. Late psychological evaluation has been studied in many reports on subdural hematomas but generally no distinction has been made between acute or chronic lesions Gutierrez in his pediatric series notes an I. Q. over 80 in 72.7% of the cases in the surgical group and 25% in the non surgical group. Hayakawa points out that the cases with a low I. Q. below 80 were 6 of a total 11 cases (54.5%).

In conclusion one can say that acute subdural hematomas in children have a lower mortality rate than in adults but the quality of survivors is not as favourable as generally expected.

## B. Extradural Hematomas

Classically posttraumatic extradural hematomas in children are infrequent and very few series can be found in the literature. Publications in children concern generally short series or case reports. The explanation of this rarity is not clear, since the incidence of head injuries in children is higher than in adults and the pathological study of the dura and the skull in childhood demonstrates with accuracy the importance of the vascularization. In a previous study we have illustrated by intravascular injection of the dura in infants, the significant richness of this vascularization not only at the level of the meningeal arteries but also in every surface of the dura. At the same time we have mentioned the high diploic vascularization in infants or in young children, explaining the frequent bone origin of bleeding into the extradural space. Extradural hematomas in children, more commonly than in adult, are due to venous hemorrhage, from emissary veins, or dural veins.

Adherences between bone and the dura, especially at the level of the sutures, have been considered as another anatomical feature to explain the rarity of extradural hematomas in children. We cannot agree with this option since firm adherences between bone and dura at a distance from the sutures, are more rare in children than in adults. In infants the only attachment of the dura and the bone is at the level of the coronal sutures. In older children many extradural hematomas are extensive and cross the sutural level.

In order to have a better consideration of the main characteristics of extradural hematomas in children five series will be studied which represent 379 cases [Matson 1969; 44 cases of children under 12 years of age, Hendrick 1964: 40 cases, Arseni (1980) 61 cases under 16 years of age, Mazza: 62 cases under 15 years of age and our series of 172 cases under 15 years of age].

## Incidence

Considering the number of head traumas in children, extradural hematomas represent a proportion of 0.9% to 3%.

Campbell (1951) gives the same proportion (1.8%) but Svendsen mentions a proportion of 3.7%. Finally it is important to mention that the

|                    | Number of head traumas | Number of EDH |
|--------------------|------------------------|---------------|
| Matson (1969)      | 3,053                  | 40            |
| Hendrick (1964)    | 4,465                  | 40 (0.9%)     |
| Arseni (1980)      | 4,739                  | 61 (1.3%)     |
| Mazza (1982)       |                        | 62 (3%)       |
| Pang (1983)        | 813                    | 45 (5.5%)     |
| Our series (1984)  | 11,200                 | 172 (1.5%)    |

proportion of extradural hematomas in children is nearly the same as in adults (between 1.5 to 3.5%).

Considering the incidence of pediatric cases in extradural hematoma series we see the following figures:

|                          | Number of EDH | Children |
|--------------------------|---------------|----------|
| McKissock (1960)         | 190           | 31%      |
| Pia (Gerlach) (1967)     | 125           | 22%      |
| Jamieson (1968)          | 167           | 14%      |
| Marseille series (1984)  | 648           | 26.5%    |

## Age

Extradural hematomas in the newborn are exceptional and are generally discovered at autopsy (3 among 134 autopsies for Takagi).

Extradural hematomas in infants are rare. McLaurin and Ford in 1963 did not find any infant in a series of 47 children. McKissock found 6 infants in a series of 125 cases. In our series of 172 extradural hematomas in children, infants represent 26 cases (15%).

Extradural hematomas occurring in children under the age of one are rare: 3 among 40 pediatric cases for Hendrick, 10 among our 172 cases.

The majority of pediatric extradural hematomas are seen in children over 15 years and especially after 10 years.

| Age   | Matson       | Mazza (62 cases) | Our series (172 cases) |
|-------|--------------|------------------|------------------------|
| 0–2   | 17 (38.6%)   | 8 (12%)          | 26 (15%)               |
| 2–12  | 27           | 22               | 94                     |
| 12–15 |              | 32               | 52                     |

## Sex

As in adults the sex incidence in children is higher in males, but the difference is much lower in children under 2 years old.

In our series among 26 cases of extradural hematomas in infants, 15 were boys and 11 were girls. The sex distribution in three series is shown in this figure.

|  | Matson (44 cases) | Mazza (62 cases) | Our series (172 cases) |
|---|---|---|---|
| Boys | 31 (70%) | 49 (79%) | 134 (78%) |
| Girls | 13 (30%) | 13 (21%) | 38 (22%) |

## Etiology

The main cause of extradural hematoma in children is a fall (more than 50% of the cases) but the proportion of traffic accident remains quite high (40–50%). In Matson's series the low incidence of traffic accidents can be explained by the fact that he has considered children under 12 years old only.

|  | Matson | Mazza | Our series |
|---|---|---|---|
| Fall | 72% | 50% | 62% |
| Road accident | 11% | 47% | 42% |
| Others | 17% | 3% | 6% |

## Localization (Table 2)

It is common to said that extradural hematomas in children are well localized and do not pass the level of the sutures. In a previous series of 96 cases we have reported 45, which were extensive covering near all the hemisphere. In our actual series we confirm this proportion. Among 172 cases, 94 were localized hematomas (54.6%) and 78 were extensive (45.4%). Arseni found nearly the same proportion of extensive hematomas (48.5%) and also Goutelle (44%). We must point out the proportion of extensive hematomas in infants (52.4%). Consequently it is difficult to admit that adherences between sutures and dura will limit the extension of the hematoma in young children.

Table 2. *Extradural Hematomas Localization in Five Pediatric Series*

|  | Goutelle 25 cases | Harwood-Nash 40 cases | Arseni 61 cases | Mazza 62 cases | Our series 172 cases |
|---|---|---|---|---|---|
| Frontal | 20% | 12% | 3.3% | 30% | 15% |
| Temporal | 32% |  | 42% |  | 27.6% |
| Parietal |  | 81% | 0% | 66% | 8.6% |
| Occipital |  |  | 0% | 3.2% | 0.5% |
| Posterior fossa |  | 7% | 3.2% | 1.6% | 3% |
| Parieto-temporal | 24% |  | 21.3% |  | 17.8% |
| Fronto-temporal | 12% |  | 18% |  | 6.3% |
| Hemispheric | 8% |  | 11.5% |  | 4.6% |

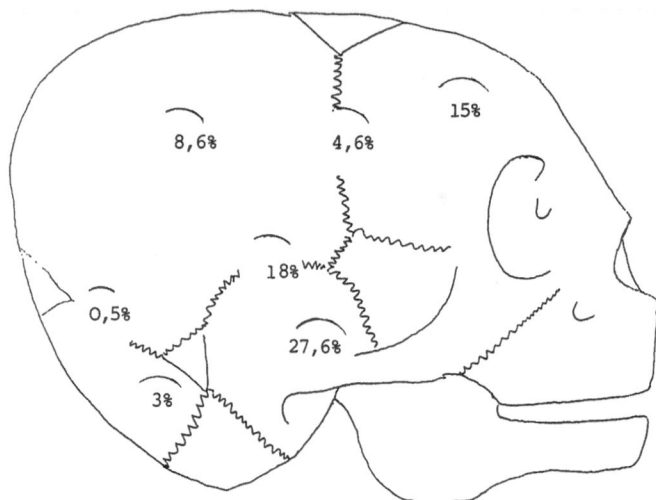

As in adults, the classical temporal localization remains the most frequent as well in infants than in older children. Limited temporal hematomas represent 30 to 40% of the cases. Considering now hematomas occupying partially or exclusively the temporal space, we see that they represent 81% for Harwood-Nash, 81% for Arseni, 66% for Mazza and 68.4% in our series. Basal hematomas are not rare in children (12 among 47 temporal hematomas in our series). Their evolution is generally acute and the mortality remains quite high.

The incidence of frontal hematomas in children is notable in many series (20% for Goutelle, 12% for Harwood-Nash, 15% in our series, 30% for Mazza). Frontal localization is much more frequent at the pediatric age:

70%. In our series an extradural hematoma was partially or exclusively situated in the frontal region in 27.9% of the cases. In 4 cases frontal hematomas were bilateral.

The occipital localization is very rare in children (no one for Arseni, 1 case for us, 2 cases for Mazza). Among 18 extradural occipital hematomas in the Marseille's series, only one was a pediatric case.

Extradural hematomas of the posterior fossa in children are infrequent but the incidence is certainly higher since its diagnosis remains difficult and the mortality is important. Now with the CT scan the detection has become easier. Incidence of posterior fossa hematoma is situated between 1.6 to 7%. Jamieson in a series of 167 cases at all ages, mentions that among the 12 hematomas located in the posterior fossa, 5 were pediatric cases. In our series we have found 5 cases, two of them in infants. In two other cases the hematoma was infra- and supratentorially situated at the same time.

The hemispheric hematomas, which cross two sutures, are not exceptional. In our series we have found 8 cases of such extensive hematomas (4.6%). They represent 8% for Goutelle and 11.5% for Arseni.

Bilateral hematomas can be found in the frontal region or in the vertex. We have found 6 cases of bilateral extradural hematomas in our series. Four of them were biparietal, one crossing the midline.

Extradural hematomas presenting in two different intracranial compartments are exceptional. Cervantes in 1983 has presented a case of both temporal and posterior fossa hematomas in a 16-year-old girl.

## Clinical Signs (Table 3)

*Consciousness*

An immediate disturbance of consciousness is present in 53% of 330 cases of the literature (Goutelle 40%, McKissock 30%, Matson 25%, Mazza 73%, our series 55%).

In our series 26% of children presented a brief loss of consciousness and 20% an initial coma. The duration and the severity of this initial loss of consciousness are not always precise in injured children. We must mention that there is no relation between the importance of the immediate disturbance of consciousness and the severity of the head injury. 82 children in our series (48%) did not present any initial disturbance of consciousness. In infants this percentage is much more important.

Later, a coma is present in 60% of the cases (Goutelle 50%, McKissock 60%, Matson 60%, Mazza 80%, our series 52%). A lucid interval is present in our series in 88 cases (51%). In only one other series is a delayed loss of consciousness mention (48.7% for Hendrick). The duration of the lucid interval is generally short, less than 24 hours. In posterior fossa hematomas a double lucid interval has been described with a delayed diagnosis of the lesion (Parkinson). Practically it is important to note that the classical

M. Choux:

Table 3. *Clinical Findings in Seven Series*

| | | Initial loss of consciousness | Coma | Lucid interval | Motors signs | Unequal pupils | Vomitings | Convulsions |
|---|---|---|---|---|---|---|---|---|
| Campbell | (20 cases) | | 50% | | 65% | 50% | | 10% |
| Goutelle | (25 cases) | 40% | 48% | 80% | 20% | 48% | 60% | |
| McKissock | (27 cases) | 29.6% | 59% | | | | | |
| Matson | (44 cases) | 25% | 65% | | 68% | 50% | 79.5% | 0% |
| Harwood-Nash | (40 cases) | | 53.6% | 48.7% | 30% | 55% | 62.5% | 7.5% |
| Mazza | (62 cases) | 74% | 72% | 40.3% | 30% | 19% | 53% | 1.6% |
| Our series | (172 cases) | 52% | 49.5% | 51% | 40% | 36% | 55% | 8.7% |

sequence, trauma—brief loss of consciousness—true lucid interval—secondary deterioration, is precisely present in very few cases (7.3% of our cases). In the majority of the cases the evolution of the consciousness is made by drowsiness, period of confuaion or agitation, before the loss of consciousness. We must mention that one third of children in our series did not present a loss of consciousness (36% for Hendrick). 7.3% never had a disturbance of conscious level (5% for Mazza and 2.6% for Hendrick).

Considering now the different types of evolution we can distinguish four groups in relation to changes in the level of consciousness.

*In group I*, patients are always conscious until the diagnosis. They represent 2.6% for Harwood-Nash, 5% for Mazza and 10.5% for us.

*In group II*, patients are unconscious during the entire evolution. They represent 2.6% of the cases for Harwood-Nash, 21% for Mazza and 20% for us.

*In group III*, patients present with drowsiness or confusion until treatment. An initial loss of consciousness can be present or not. They represent 33.3% of the cases for Harwood-Nash, 18% for us.

*In group IV*, patients had an initial loss of consciousness, a lucid interval and then deteriorated. The incidence of this group is 48.7% for Harwood-Nash, 40% for Mazza, 51% for us. We have mentioned previously that what is generally called a lucid interval is a period where the patient is not in a comatous state but in the majority of the cases drowsiness or confusion are noted. A true lucid interval remains uncommon (7% in our series).

Delayed extradural hematomas have been described in children. One should pointed out the frequency of a hemorrhage of venous origin in "chronic" extradural hematomas. In young children an associated sub-periosteum hematoma which communicates with the extradural hematoma through a fracture, can explain a prolonged clinical course. We have noted this fact in two of our cases and Iwakuma has mentioned the same possibility.

## Neurological Signs

Localizing signs are pyramidal or ocular. Significant pyramidal signs occurred in 46% of the cases (in 149 cases among 363 cases of the literature). The hemiparesis or hemiplegia is more often contralateral.

An ipsilateral dilatation of the pupil is one of the classical signs of an extradural hematoma but it is not encountered in every case. Its incidence in children varies from 19% (Mazza) to 50% (Campbell, Goutelle, Matson and Harwood-Nash). We have encountered a mydriasis in 36% of our cases.

## Other Clinical Signs

Recurrent vomiting is common to all pediatric head injuries but they are significantly more frequent in cases of extradural hematoma (between 53 to 80% of the cases), than in subdural hematoma or in brain damage.

A low red blood cell count (the anemic clinical type) existed in our series in 6 infants.

A blood loss in small children is significant enough to cause shock which can be masked by signs of intracranial hypertension. An important bradycardia at the moment of deterioration was present in our series in 19 cases (11%). Matson found it in one case (2.3%) and Goutelle in 5 cases (20%). In infants a bradycardia is not more frequent (10% in our series).

Convulsions are not exceptional in cases of extradural hematoma in children. Considering preoperative manifestations, their incidence is represented by 8.7% in our series (10% for Campbell, 7.5% for Harwood-Nash). Matson does not mention this sign in his series.

An extradural hematoma may be associated with a cephalhematoma in neonates and even, both hematomas can communicate. This very unusual situation has been described by Aoki in a newborn baby who presented with a cephalhematoma and a depressed skull fracture below. CT scan revealed an isodense extradural hematoma which communicated with the cephalhematoma through the skull fracture. We have found the same condition in two infants of 4 and 9 months old.

## Diagnostic Aids

*A. Plain X-rays.* A fracture is not always present in skull X-rays. The fracture sometimes can be difficult to visualize and some children are operated in emergency or without skull X-rays. We have mentioned in our first series of 104 cases that in 19% of the cases the fracture was not visualized by X-rays but was found at surgery. Mazza points out the same figure since among 15 cases with negative skull X-rays, in 6 of them a fracture was discovered at operation.

It seems that in children the absence of fracture is more common than in adults. The incidence of fractures in cases of extradural hematomas is indicated in Table 4.

Table 4. *Fracture and Extradural Hematoma*

|              | Fractures | Proportion of depressed fractures |
|--------------|-----------|-----------------------------------|
| McKissock    | 79%       |                                   |
| Goutelle     | 56%       |                                   |
| Matson       | 72%       |                                   |
| Harwood-Nash | 40%       | 50%                               |
| Arseni       | 75%       |                                   |
| Mazza        | 72.6%     |                                   |
| Our series   | 72%       | 13.7%                             |

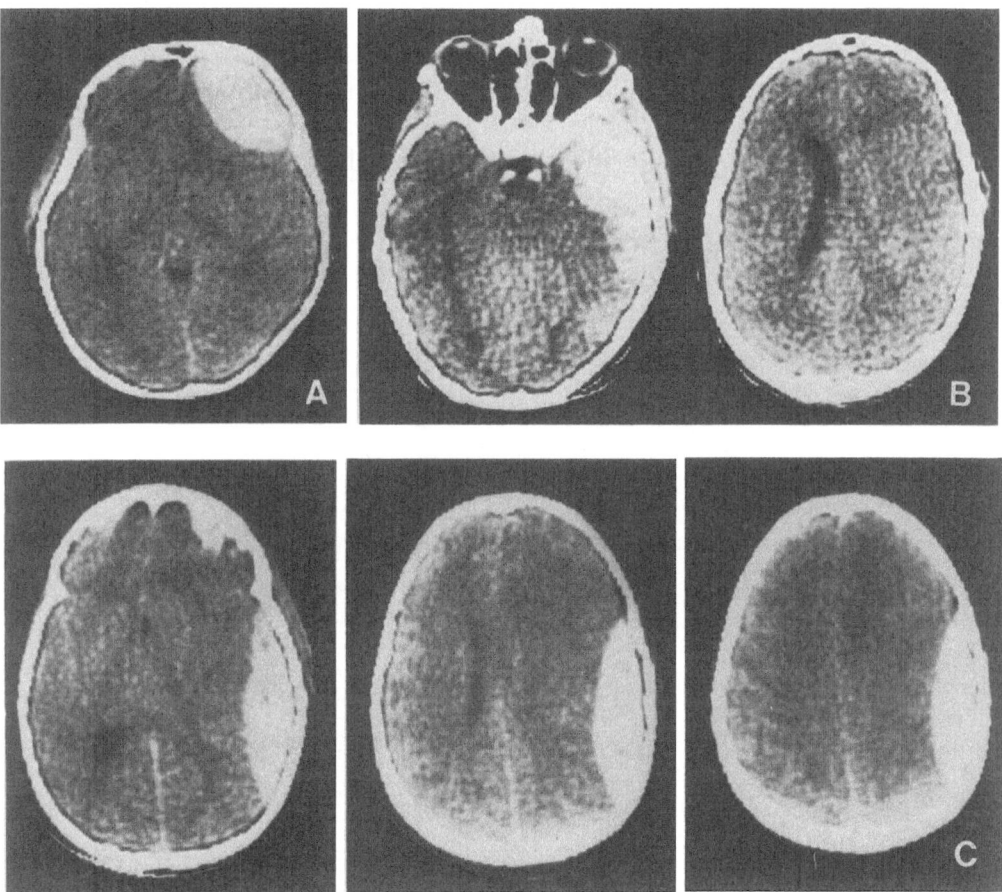

Fig. 7. CT scan aspects of extradural hematomas. A) Right frontal hematoma. Left parietal fracture. B) Acute subtemporal hematoma with a 30-minute lucid interval. C) Right parietal extradural hematoma. D) Posterior fossa extradural hematoma with a vertical occipital fracture

We find the same proportion of fractures in children under or after 2 years old. Concerning the type of fracture, depressed fractures represent 50% of the cases for Harwood-Nash but only 13.7% in our series.

We have noted that in 7.5% of our cases the location of the hematoma did not correspond to that of the fracture. We have observed 2 hematomas contralateral to the fracture and 11 homolateral hematomas which were not underlying the fracture. We must point out the necessity of repeated plain X-rays of the skull, especially in infants to detect an evolving splitting of the sutures which occurs in 20% of the cases. The main conclusion of this chapter can be that the absence of fracture does not exclude the possibility of an EDH consequently the clinical evaluation is far more significant.

*B.* CT scan (Fig. 7) is now the first and the main method to detect an extradural hematoma. It gives the exact localization, the extension, the density and the volume of the hematoma and shows the existence of an

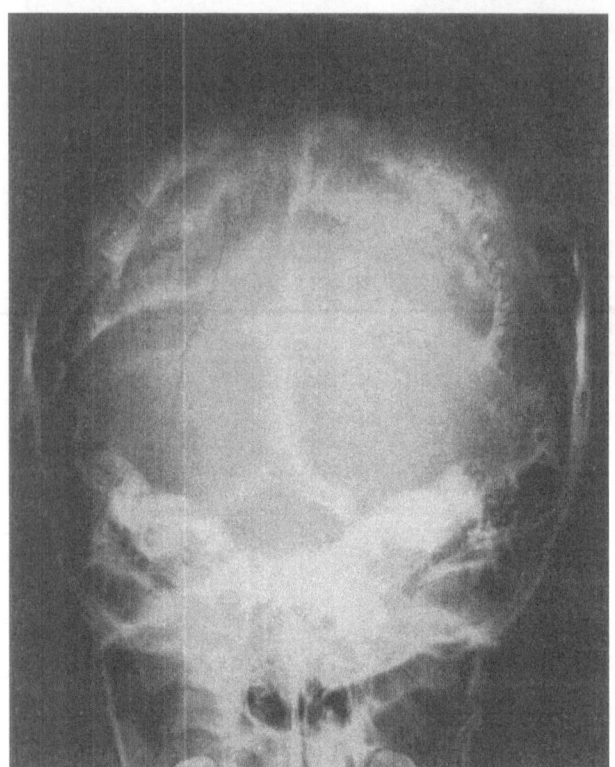
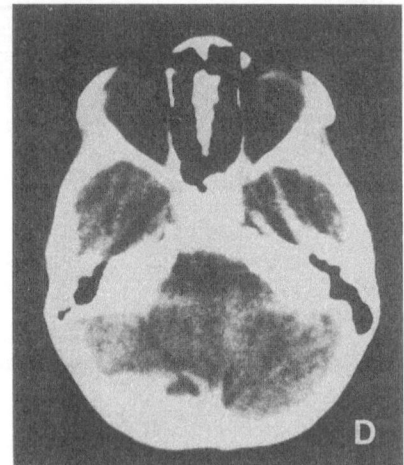

Fig. 7 D

associated brain lesion. Prior to the CT scan, cerebral angiography was performed in 74 children in our first series of 104 cases. Since 1975 in our department only 6 angiographies were performed among 68 cases of extradural hematomas. With the advent of the CT scan an increasing number of unjured children with minor neurological symptoms were scanned. A relatively high proportion of asymptomatic hematomas have been found as well as unusually situated extradural hematomas.

Now the CT scan permits identification of the stage of the hematoma as Zimmerman and Bilaniuk have recently described. Type I (acute hematoma) with a heterogeneous clot represents the most frequent in children (62% in our series). Type II (subacute hematoma) with a homogeneous blood density represents 25% of our cases. Type III (chronic hematoma) with a low-density collection and a contrast-enhanced membrane represents 13%.

## Treatment

An injured child who develops an extradural hematoma can deteriorate quickly, especially young children. It is logical to recommend a clot evacuation in emergency. Trowbridge in 1954 and Burrres in 1979 express doubt about the need for craniotomy in patients with no objective deficits.

Weaver in 1981 mentions a spontaneous resolution of two epidural hematomas. Moreover, with the advent of CT a large number of extradural hematomas, sometimes extensive, have been discovered in children presenting mild symptoms and a normal level of consciousness.

Recently Pang has discussed the indication for immediate operative intervention in a series of 11 children who were neurologically normal. The extradural hematoma was discovered 4 hours to 6 days after the trauma. Nine children recovered without surgery and the resorption of the extradural clot was similar to that of the chronic subdural hematoma.

We do not deny the interest of such publications and it is true that some extradural hematomas can reasorb spontaneously without worsening of the clinical status. If we consider the low incidence of asymptomatic hematomas with normal consciousness in children and the large number of children who deteriorate rapidly, sometimes in a few minutes, especially in infancy, we are doubtful to promote a nonsurgical management of extradural hematomas. Such an attitude in neurosurgical centers which are sensitive to traumatic problems, could be dangerous in many others centers. Moreover, we must emphasize that there is no surgical mortality in cases of asymptomatic extradural hematomas in children.

## Surgical Treatment

We recommend a large bone flap in all cases since it is clear that burr holes are insufficient to evacuate a consolidated or extensive hematoma and inconvenient to find the bleeding point (Fig. 8). Nevertheless, we must emphasize that a burr hole can be useful in very acute cases, not only to discover an extradural hematoma but also to evacuate it, partially, before performing a bone flap. Seven children in our series have been saved with this technique. CT data will define the exact localization of the bone flap and its extension. After the skin opening it is possible to discover a skull fracture invisible in X-rays. After the opening of the bone flap the management of an extradural hematoma will follow four steps: evacuation of the clot, treatment of the bleeding point, detection of an associated brain lesion or a subdural collection by an incision of the dura and hanging of the dura to avoid a recurrence of the clot.

*Bleeding point* (Table 5). Usually the bleeding point is located, especially when the source is arterial. This occurs in 40 to 60% of the cases. The commonest source of bleeding is the posterior branch of the middle meningeal artery, more than the trunk of the meningeal artery. It is important to note that an arterial source of bleeding is not more frequent when a fracture is present.

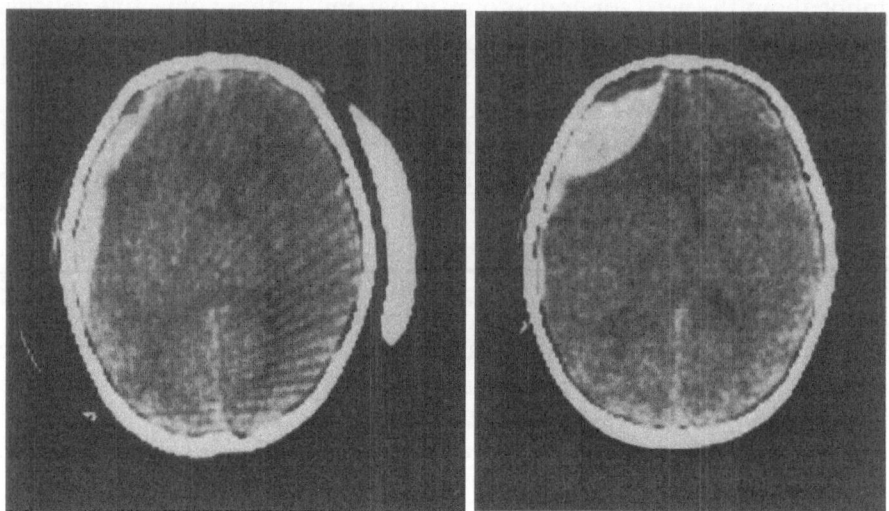

Fig. 8. Road accident in a 14-year-old boy. Drowsiness left cerebral contusions with an extradural hematoma. Burr hole drainage. One day later large frontal extradural hematoma

In a few cases there is a diffuse bleeding from the dura, sometimes along the course of meningeal vessels. In these cases a fracture is often the cause of a dural dilaceration. A dural bleeding point is found between 9 to 13% of the cases. Extradural hematoma of osseous origin only, is rare in the literature. Nevertheless, we have found in our series 20 cases (11.6%) with bleeding originated from a fracture, generally a large one. A venous origin of the bleeding, from a sinus or from an emissary veins, occurs in 7 to 11% of the cases. In our series we have 5 cases of extradural hematomas with a sinus lesion. In one case it was the sagittal sinus with a bilateral parietal hematoma. In the four other cases the hematomas were supra and infratentorially situated with a lesion of the lateral sinus.

*Associated lesions:* extradural hematomas can be associated with underlying lesions. In our series the incidence of an associated lesion is less important in children (26%), than in adults (40%). Mazza mentions an incidence of 38%.

Table 5. *Bleeding Points*

| | Meningeal artery | Dura | Osseous | Sinus vein | Unknown or not stated |
|---|---|---|---|---|---|
| Goutelle (25 cases) | 13 (52%) | | 2 (8%) | 3 (12%) | 7 |
| Matson (44 cases) | 26 (59%) | 6 (13.6%) | | 3 (6.8%) | 9 |
| Mazza (62 cases) | 37 (59%) | 4 (9%) | | 7 (11.2%) | 13 |
| Our series (172 cases) | 67 (39%) | 17 (10%) | 20 (11.6%) | 14 (8.1%) | 54 (31%) |

A brain contusion is present in 9.3% of our cases. Arseni mentions an incidence of 62% but in his series 65% of contusions are minor lesions. A subdural hematoma can be associated with brain contusion (in 16% for Mazza and 10% for us). A true subdural hematoma is more rare. A compounding of the fracture associated with an extradural hematoma is very exceptional (one case in our series). We have observed also a carotid cavernous fistula associated with a frontal hematoma.

Table 6. *Associated Lesions*

|  | Subdural hematoma | Subdural hematoma contusion | Contusion | Intracerebral hematoma |
|---|---|---|---|---|
| Goutelle 25 cases | 1 |  | 1 |  |
| Arseni 61 cases |  |  | 38 (62%) |  |
| Mazza 62 cases | 3 (4.8%) | 10 (16%) | 11 (17%) |  |
| Our series 172 cases | 11 (6.3%) | 18 (10.5%) | 16 (9.3%) |  |

*The volume* of the hematoma is not always in relation to the severity of the clinical manifestations, especially in infants. The volume of the hematoma is usually more important in infants than in older children. In addition, the hematoma is generally more voluminous in children than in adults. In our series we have found 56 (32.5%) very large hematomas (more than 150 cc), 81 (47%) extensive hematomas (100 cc) and 35 (20.5%) small hematomas.

## Results

The comparison of results from different series is difficult since the material from one to another is quite different. Many large series date from different periods and one must stress the results before CT and since the CT.

The overall mortality rate in the literature is shown in Table 7. Considering the major series, the true mortality during the first month after surgery is situated between 10 to 15 percent. There is no relation between age and mortality. Temporal and especially subtemporal hematomas have the highest mortality rate. In our series 50 percent of children with associated underlying brain lesions have had a fatal evolution. Mazza found nearly the same proportion (42 percent). In our series there is no significant difference in the mortality before the CT era and the present.

As stressed by other authors, morbidity is significantly lower in children and especially in patients under the age of 10. Factors for a bad prognosis are the clinical history (initial coma and short free interval), the presence of associated brain lesions, and the circumstances of trauma (especially the delay of transpiration, in cases of accident occurring far from a Neuro-surgical Department).

Table 7. *Mortality*

| | |
|---|---|
| McKissock | 7% |
| Goutelle | 12% |
| Fenelon | 9% |
| Gallagher | 8% |
| Masson | 9% |
| Harwood-Nash | 10% |
| Mazza | 17% |
| Our series | 14% |

In our series a mild secondary disability exists in 8 percent of the cases and a severe disability in 4 percent. It is interesting to note that EEG remains abnormal in 8 percent of patients (12 percent for Mazza), even if epileptic manifestations are rare.

## How It Should Be Done

*I. Posttraumatic extracranial hematomas* must be separated theoretical-ly, into subcutaneous (between the skin and the galea), subgaleal (between the galea and the periosteum) or cephalhematoma (between the periosteum and the skull). Diagnosis of these three varieties may be clinically difficult, except for cephalhematoma in neonates, when it presents as a bilateral, separated and parietal swelling of the scalp.

Practically these three types of "subcutaneous" hematomas are iden-tically managed, since puncture by needle or evacuation must be prohibited. Secondary infection is the main risk of a puncture.

An extensive hematoma in infants may cause anemia and a large aspiration of such a hematoma can worsen shock manifestations. Quite often the aspiration of a "subcutaneous" hematoma is followed by an immediate recurrence of the hemorrhage.

Consequently, these superficial hematomas are more often a visible manifestation of a head trauma, than a posttraumatic complication needing surgical management.

*II. Acute or subacute subdural hematomas in children* are much more rare than the classical chronic subdural hematoma. They are certainly more rare in children than in adults.

Generally they are localized in the supratentorial compartment, but posterior fossa subdural hematomas are not exceptional in children, especially in neonates after birth injury.

In the new-born, acute or subacute subdural hematomas may lead to signs of shock, distress, focal seizures and retinal hemorrhage. The CT scan will confirm the diagnosis and also the existence of an associated brain contusion.

In many cases emergency treatment is needed.

Subdural taps will be at the same time a method of diagnosis and a treatment. In acute cases or in neonates in bad conditions evacuation, by subdural tap of some quantity of blood could help to pass a critical period. In contrast with a chronic subdural effusion, a puncture of the fontanelle, can ignore an acute subdural hematoma located in the temporal or the parieto-occipital region.

In some cases a dense subdural hematoma will not be evacuated by a subdural tap and a trepan is necessary. It will permit a complete evacuation of the clot and a fluid drainage of the subdural space. In the majority of the cases a bone flap is not necessary.

*III. An extradural hematoma* in children must be evacuated in an emergency, especiall in young children. A spontaneous resolution of some epidural hematomas has been described but, considering that a child can suddenly deteriorate, we are doubtful of promoting a nonsurgical management of extradural hematomas.

Burr holes are insufficient to evacuate an extensive or a consolidated hematoma. Nevertheless a burr hole may be useful in very acute cases, to discover a hematoma and to evacuate it. In these cases the burr hole is situated in the lower temporal region over the meningeal vessels. In cases of absence of a hematoma another burr hole will be performed in the posterior-partietal region.

In other cases, when a CT scan has confirmed the diagnosis and given the exact situation and extension of the hematoma, a large bone flap will be done. Often a fracture is encountered at the level of the bone flap.

The four surgical stages are: evacuation of the clot, treatment of the bleeding point (arterial in 40 to 60 percent of the cases, dural in 10 percent, and osseous in 10 percent), detection of an associated brain lesion (subdural hematoma, brain contusion) and hanging of the dura to avoid a recurrence of the clot.

## References

1. Abroms, I. F., McLennan, J. E., Mandell, F., 1977: Acute neonatal subdural hematoma following breach delivery. Amer. J. Dis. Child. *131*, 192−194.
2. Adeloye, A., Odeku, I. E. L., 1975: Subgaleal hematoma in head injuries. Int. Surg. *60*, 263−265.
3. Alvarez-Garijo, J. A., Gomila, D. T., Aytes, A. P., Mengual, M. V., Martin, A. A., 1981: Subdural hematomas in neonates. Child's Brain *8*, 31−38.
4. Aoki, N., 1983: Epidural hematoma communication with cephalhematoma in a neonate. Neurosurgery *13*, 55−57.
5. Arkins, T. J., McLennan, J. E., Winston, K. R., Strand, R. D., Suzuki, Y., 1977: Acute posterior fossa epidural hematomas in children. Amer. J. Dis. Child. *131*, 690−692.
6. Arseni, C., Horvath, L., Ciurea, A. V., 1980: Patologia neurochirurgicala infantila. Editura academiei republicii socialiste. Romania 321−327.
7. Bricolo, A. P., Pasut, L. M., 1984: Extradural hematoma. Toward zero mortality. Neurosurgery *14*, 8−11.
8. Burres, K. P., Hamilton, R. D., 1979: Chronic extradural hematoma. Case report. Neurosurgery *4*, 60−62.
9. Caffey, J., 1946: Multiple fractures in the long bones of infants suffering from subdural hematomas. Amer. J. Roentg. *56*, 163.
10. Caffey, J., 1972: On the theory and practice of shaking infants. Amer. J. Dis. Child. *124*, 161.
11. Campbell, J. B., Cohen, J., 1951: Epidural hemorrhage and the skull of children. Surg. Gynec. Obstet. *92*, 257−280.
12. Cantu, R. C., 1971: Complications of long hair. Lancet 1−350.
13. Capon, N. B., 1922: Intracranial trauma in the newborn. J. Obstetrics and Gynaecology of the British Empire. *29*, 572−590.
14. Carcassonne, M., Choux, M., Grisoli, F., 1977: Extradural hematomas in infant. J. Pediat. Surg. *12*, 69−73.
15. Choux, M., Grisoli, F., Peragut, J. C., 1975: Extradural hematomas in children. 104 cases. Child's Brain *1*, 337−347.
16. Cervantes, L. A., 1983: Concurrent delayed temporal and posterior fossa epidural hematomas. J. Neurosurg. *59*, 351−353.
17. Coblentz, R. G., 1940: Cerebellar subdural hematoma in infant 2 weeks old with secondary hydrocephalus. Operation with recovery. Surgery *8*, 771−776.
18. Craig, W. S., 1938: Intracranial hemorrhage in the newborn. Arch. Dis. Child. *31*, 89.
19. Esparza, J., Portillo, J. M., Mateos, F., Lamas, E., 1982: Extradural hemorrhage in the posterior fossa in the neonate. Surg. Neurol. *17*, 341−343.
20. Faber, M., 1976: Massive subgaleal hemorrhage: a hazard of play-ground swings. Clin. Pediat. *15*, 384−385.
21. Falfo, Ce., San Filippo, J. A., Vartany, A., 1981: Subgaleal hematoma from hair combing. Pediatrics *68*, 583−584.
22. Fenelon, J., 1967: L'hématome extradural. Thèse Bordeaux, France.
23. Gerlach, J., Jensen, H. P., Koos, W., Kraus, H., 1967: Pedriatische Neurochirurgie. Stuttgart: G. Thieme.

24. Goutelle, A., Lapras, C., Dechaume, J. P., Chadensson, O., 1960: L'hématome extradural traumatique de l'enfant—à propos de 25 observations. Pediatrie *25*, 21–30.

25. Gresham, E. L., 1975: Birth trauma. Pediatrics clin. North. Amer. *22*, 317–328.

26. Guthkelch, A. N., 1971: Infantile subdural hematoma and its relationship to whiplash injuries. Brit. Med. J. 430.

27. Gutierriez, F. A., Raimondi, A. J., 1975: Acute subdural hematoma in infancy and childhood. Child's Brain *1*, 269–290.

28. Hahn, Y. S., Raimondi, A. J., McLone, D. G., Yamanouchi, Y., 1983: Traumatic mechanisms of head injury in child abuse. Child's Brain *10*, 229–241.

29. Hamlin, H., 1968: Subgaleal hematoma caused by hairpull. JAMA *204*, 129.

30. Harwood-Nash, D. C., 1973: Cranio-cerebral trauma in children. Current Prob. in Radiol. *3*, 11–42.

31. Hayakawa, I., Fujiwara, K., 1985: Acute traumatic subdural hematoma in children and its late results after surgery. Child's Brain (in preparation).

32. Hendrick, E. B., Harwood-Nash, D. C. F., Hudson, A. R., 1964: Head injuries in children: a survey of 4,465 consecutive cases at the hospital for thick children, Toronto, Canada. Clin. Neurosurg. *II*, 46–65.

33. Ingraham, F. D., Matson, D. D., 1944: Subdural hematoma in infancy. J. Pediat. *24*, 3–37.

34. Iwakuma, T., Brunngraber, C. V., 1973: Chronic extradural hematomas; a study of 21 cases. J. Neurosurg. *38*, 488–493.

35. Jamieson, K. G., Yelland, J. D. N., 1968: Extradural hematoma report of 167 cases. J. Neurosurg. *29*, 13–23.

36. Kaufman, H. K., Sadhu, V. K., Handel, S. F., Cohen, G., 1980: Isodense acute subdural hematoma. J. Comput. Assist. Tomogr. *4*, 557–559.

37. Kempe, C. H., Silverman, F. N., Steele, B. F., Drogenmueller, W., Silver, H. K., 1962: The battered child syndrome. J. Amer. Med. Ass. *181*, 17–24.

38. Kendall, N., Woloshin, H., 1952: Cephalhematoma associated with fracture of the skull. J. Pediat. *41*, 125–132.

39. Kuban, K., Winston, K., Bresnan, M., 1983: Childhood subgaleal hematoma following minor head trauma. Amer. J. Dis. Child. *137*, 637–640.

40. Larroche, J. C., 1977: Developmental Pathology of the Neonates. Amsterdam: Excerpta Medica.

41. McClelland, C. Q., Rekate, H., Kafman, B., Persse, L., 1980: Cerebral injury in child abuse: a changing profile. Child's Brain *7*, 225–235.

42. McHenry, T., Girdany, B. R., Elmer, E., 1963: Unsuspected trauma with multiple skeletal injuries during infancy and childhood. Pediatrics *31*, 903.

43. McKissock, W., Taylor, J. C., Bloom, W. T., Till, K., 1960: Extradural hematoma: Observations on 125 cases. The Lancet *2*, 167–172.

44. McLaurin, R. L., Ford, L. E., 1964:: Extradural hematoma. Statistical survey of 47 cases. J. Neurosurg. *21*, 364–371.

45. Matson, D. D., 1969: Neurosurgery of Infancy and Childhood, ed. 2, pp. 316–327. Springfield, Ill.: Ch. C Thomas.

46. Mazza, C., Pasqualin, A., Feriotti, G., da Pian, R., 1982: Traumatic extradural heamatomas in children. Experience with 62 cases. Acta Neurochir. (Wien) *65*, 67 – 80.

47. Mealey, J. R., 1968: Pediatric Head Injuries. Springfield, Ill.: Ch. C Thomas.

48. Merry, C. J., Stuart, G., 1979: Extradural hematoma in the neonate. Case report. J. Neurosurg. *51*, 713 – 717.

49. Mori, K., Handa, H., Munemitsu, H., Oda, Y., Hashimoto, N., Kojima, M., 1983: Epidural hematomas of the posterior fossa in children. Child's Brain *10*, 130 – 140.

50. Ommaya, A. K., Faas, F., Yarnell, P., 1968: Whiplash injury and brain damage. J. Amer. Med. Ass. *204*, 285.

51. Pang, D., Horton, J. A., Herron, J. M., Wilberger, J. E., Vries, J. K., 1983: Nonsurgical management of extradural hematomas in children. J. Neurosurg. *59*, 958 – 971.

52. Pape, K. E., Wigglesworth, J. S., 1979: Hemorrhage Ischemia and the Prenatal brain. Suffolk, England: Lakenham Press 61-75 LTD.

53. Parkinson, D., Hunt, B., Shields, C., 1971: Double lucid interval in patients with extradural hematomas of the posterior fossa. J. Neurosurg. *34*, 534 – 536.

54. Ponte, C., Remy, J., Christiaens, J. L., Bonte, C., Lacombe, A., Lefevre, P., 1971: Hematomes intra-cérébral et sous-dural chez un nouveau-né. Arch. Franç. Pediat. *28*, 267 – 276.

55. Potter, E. L., Craig, J. M., 1976: Pathology of the Fetus and the Infant. Chicago Year Book Medical, Publ. London: Lloyd-Luke.

56. Robinson, R. J., Rossiter, M. A., 1968: Massive subaponeurotic hemorrhage in babies of African origin. Arch. Dis. Child. *43*, 684 – 687.

57. Rosenvonn, J., Gjerris, F., 1978: Long-term follow-up review of patients with acute and subacute subdural hematomas. J. Neurosurg. *48*, 345 – 349.

58. Saeki, N., Hinokuma, K., Vemura, K., Makino, H., 1979: Subacute bilateral epidural hematoma in an infant. Surg. Neurol. *11*, 67 – 69.

59. Schipke, R., Reige, D., Scoville, W., 1954: Acute subdural hemorrhage at birth. *14*, 468 – 474.

60. Schwartz, P., 1961: Birth Injuria of the New-born. Basel: S. Karger.

61. Scott, M., 1936: Non traumatic spontaneous subaponeurotic hematoma its probable relation to atypical scurvy. JAMA *107*, 348 – 350.

62. Shapiro, K., 1983: Pediatric Head Trauma. Futura Publishing Comp. N. Y.

63. Sjovall, A., 1936: Le cephalhématome des nouveaux-nés. Acta Obstet. Gynec. Scand. *15*, 443.

64. Sparacio, R. R., Khatib, R., Cook, A. W., 1971: Acute subdural hematoma in infancy. N. Y. State J. Med. *71*, 212 – 213.

65. Stanley, L., Bascour, A., 1961: Giant cephalhematoma of newborn. Amer. J. Dis. Child. *101*, 170 – 173.

66. Sulama, M., Vera, P., 1952: An investigation into the occurrence of perinatal subdural hematoma; its diagnosis and treatment. Acta Obstet. Gynecol. Scand. *31*, 400 – 412.

67. Suzuki, J., Aihara, H., Suzuki, S., 1970: Investigation of acute subdural hematoma in infancy. Brain Nerve *22*, 43 – 50.

68. Svendsen, V., 1972: Epidural hematoma in children. Excerpta Medica Neurology and Neurosurg. *25*, 462−463.
69. Takagi, T., Nagai, R., Wakabayah, S., Mizawa, I., Hayashi, K., 1978: Extradural hemorrhage in the newborn as a result of birth trauma. Child's Brain *4*, 306−318.
70. Takagi, T., Fuluoka, H., Wakabayashi, S., Nagai, H., Shibata, H. T., 1982: Posterior fossa subdural hemorrhage in the newborn as a result of birth trauma. Child's Brain *9*, 102−113.
71. Tan, K. L., 1970: Cephalhematoma. Aust. N. Z. J. Obstet. Gynecol. *10*, 101.
72. Till, K., 1968: Subdural hematoma and effusion in infancy. Brit. Med. J. 400−402.
73. Trowbridge, W. V., Porter, R. W., French, J. D., 1954: Chronic extradural hematomas. Arch. Surg. *69*, 824−830.
74. Zander, E., Campiche, R., 1974: Extradural hematoma. Advances and Technical Standards in Neurosurgery (Krayenbühl, H., *et al.*, eds.), Vol. 1, pp. 121−139. Wien-New York: Springer.
75. Zelson, C., Lee, S. J., Pearl, M., 1974: The incidence of skull fractures underlying cephalhematoma in newborn infants. J. Pediat. *85*, 371−373.
76. Zimmerman, R. A., Bilaniuk, L. T., 1981: Computed tomography in pediatric head trauma. J. Neuroradiol. *6*, 332−341.
77. Zimmerman, R. A., Bilaniuk, L. T., 1982: Computed tomographies staging of traumatic epidural bleeding. Radiology *144*, 809−812.
78. Zucarello, M., Pardatscher, K., Andrioli, G. C., 1981: Epidural hematomas of the posterior cranial fossa. Neurosurgery *8*, 434−437.

# Intracranial Pressure Monitoring: Theory and Practice

L. F. MARSHALL

Division of Neurosurgery H-893, University of California Medical Center,
San Diego, California (U.S.A.)

With 7 Figures

## Contents

Intracranial dynamics have been of interest to scientists and clinicians for more than two hundred years. Descriptions of the factors governing the relationship between pressure and volume within a closed space such as the head have been the subject of a large body of both experimental and clinical investigation which has contributed much to our understanding of pathological states of increased intracranial pressure (ICP).

It is appropriate to begin with the tremendous contributions of Monro and Kellie who described the relationship of volume and pressure within the intracranial space[9, 24]. Based on these observations, Burrows sometime later concluded that the volume within the intracranial space can in fact change under a variety of conditions and that these changes must in order to be compensated for be accompanied by reciprocal changes in the volume of those compartments in which such changes can occur, *i.e.,* the cerebral spinal fluid, the brain tissue itself and, most frequently, brain blood volume[4]. Early in the twentieth century, Cushing in a classic monograph described the relationship between heart rate, blood pressure and what he termed intracranial tension[5]. Finally, Weed *et al.,* carried out a series of experiments which were designed to test the Monro-Kellie doctrine[32]. When these experiments were reported, the scientific basis for much that has transpired since had been developed.

The application of the basic pathophysiology to clinical practice was brought about primarily by the efforts of workers in two countries, *i.e.,* Lundberg working in Sweden and Guillaume and Janny working in France[7, 15]. When these investigators demonstrated that the ICP could be safely measured and continuously recorded for prolonged periods, the modern era of ICP research had begun.

Lundberg's accomplishments were many, but perhaps the two most important were[1] his demonstration that ICP monitoring could be performed safely for long periods of time and[2] that extremely useful information about dynamic changes within the intracranial space was easily obtained from this simple measurement. Lundberg described several types of changes in ICP which he called waves. A waves are those that are almost certainly due to fluctuations in brain blood volume and are characterized by steep increases in ICP to a plateau lasting from 2 to 15 minutes and during which the ICP rises from 15 to 50 mm Hg. In our experience, following such pressure waves the ICP does not return to baseline but appears to be set at a level slightly above that point. Lundberg hypothesized that these waves would warn of potentially fatal changes in ICP and that plateau waves were indicants of the patient having reached a point on the volume pressure curve (Fig. 1) where even small increases in intracranial volume would result in herniation and irreversible brain damage. The classical relationship for volume and pressure demonstrated in the curve illustrates the fact that initially with small increments in volume there is little change in pressure within the intracranial space but that, at some point, the spatial reserves of the intracranial compartment are completely utilized and even a small further increase in volume results in a dramatic rise in ICP. This compensatory capacity of the intracranial space has been called its compliance. Thus, as the volume within the intracranial space increases, the compliance decreases.

The second wave that Lundberg described are B waves which are characterized by much shorter and much less dramatic rises in ICP. They appear to be fluctuations associated with respiration and are clearly pathological. Finally, Lundberg describes C waves or what have been subsequently termed arterial Traube-Herring waves. While most consider them to be of less significance, as more aggressive therapy for intracranial hypertension became more common these waves as well as the steepness of the pulse pressure have been relied upon by some to indicate the need for more aggressive therapy.

Following on the work of Lundberg and Guillaume and Janny, Langfitt, in the mid1960s, began to describe the response of the brain to intracranial

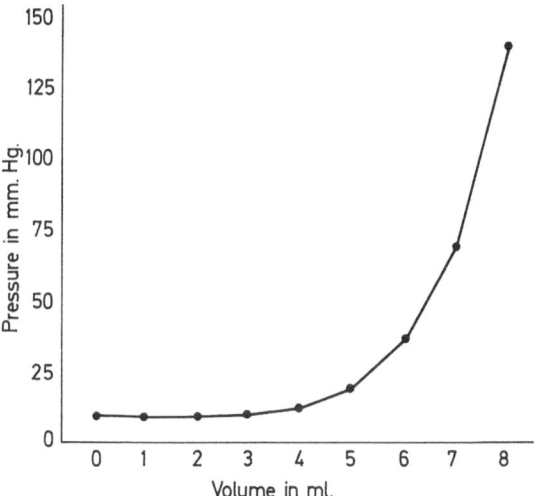

Fig. 1. The classical relationship between volume and pressure is illustrated

mass lesions[12, 13]. He demonstrated that brain swelling occurred frequently following the "evacuation" of such mass lesions. The possibility that ICP could become elevated because of brain swelling following removal of an intracranial mass was a relatively new concept. ICP elevations occurring after the brain had been decompressed raised the possibility that the detection of such events would not occur until irreversible signs of brainstem compression had occurred and that ICP monitoring which had been shown to be safe might be useful in detecting premonitory rises in ICP prior to irreversibly fatal ones.

Since that time literally thousands of articles have been published on intracranial dynamics and ICP. The proliferation of articles was a reflection of the fact that clinical interest in the measurement of ICP increased tremendously as did interest in the role of therapy for intracranial hypertension. Prior to the early 1970s ICP rises were treated almost universally on the basis of clinical grounds and often when signs of transtentorial herniation such as pupillary dilitation or major disturbances in ventilation had already occurred. The elaboration by Miller on the previous work of Ayala and Lofgren on volume/pressure relationships demonstrated that patients could be at risk who appeared to be in relatively good clinical states and this further peaked the interest of neurosurgeons monitoring ICP[1, 14, 22].

Miller developed quantitative descriptions of each patient's volume/pressure relationship (the VPR). In the initial description, 1.0 cc of fluid was rapidly injected through a ventricular catheter into the ventricle and the rise in one second in ICP which this produced was recorded. If the ICP is in excess of 20–25 mm Hg, this test should not be utilized as the introduction of even a small volume of fluid might precipitate catastrophe in such patients. Initially, it was felt that when a rise of less than 3–4 mm Hg was elicited in response to the 1 cc fluid challenge that one could conclude that the patient had quite good cerebral compliance implying that there was at least some reserve before decompensation would occur. In some instances, however, our clinical experience suggested that smaller volume pressure changes are significant. This has been particularly true in patients treated with high doses of barbiturates for uncontrolled intracranial hypertension and in whom satisfactory control of the ICP had thought to have been achieved. Thus while on theoretical grounds the volume pressure relationship is extremely useful, it has been somewhat less helpful in the clinical setting.

Despite the clinical limitations of the volume pressure response, the fact that patients who appeared clinically "safe" from intracranial hypertension might be in jeopardy further increased the interest of neurosurgeons in ICP monitoring. Although some continued to argue that the utility of ICP monitoring has been exaggerated and that patients could be managed equally well without ICP monitoring, such arguments appeared illogical based on the fact that the pressure within the intracranial space cannot be known without measurements and that premonitory rises are often seen before fatal plateau waves. This does not mean that monitoring should be unintelliently applied nor that all patients with significant neurosurgical problems require monitoring. Rather, if ICP elevations are likely to complicate the course of a patient with a significant head injury and such ICP changes need therapy, ICP recording can be extremely useful to rationally guide therapy and avoid potential iatrogenic errors. It is the purpose of this discussion to describe the techniques of ICP monitoring and their clinical applications.

However, before dealing with the techniques of ICP monitoring, it appears appropriate to delineate some of the theoretical problems as well as issues which have arisen as ICP monitoring has evolved. Despite the large body of work published which supports the utility of ICP monitoring in the management of severely head injured patients, there is still hesitancy on the part of many neurosurgeons to monitor ICP. This is due, in part, to the invasiveness of the procedure and also because ICP is not elevated in all instances of head injury, which has made some neurosurgeons reluctant to monitor patients unless they could be relatively certain that targeted populations could be identified. Thus, those of us in the academic neurosurgical community have been forced, and appropriately so, to generate specific requirements that should be met prior to the institution of ICP monitoring. While such requirements apply to monitoring in general, they are especially well suited to judging the appropriateness of ICP monitoring in brain injury.

## Prerequisites for Monitoring

The first requirement that must be met by any monitoring tool is that the parameter to be measured plays an important role in the pathophysiology of the disease process. Miller and Becker demonstrated some years ago that ICPs in excess of 20 mm Hg, which using standard methods could not be controlled, had always proved to be fatal in patients suffering severe head injury[23]. Over one half of the fatalities in the Richmond series published in 1977 were the result of uncontrolled ICP and in our experience one half of the fatalities from head injury were also due to uncontrolled ICP[17]. Of the approximately 35,000 patients who suffer severe head injury and die in hospitals in the United States, approximately one half will die from elevated ICP. Thus, the first requirement for monitoring, namely that the parameter to be measured plays an extremely important role in determining the outcome in patients with severe head injuries has been met.

The second requirement is that the monitoring technique to be utilized is reliable and has few false negatives and false positives. This criteria is certainly met by the intraventricular catheter and, in experienced hands, by the subarachnoid screw although, as we discuss later, there is a higher failure rate with the latter device.

Third, abnormalities in the parameter to be measured must be sufficiently frequent to justify patient invasion. Bruce and his colleagues, in a large series of pediatric head injuries, demonstrated that 80% of the patients had elevated ICP which required therapy[3]. In a more recent preliminary report, Eisenberg, in reviewing the experience of the National Pilot Traumatic Coma Data Bank, noted that over half of the patients in this national collaborative study had ICPs of over 30 mm Hg some time during their course[6]. Thus, one can conclude that ICP elevations are very frequent in severely head injured patients and this satisfies the third requirement.

The fourth requirement is that there be no noninvasive method available to detect elevations in ICP. Although CT scanning is extremely useful in assessing the structural integrity of the brain and can further delineate specific subsets of patients with severe head injury who are likely to have high ICP, CAT scanning is not absolutely reliable and it lacks the dynamic characteristics which are available from continuous ICP monitoring.

Our own experience and that of others has clearly shown that reliance on the vital signs to detect changes in ICP is completely unreliable[16]. In patients in whom the ICP exceeded 30 mm Hg, changes in the vital signs which would have been useful in guiding ICP therapy occurred in less than 25% of the patients. It is obvious that, at least in theory, a noninvasive method to continuously record the ICP would be extremely desirable. To date, radiotelemetric devices which sit on the outside of the skull have not shown the reliability necessary for long term patient management. Furthermore, the intraventricular catheter allows for ventricular drainage, a technique which is frequently useful and occasionally life saving in patients with elevated ICP. Thus, there are potential disadvantages of a noninvasive method of ICP monitoring which does not permit ventricular drainage.

The fifth and final requirement is that the technique to be utilized be sufficiently safe that the risk is substantially less than the benefit to be derived. Although the specific complications of ICP monitoring are discussed later, it is important to note here that in our experience and in the experience of others the risks of ICP monitoring have been quite low and, therefore, one can say with a reasonable degree of certainty that the risk benefit ratio is significantly shifted toward the benefit side.

### Indications for Monitoring

The largest experience in continuous monitoring of the ICP has been in patients suffering head injury. Thus, it is in this group of patients that criteria for monitoring have been best defined. Most neurosurgeons with a large trauma experience have advocated continuous monitoring of the ICP in patients in whom the Glasgow Coma Scale score is 8 or less following resuscitation. These patients have been shown to be at substantial risk of dying with a reported mortality rate of approximately 10–25% in patients with Coma Scale scores of 8 and mortality progressively increasing as the severity of injury increases.

We have modified this philosophy by ommiting monitoring in patients in whom the Coma Scale score is 7 or 8 and in whom the CT scan is normal, provided that those patients have no other major system injuries. In our experience and that of the group in Richmond, these patients have an extremely low incidence of intracranial hypertension, certainly less than 5%, and, thus, the risk approaches the potential benefit[10]. The CT scan must, however, be entirely normal. In Fig. 2 the basal cisterns as they are seen under normal circumstances are shown. In Fig. 3, a compressed basal cistern, often the sole radiographic sign of intracranial hypertension present

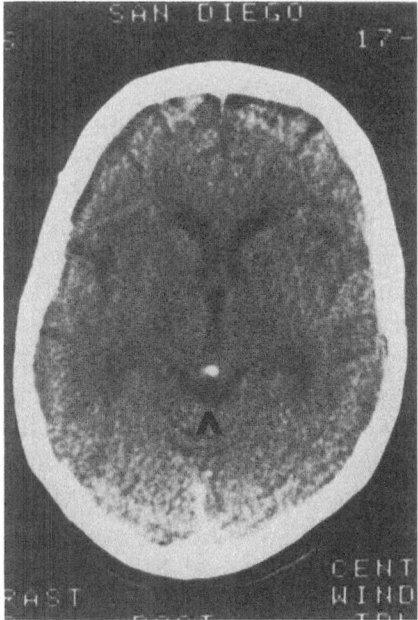

Fig. 2. Normal basal cisterns are shown

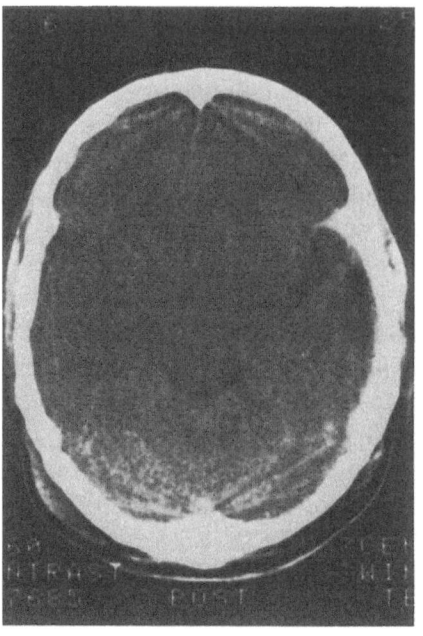

Fig. 3. The basal cisterns are compressed when compared to Fig. 2. This indicates a substantial risk of elevated ICP

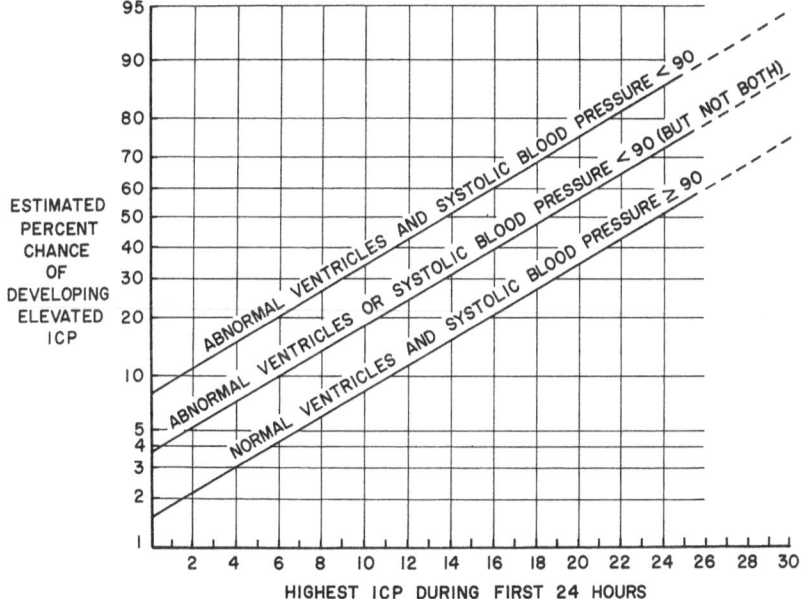

Fig. 4. The influence of systemic hypotension and asymetrical ventricles on delayed elevations of ICP are shown

or pending, is shown. If the basal cisterns are well seen and there is no evidence of shift or brain contusion, then monitoring, in our view, is not likely to aid management. We must emphasize, however, that in patients in whom systolic hypotension or hypoxia have occurred prior to or during resuscitation, that ICP monitoring is necessary. In a recent publication, Klauber et al., have demonstrated that the presence of ventricular asymmetry and of systolic hypotension during the first 24 hours following injury increases the probability of the ICP exceeding 30 mm Hg 24 to 72 hours following injury substantially[11]. This is illustrated in Fig. 4. In a relatively brief report, Harr, in a series of patients in whom blood gases were collected prior to hospitalization, demonstrated that prehospital hypoxia was associated with a much greater frequency of late ICP rises as well as with much higher ultimate ICPs[8]. One must take great care, therefore, in the selection of patients with severe head injuries in whom monitoring can be excluded and the admonitions regarding patients who have suffered systemic compromise following their injury must be heeded.

It is also appropriate to note that monitoring should be omitted in patients who are considered to be untreatable because of the severity of their head injury. We will not monitor patients whom we do not intend to treat vigorously. Such a decision does not rest on the absence of brain stem reflexes and motor flaccidity, rather we depend on the overall prognosis of the patient and may choose not to monitor an elderly patient where overwhelming systems injuries are present.

## Is ICP Monitoring Clinically Useful?

Despite the worldwide increase in ICP monitoring in the care of head injured patients, debate continues unabated regarding the clinical utility of such monitoring. Publications have recently appeared reporting mortalities in unmonitored patients similar to those reported from institutions which practiced aggressive therapy for intracranial hypertension based on ICP monitoring[26]. In part this debate is somewhat spurious as those institutions reporting good results without monitoring have not been subjected to the intense scrutiny of the major head injury centers and the series reported have been relatively small. Moreover, there is some large body of evidence which suggests that not only does the rational management of intracranial hypertension improve outcome, but that the incidence of uncontrolled ICP, which in our experience has almost invariably lead to fatality, can be substantially lowered with early treatment[2].

Evidence that one cannot determine the level of ICP which is potentially deleterious for an individual patient comes from several sources. The recent demonstration from our group that the oval pupil (Fig. 5) is a transitional sign indicating brain stem compression because of transtentorial herniation is of interest as almost one half of the patients in whom this finding developed had ICPs under 30 mm Hg. In fact, three patients had ICPs of less than 20 mm Hg. Once we recognized the probability of brain stem compression in such cases at low pressure we became much more aggressive in the therapy of these patients and treated them at levels of 15–20 mm Hg in order to avoid this ominous sign. Since that time it has become evident that there are patients who will tolerate only extremely modest levels of intracranial hypertension and that they need early aggressive therapy to produce good control of the ICP. Bellegarrigue and Ducker, in reviewing

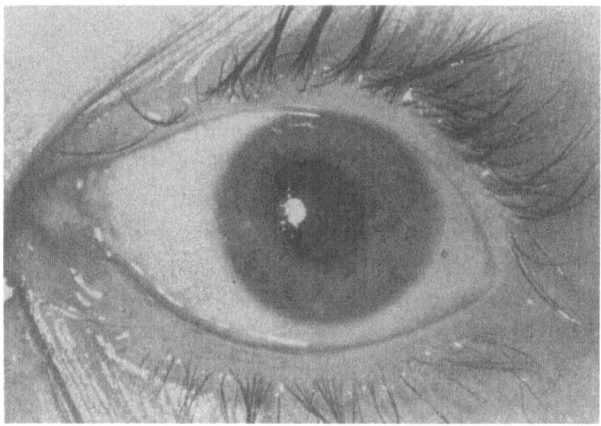

Fig. 5. The oval pupil associated with modest elevations is shown

the experience at the Maryland Institute of Emergency Medicine, observed that the incidence of intracranial hypertension exceeding 25 mm Hg fell from 34% in their initial series to 12% in their latest series[2]. As there is a direct correlation between the ability to reduce the ICP below 25 mm Hg and outcome, it is extremely tempting to conclude that the policy of earlier intervention, *i.e.,* therapy for ICP above 25 mm Hg in the first series and at pressures above 15 mm Hg in the last series was responsible for the improved outcomes reported.

If this conclusion is correct, it is further support for the utility of ICP monitoring. Certainly one could not begin therapy at these levels if one does not measure the ICP. Clinical signs in the comatose head injured patient are not likely to be useful to detect relatively small rises in ICP above 15 mm Hg. Furthermore, the use of sedation and muscle relaxants has become common in order to allow for improved ventilation and the blunting of noxious stimuli in such patients and is another reason why ICP monitoring is necessary. If one needs to sedate and ventilate these patients, the clinical examination is lost and ICP monitoring provides a reliable guide to intracranial events. For example, modest rises in ICP can be the first sign of a delayed traumatic intracranial hematoma. Thus, for the forgoing reasons, it appears that the use of intracranial pressure monitoring is emminently logical, defensible and necessary.

## ICP Monitoring and the Decision to Operate

The Glasgow group has emphasized the utility of ICP monitoring in deciding whether to operate[27]. They showed in patients with acute traumatic intracranial hematomas that if the ICP exceeds 30 mm Hg that surgical intervention was almost always necessary. In contrast, in those patients in whom the ICP remained below 20, surgical intervention was not required. This is one rational application of ICP monitoring. However, there are some potential perils with this approach. There is increasing evidence that the location of a mass lesion, and not necessarily the highest level of ICP reached, is an important and potentially crucial factor in some patients which will determine the need for surgery. Specifically, isolated frontal contusions producing modest elevations in ICP may be much less dangerous than an equivalent lesion in the medial portion of the temporal lobe. We have observed this on several occasions and have decided to operate on patients with shifts of approximately 4–5 mm when the temporal lobe was involved, but have decided to wait in patients with mass lesions in the parietal lobe, for example, when the shift is between 5–7 mm. This clinical application of the CT scan results is important because ICP monitoring should not be seen as a tool in isolation.

## ICP Monitoring and the CT Scan

Recently, Van Dongen and his colleagues in the Netherlands have demonstrated that the appearance of the basal cisterns on the initial and subsequent CT scans is an extremely important predictor of outcome[28]. Furthermore, we have utilized the appearance of the basal cisterns to predict the likelihood of elevated ICP[28]. In that report from our Center, Toutant *et al.*, described the frequency of differing basal cistern appearance in 256 consecutive patients entered into the National Pilot Traumatic Coma Data Bank. There was a striking and progressive increase in the frequency of ICP in excess of 30 mm Hg as the appearance of the basal cisterns changed from present to absent. However, this correlation was not absolute and almost 30% of patients who had basal cisterns present on the initial CT scan had ICPs in excess of 30 mm Hg. Thus, while we as well as others are attempting to further define clinical and radiographic observations that can be used to identify patients at particular risk from elevated ICP, we have not yet reached the stage where monitoring can be omitted in the population of patients with severe head injury. One can say with a reasonable degree of certainty that the overwhelming majority of patients who have compressed or absent basal cisterns will have pathological rises in ICP which require therapy and that in these groups ICP must be monitored.

## Monitoring Techniques

The long experience and the reliability of the ventricular catheter make it the procedure of choice for the continual recording of ICP. Many neurosurgeons are somewhat reluctant to utilize intraventricular cannulation because of the risk of infection from penetration of the dura and the brain. While this is certainly a legitimate concern in the hands of those who use ICP monitoring only occasionally, for the experienced neurotraumatologist this should not be a major issue. While the ventricles can be substantially shifted and are often small, they are easily entered in approximately 95% of patients.

It is extremely important to follow a standard regimen for both placement and care of a ventricular catheter. After the appropriate area, usually the right frontal region, of the head has been shaved and prepared, we anaesthesize the skin with 1% Xylocaine with $1/_{100,000}$ Norepinephrine. The catheter is always placed, unless there is scalp injury at the site, 3 cm lateral to the sagittal sinus and directly over the coronal suture. Using a small hand held twist drill containing an $^{11}/_{64}$ inch bit cut short to prevent plunging, the skull and the dura are perforated. Others utilize a large gauge needle or a curved currette to open the dura. The catheter is then introduced into the ventricle with the catheter tip directed somewhat medially. A useful landmark is the inner canthus of the eye. We always tunnel the catheter subcutaneously (Fig. 6) and secure it in place with several 4.0 silk sutures. Zeroing of the transducer should be carried out at the level of the lateral ventricle, which can be estimated with the head in the supine position as a point 2 cm above the right ear. The transducer should be moved with the head in order to allow for accurate recording if the head is elevated or lowered.

Infection, which is the major hazard of the placement of intraventricular catheters, can be limited if meticulous care of the catheter is taken and a sterile occlusive dressing carefully applied. One should not attempt to enter the ventricles with an intraventricular catheter if three passes have failed to deliver CSF. The risk of a complication from brain penetration increases substantially with each pass and, based on our own experience, if one

cannot easily enter the ventricle it is unlikely that useful information will be
obtained from further passes.

Under some circumstances, ventricular cannulation is not appropriate.
If the ventricles cannot be visualized on CT or are extremely small and the
neurosurgeon caring for the patient feels that ventricular cannulation will
be difficult, a variety of epidural devices or the subarachnoid bold are very

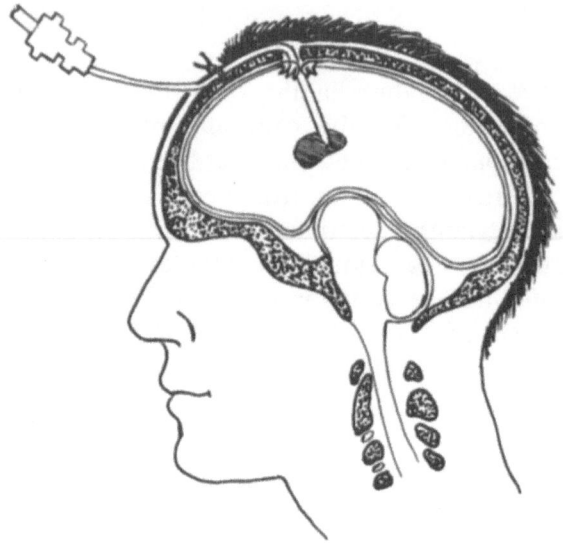

Fig. 6. The method for tunnelling of the ventricular catheter is illustrated

suitable alternatives. The subarachnoid bolt, developed by the Richmond
group in the early 1970s, is a hollow metal or plastic screw, which can be
placed through the exact same twist drill hole used for ventricular
cannulation[30]. It is dependent on open communication between the
subarachnoid space and the transducer. Thus, it is extremely important that
the dura be well perforated when this device is used. The screw offers the
advantage of not requiring brain penetration and this is reflected in the fact
that the infection rate with the subarachnoid screw is extremely low. The
subarachnoid screw must be placed on the side of the greatest swelling, not
on the contralateral side, a frequent choice for ventricular cannulation.
Once the subarachnoid bolt is in place it may require flushing to remove
debris and blood which can accumulate. This can be done initially when the
subarachnoid bolt is first introduced by flushing it directly using a small
syringe and a 22 gauge needle. Once the device is in place, however, there is
danger in introducing large volumes of fluid into the subarachnoid space.

Flushing should be carried out only by experienced personnel, and extremely small volumes, usually 0.1–0.2 cc, should be initially used. Periodic flushing, in the absence of signs of subarachnoid bolt malfunction, should be avoided.

Placement of the subarachnoid bolt through a closely fitting twist drill hole is extremely important. The device can be dislodged if it is not firmly

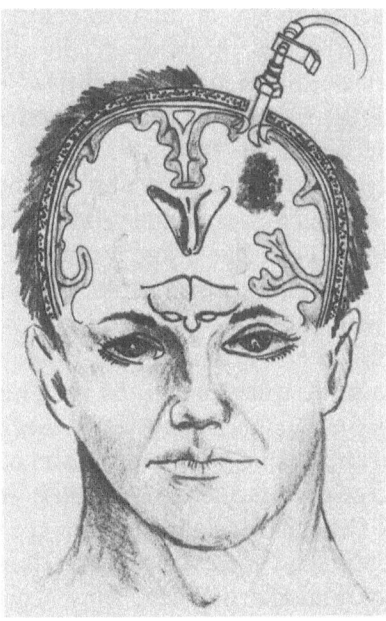

Fig. 7. The coplanar application and need for dural perforation for placement of the subarachnoid screw is shown. Note that the device is placed on the same side as the lesion

fixed into the skull and this may result not only in actual loss of the device but also in the production of false readings which may lull the nurse or physician caring for the patient into a false sense of security. It is critical that the twist drill hole be placed directly perpendicular to the dura in order to ensure that coplanar application of the hollow orifice and the subarachnoid space is obtained (Fig. 7). Aperture occlusion is much more frequent when coplanar application has not been obtained. Transducer placement is at the level of the skull, directly adjacent to the site of application. This differs from that recommended with a ventricular catheter. However, as with the ventricular catheter, the transducer should be moved if the head is raised or lowered.

In a search for improved devices to continually monitor ICP, several epidural devices have been introduced. This subject has been carefully reviewed by Wilkinson[33]. The most promising of these is the Gaeltec intracranial catheter tip pressure transducer (Medical Measurements, Inc., Hackensack, New Jersey 07601). This device has a pressure sensing diaphragm at the tip which functions as a strain gauge. A unique feature of the Gaeltec epidural device is that it can be accurately calibrated in vivo. The major disadvantage of this device is that it must be placed through a burr hole which makes the procedure somewhat more cumbersome than that required for the placement of an intraventricular catheter or sub-arachnoid screw. Nevertheless, because of the high level of reliability reported with this device and the occasional need to monitor ICP in the post-operative period, the fact that it requires a burr hole for placement is not a severely limiting factor.

The Ladd fiber optic transducer, which has been the most popular epidural device in the United States, utilizes rather small fiber optic cables to continuously record ICP. It also has the advantage of relative simplicity, but the disadvantage of requiring a burr hole for placement and, from a technical standpoint, an increased rate of drift when compared to the ventricular catheter or the Gaeltec device. The technique is relatively expensive, as the fiber optic tubes cannot be used reliably more than once. As with other epidural or subarachnoid devices, the fiber optic catheter does not permit ventricular drainage. Another epidural monitor which has been relatively recently introduced is the cup catheter. As the epidural devices become more reliable they will increasingly replace the subarachnoid bolt because they do not require penetration of the dura. It is also likely that these devices will become smaller allowing for placement through a bedside twist drill.

### Contraindications to ICP Monitoring

As neurosurgeons have become increasingly skilled in the placement of ICP monitoring devices, contraindications in the head injured population have continued to fall. As we have indicated previously, patients in whom the prognosis is hopeless should not be monitored.

Furthermore, those individuals who have evidence of severe dissemi-nated intravascular coagulopathy certainly should not be monitored with a ventricular cannula. We are reluctant to monitor ICP if the platelet count has fallen to less than 100,000, the prothrombin time is greater than twice normal or if the partial thromboplastin time is substantially increased. Under circumstances where more modest disturbances of coagulation are present we have elected to perform the procedure for placement of monitoring devices in the operating theater as opposed to our usual practice of placing it at the patient's bedside. This is because suction and better lighting are available in the operating room. Meticulous technique with perfect hemostasis is required. In patients who have substantial clotting disturbances, the release of brain tissue thromboplastin, although small from the placement of a monitoring device, may be enough to exacerbate disseminated intravascular coagulopathy. While such severe coagulation disturbances are rare, even in patients with severe head injury, this condition must be rigorously looked for in order to avoid a major iatrogenic complication.

### Technical Complications of Intracranial Pressure Monitoring

Complications resulting from the placement of ICP monitoring devices should be considered under two main categories: 1. infection[25] and 2. inaccurate or failed pressure data.

Certainly with the ventricular cannula the major risk is that of infection. In a recent study, Mayhall *et al.,* at the Medical College of Virginia, reported an infection rate of approximately 11% in patients in whom the ICP was continuously monitored using the ventricular cannula[19]. From that study several very useful suggestions regarding the use of ventricular cannulas were made. If this device is used, a new twist drill should be placed and the catheter changed every five days. This is a reflection of the fact that risk of infection increases substantially with increasing time of catheter placement and that changing the catheter appears to restart the clock in such patients. In our own hands, the risk of infection with a ventricular catheter is less than 5% with a ventricular catheter. We have had only one fatal infection in the last six years. In an additional 2 patients, infection was responsible for persistent hydrocephalus which required shunting, in the others the infections were benign and treated by removal of the catheter and a ten day course of intravenous antibiotics. Staphylococcus epidermatis continues to be the most frequent organism cultured in such patients. Unfortunately, there is no evidence that prophylactic antibiotics reduce the risk of infection in patients in whom a ventricular catheter is employed. While most centers routinely utilize such prophylaxis, a controlled clinical trial would be extremely useful in assessing its efficacy.

There are several important points that can be made regarding the incidence of infection. It is our impression that the subcutaneous tunnelling of the catheter is extremely important in reducing the incidence of infection. Drainage systems which are closed and empty from the bottom of a bag which is located a substantial distance from the head of the patient are superior to those which require frequent changing of the collection system.

The incidence of infections of a serious nature with the subarachnoid or epidural recording devices is extremely low and is almost of no real clinical significance. Skin slough can occasionally occur if a subarachnoid bolt is snugged too tightly to the scalp, but this problem is easily avoidable as one gains experience with the technique.

## Hemorrhage

Hemorrhagic complications from the placement of a ventricular catheter or subarachnoid bold have been discussed previously. In our experience in over 500 patients, serious hemorrhage did not occur from placement of either of the devices in patients where the platelet count has exceeded 100,000 and there have not been severe abnormalities of prothrombin time or partial prothromboplastin time. In the experience of Winn *et al.*, at the University of Virginia, in over 650 patients who underwent placement of a subarachnoid bolt, there was not one significant subdural intracranial hemorrhage[34].

## Inaccurate Data Recording

The ventricular catheter remains the most reliable method for continuous recording of the ICP. The incidence of damping and inaccurate data collection is extremely low with this device. While it may occasionally plug in patients with small ventricles because of debris, this, in experienced hands, is a relatively minor problem. Data loss, however, with the subarachnoid bolt is a much more substantial problem. In a recent study, Mendelow *et al.*, demonstrated in a substantial number of cases that, as the ICP rose, the subarachnoid bolt became less and less accurate in detecting such rises and, indeed, could be misleading in the face of signs of intracranial catastrophe[21].

Fluid damping and complete occlusion of the subarachnoid screw are significant problems and merit further discussion. In our own Center, herniation has occurred in 3 patients when what appeared to be good wave form and a low ICP were recorded with a subarachnoid screw. When ventricular cannulation was performed, these patients had extremely high ICPs at the time that their neurologic status had precipitiously declined. In each of these cases, CT scanning demonstrated transtentorial herniation which further supported the contention that the subarachnoid device had failed to accurately reflect intacranial events.

In patients with severe diffuse swelling, which occasionally occurs in head injury, subarachnoid screw occlusion is not infrequent. In patients in whom massive shift has occurred, problems with the accuracy of the subarachnoid screw, as has been noted earlier, are substantial and if the ventricles can be visualized, consideration should be seriously given to the placement of a ventricular catheter. While accurate recordings can be obtained, in approximately three quarters of the patients with severe head injury who are monitored with this device a 25% failure rate is substantially higher than one would like.

A second major technical problem is the fact that there appear in some patients to be multiple compartments within the intracranial space when a mass lesion is present. While neurosurgeons have recognized for decades that bicompartmental syndromes may develop in patients who have supratentorial or infratentorial masses with subsequent obstruction of communication between those two compartments, particularly when transtentorial herniation has occurred with a supratentorial mass, little attention has been paid to multiple compartmental pressures within the supratentorial space.

Utilizing bilateral subarachnoid screws and a ventricular catheter, we have recorded ICP continuously in 11 patients in whom a mass lesion was present. In general, recording from the involved hemisphere demonstrates substantially higher pressures, often exceeding those recorded on the contralateral side by 5 mm Hg or more. It has been shown by others that the subarachnoid screw is likely to yield higher and more accurate pressures when pressure is recorded over the hemisphere in which a mass lesion is present, although acute recordings from the contralateral hemisphere can often be obtained[31]. The fact that pressures recorded from the contralateral side are often lower and substantially different from those on the side of the mass lesion indicates that there are different compartments within the intracranial space. This observation is important for it suggests that in patients with substantial shift from a mass lesion that differential pressures will occur and that a false sense of security may be generated even when the monitor is placed over the site of the mass when a subarachnoid screw is used.

The problem is made more complex by recent clinical observations. These have suggested that not only is the level of pressure important but equally or even more important is the location of the mass lesion responsible for the rise in ICP. We have observed the oval pupil, a definite sign of brain stem compression in 3 patients with ICPs under 20 mm Hg[18]. In every instance the mass was located in the temporal region. This is a clear demonstration of the fact that ICP data should not be viewed in isolation but must be interpreted in the light of other information regarding the patient's intracranial dynamics.

## ICP Monitoring in the Future

The theory and practice of ICP monitoring has been described. It is important to recognize, however, that ICP monitoring is a relatively crude guide to the adequacy of brain perfusion and to the efficacy of treatment for severe head injury. What one is really interested in is the adequacy of brain function and perfusion which could be better assessed by electrophysiological and metabolic parameters. Unfortunately, these are not yet available in a serial fashion and ICP measurements are the best index to date of the dynamic events which characterize head injury.

The data obtained from continuous recording of the ICP should be seen as one part of the data base which guides rational decision making. The future is likely to be characterized by combined modalities, including somatosensory and brain stem evoked potentials, serial CT scanning, and NMR imaging of brain and metabolites as well as the analysis of ICP both in terms of its absolute level as well as the form and trend of the pulse pressure. Much more sophisticated analysis of ICP, as well as other parameters, will be required if we are to make substantial advances in the treatment of severe head injury and other intracranial catastrophes. The tremendous capacity of modern computer systems and microprocessors should permit such analyses.

Despite the fact that ICP monitoring has contributed to both our understanding of the pathophysiology and to the rational therapy of patients suffering severe head injury, it is a limited tool and one whose importance should neither be over or underemphasized. It is unlikely, at least in the next decade, as alternatives become available for the continuous monitoring of the severely head injured patient, that they will supplant ICP monitoring. Rather, their success or failure will be judged on their ability to augment the substantial information which can already be derived from ICP monitoring.

## References

1. Ayala, G., 1923: Über den diagnostischen Wert des Liquordruckes und einen Apparat zu seiner Messung. Z. Neurol. Psychiat. 84, 42–95.
2. Bellegarrigue, R., Ducker, T. B., 1983: Control of intracranial pressure in severe head injury. In: Ishii, S., Nagai, H., Brock, M. (eds.): ICP V. Berlin-Heidelberg-New York: Springer.
3. Bruce, D. A., Schut, L., Bruno, L. A., Wood, J. H., Sutton, L. N., 1978: Outcome following severe head injuries in children. J. Neurosurg. 48, 679–688.
4. Burrows, G., 1846: Disorders of the Cerebral Circulation. London.
5. Cushing, H., 1902: Some experimental and clinical observations concerning states of increased intracranial tension. Amer. J. Med. Sci. 124, 375–400.
6. Eisenberg, H. M., Cayand, C., Papanicolaou, A., et al., 1983: The effects of three potentially preventable complications on outcome after severe closed head injury. In: Ishii, S., Nagai, H., Brock, M. (eds.): ICP V. Berlin-Heidelberg-New York: Springer.
7. Guillaume, J., Janny, P., 1951: Monometric intracranienne continue; interet physio-pathologique et clinique de la methode. Presse Med. 59, 953–955.
8. Haar, F. L., Phillips, S., Huchtor, J. I., 1981: The incidence and significance of early hypoxemia on head injury patients. Trans. Amer. Assoc. Neurosurg.: Boston.
9. Kellie, G., 1824: An account of the appearances observed in the dissection of two of the three individuals presumed to have perished in the storm of 3 D, and whose bodies were discovered in the vicinity of Leith on the morning of the 4th

November 1821 with some reflections on the pathology of the brain. Trans. Med. Chir. Sci., Edinburgh *1*, 84–169.

10. Kishore, P. R. S., Lipper, M. H., Becker, D. P., 1982: Correlations of intracranial pressure and computerized tomography findings in severe head injury. In: Grossmon, R. G., Gildenberg, P. L. (eds.): Head Injury: Basic and Clinical Aspects. New York: Raven Press.

11. Klauber, M. R., Toutant, S. M., Marshall, L. F., 1984: A model for predicting delayed intracranial hypertension following severe head injury. J. Neurosurg. *61*, 695–699.

12. Langfitt, T. W., Kassell, N. F., Weinstein, J. D., 1965: Cerebral blood flow with intracranial hypertension. Neurology *15*, 761–773.

13. Langfitt, T. W., Weinstein, J. D., Kassell, N. F., 1966: Vascular factors in head injury: Contribution to brain swelling and intracranial hypertension. In: Caveness, W. F., Walker, A. E. (eds.): Head Injury, Conference Proceedings, pp. 172–194. Philadelphia: Lippincott.

14. Lofgren, J., von Essen, G., Zuenon, N. N., 1973: The pressure volume curve of the cerebrospinal fluid space in dogs. Acta Neurol. Scand. *49*, 557–574.

15. Lundberg, N., 1960: Continuous recording and control of ventricular fluid pressure in neurosurgical practice. Acta Psychiatr. Neurol. Scand. (Suppl.) *149*, 1–193.

16. Marshall, L. F., Smith, R. W., Shapiro, H. M., 1978: The influence of diurnal rhythms in patients with intracranial hypertension: Implications for management. Neurosurg. *2*, 100–102.

17. Marshall, L. F., Smith, R. W., Shapiro, H. M., 1979: The outcome with aggressive treatment in severe head injuries. Part I: The significance of intracranial pressure monitoring. J. Neurosurg. *50*, 20–25.

18. Marshall, L. F., Barba, D., Toole, B. M., Bowers, S. A., 1983: The oval pupil: clinical significance and relationship to intracranial hypertension. J. Neurosurg. *58*, 566–568.

19. Mayhall, C. G., Archer, N. H., Lamb, V. A., 1984: Ventriculostomy-related infections: A prospective epidemiological study. N. Engl. J. Med. *310* (*9*), 553–559.

20. McGraw, C. P., 1976: Continuous intracranial pressure monitoring: Review of techniques and presentation of method. Surg. Neurol. *6*, 149–155.

21. Mendelow, A. D., Rowan, J., Murray, L., *et al.,* 1983: A clinical comparison of subdural screw pressure measurements with ventricular pressure. J. Neurosurg. *58*, 45–50.

22. Miller, J. D., Garibi, J., Pickard, J. D., 1973: Induced changes of cerebrospinal fluid volume-effects during continuous monitoring of ventricular fluid pressure. Arch. Neurol. *28*, 265–269.

23. Miller, J. D., Becker, D. P., Ward, J. D., Sullivan, H. G., Adams, W. E., Rosner, M. J., 1977: Significance of intracranial hypertension in severe head injury. J. Neurosurg. *47*, 504–516.

24. Monro, A., 1783: Observations on the Structure and Function of the Nervous System. Edinburgh: Creech and Johnson.

25. Smith, R. W., Alksne, J. F., 1976: Infections complicating the use of external ventriculostomy. J. Neurosurg. *44*, 567–570.

26. Stuart, G. G., Merry, G. S., Smith, J. A., Yelland, D. N., 1983: Severe head injury managed without intracranial pressure monitoring. J. Neurosurg. *59*, 601–605.
27. Teasdale, G., Galbraith, S., Jennett, B., 1980: Operate or observe? ICP and the management of the "silent" traumatic intracranial haematoma. In: Shulman, K., Marmarou, A., Miller, J. D., Becker, D. P., Hochwald, G. M., Brock, M. (eds.): Intracranial Pressure IV. Berlin-Heidelberg-New York: Springer.
28. Toutant, S. M., Klauber, M. R., Marshall, L. F., *et al.,* 1984: Absent or compressed basal cisterns on first CT scan are ominous predictors of outcome in severe head injury. J. Neurosurg. *61*, 691–694.
29. Von Dongen, K. J., Braakman, R., Gelpke, G. J., 1983: The prognostic value of computerized tomography in comatose head injured patients. J. Neurosurg. *59*, 951–957.
30. Vries, J. K., Becker, D. P., Young, H. F., 1973: A subarachnoid screw for monitoring intracranial pressure. Tech. Note. J. Neurosurg. *39*, 416–419.
31. Weaver, D. D., Winn, H. R., Jane, J. A., 1982: Differential intracranial pressure in patients with unilateral mass lesions. J. Neurosurg. *56*, 660–665.
32. Weed, L. H., 1929: Some limitations of the Monro-Kellie hypothesis. Arch. Surg. (Chicago) *18*, 1049–1069.
33. Wilkinson, H. A., 1982: Intracranial pressure monitoring: Techniques and pitfalls. In: Cooper, P. (ed.): Head Injury. Baltimore: William and Wilkins.
34. Winn, H. R., Dacey, R. G., Jane, J. A., 1977: Intracranial subarachnoid pressure recording: Experience with 650 patients. Surg. Neurol. *8*, 41–47.

# Prediction of Outcome After Head Injury—A Critical Review

J. D. MILLER

Department of Surgical Neurology, Western General Hospital, Edinburgh (U.K.)

With 1 Figure

## Contents

## Introduction

For many hundreds of years, while doctors had little to offer in the way of therapy, their chief value to society lay in their ability to predict the outcome of diseases or injuries. Such predictions were based largely on personal experience, then supplemented by the written experience of others. During the past ten years a large number of reports have appeared in which the outcomes of head injuries of different but specified degrees of severity have been the principal topic. Outcome has been correlated with the status of patients on admission and considerable strides have been made in the methods of predicting outcome of head injury of a given degree of severity. Indeed, the lessons learned in these predictive exercises are now being applied with profit to the study of outcome following subarachnoid hemorrhage, ischemic stroke, intracranial infections and posthypoxic brain damage.

It is important to be clear whether outcome is being predicted in a group of patients (the proportion of anticipated survivors or mortality) or in the individual patient (the chance of survival or death) (Jennett *et al.* 1976). It is also important to specify whether prediction is to be limited to death versus survival or whether it is wished to predict the extent of disability following injury.

What is the value of predicting the outcome from a head injury of specified severity? There are numerous advantages. The triage of patients, allocation of staffing and equipping priorities, diagnostic measures and management protocols, can all be based on firm factual information rather than opinion. Counselling of families and arrangements for rehabilitation can be carried out early after injury in the most appropriate patients. Probably the most valuable contribution is in the identification of those pathophysiological factors that are most important in determining a particular outcome. In this way the critical importance for outcome of intracranial hematomas has been firmly established. Newer management strategies or therapies can be directed to those adverse pathological factors and the patients in whom they are most likely to operate. Series of patients from different centres, or subjected to different treatments, may be compared critically using this information and it is even possible to adjust data so as to ensure comparability of patient populations. In this way the impact of new treatments on the outcome of head injury can be fairly evaluated.

In this chapter the various steps involved in making outcome predictions and validating them are outlined. The importance for prognosis of the key individual factors is discussed and the current status of outcome prediction is reviewed.

## Steps Required to Determine Outcome in Individual Patients (Table 1)

### A. Defining the Patient Population

One of the reasons it has been so difficult to compare different series of head-injured patients in the past is that insufficient information was given in the publication to determine how badly the patients had been injured. Obviously, very few in a series of fully conscious head injured patients

Table 1. *Steps Required for Prognosis in Head Injury*

---

1. Define and limit the patient population
2. Describe the patient
   — age and sex
   — conscious level
   — brain stem function
   — early systemic insults
   — intracranial hematoma
   — raised intracranial pressure
3. Define the outcome
4. Form a database
5. Develop a prognostic algorithm
6. Test it prospectively (new patients)

---

would be expected to die, whereas up to 50 percent of a series of comatose head injured patients will succumb; comatose patients with one set of clinical features may have a 20 percent mortality while 80 percent of comatose patients with other clinical features will die. The overall mortality rate in any given series of comatose head injury patients is therefore dependent on the patient mix. Patients who have sustained missile injuries of the head are usually separated from those who have sustained blunt head injuries involving acceleration or deceleration of the entire head or head and body because the locations and extent of brain damage are often so different.

### B. Recording the Preinjury Factors of Importance

All doctors recognise intuitively that younger patients tend to have a better outcome from head injury than older patients; age is a most important prognostic factor and must be recorded exactly. Most head injuries occur in males but, as will be explained below, there are additional reasons why recording the sex of the patient is important. Of major importance in the prediction of disability after head injury is the psychosocial status of the patient and the presence of any previous brain lesion, whether due to prior injury or disease.

*C. Describing the Neurological Status of the Patient on Entry to the Series*

The major advance in this area has been the widespread acceptance of the need to use objective, reliable terminology to define the neurological status of patients and nowhere is this better exemplified than in the design, testing and gradual acceptance of the Glasgow coma scale as a worldwide

| *Eye opening* | *Best motor response* | *Verbal response* |
|---|---|---|
| 4 Spontaneous | 6 Obey commands | 5 Orientated |
| 3 To command |  | 4 Disoriented (confused) |
| 2 To pain |  | 3 Words |
| 1 Nil | 5 Localize pain | 2 Sounds |
|  | 4 Normal flexor | 1 Nil |
|  | 3 Abnormal flexor (decorticate) |  |
|  | 2 Extensor (decerebrate) |  |
|  | 1 Nil |  |

Fig. 1. Glasgow coma scale. International definition of coma includes all states below line. Severe head injury defined as 8 or less total score on GCS. Moderate head injury defined as 9 to 12 total score on GCS. Minor head injury defined as 13 to 15 total score on GCS

standard for description of conscious level in head injured patients. The coma scale, based on three separate scales describing eye opening, verbal response and the best motor response to standardised stimuli was proposed ten years ago by Teasdale and Jennett (1974). Before publication, the scale had been refined and extensively tested within their department by the systematic study of a large number of observers describing patients they had examined themselves or films of patients being examined by a third party (Fig. 1). Teasdale and his colleagues have shown that the terminology of the Glasgow coma scale is helpful and reliable, with an extremely low level of inter-observer error (Teasdale *et al.* 1978).

The Glasgow coma scale has been criticised both for being too simple and for being too complex but its widespread adoption by neurosurgeons, accident surgeons, nurses and ambulance crews in countries all over the world indicates that the scale represented a useful compromise and creates a powerful argument for its continued use.

The principles embodied in the Glasgow coma scale, of precision of definition, and use of exclusive terminology (placing the patient in one category automatically ensures that he cannot be in any other category) have been extended to descriptions of other important parts of the neurological examination, particularly the pupil size and light response.

## D. Other Injury Related Factors

The adverse influence of low arterial pressure or hypoxaemia on head injury outcome has long been recognized and should be recorded and included in the data used to formulate a prognosis. The importance of the highest level of intracranial pressure is now also recognized in this respect, as are the findings on CT scan.

Finally, because of the considerable importance of the presence of an intracranial hematoma for outcome, the information as to whether such a lesion is present and whether it requires surgical evacuation, must be included. The time-related evolution of head injury patients towards deterioration or recovery is also important. When a patient's clinical status is described, the data should be linked to a clear statement of the time this was obtained, for example on admission after resuscitation, or six or 24 hours after injury or the onset of coma. In addition it is important to note whether coma has been present from the time of impact or whether the comatose state represents a deterioration in neurological status as exemplified in the concepts of "lucid interval" and "talk and die" patients. It is in such cases that the factor of time is most important.

## E. Definition and Recording of Outcome

This has proved to be one of the most difficult exercises in the formulation of prognostic algorithms. Using the same pragmatic, reductionist approach Jennett and Bond (1975) advocated a Glasgow outcome scale

Table 2. *Glasgow Outcome Scale* (Jennett and Bond 1975)

| | |
|---|---|
| Good recovery<br>Moderate disability | independent |
| Severe disability<br>Permanent vegetative state | dependent |
| Death | cerebral cause<br>systemic cause |

soon after the introduction of the coma scale (Table 2). This outcome scale was a fivepoint one in which "good recovery" was defined as a return to the previous level of employment or occupation, regardless of persisting minor neurological deficits. "Moderate disability" was defined as a state in which the patients had obvious neurological or psychosocial deficits but were independent for the activities of daily living, able to look after themselves at home, and possibly able to undertake some form of occupation but not at the preinjury level. "Severe disability" was defined as a state in which the patients, who might be at home or remaining in hospital, required the assistance of others to undertake the activities of daily living. In other words, such patients were dependent, as distinct from the independent status of "good recovery" or "moderately disabled" patients. The fourth outcome category was the "permanent vegetative state", defined by Jennett and Plum (1972) as a state in which there could be spontaneous eye-opening, sleep/wake cycles but no evidence of recognition or appropriate responsiveness to changes in the environment. Such patients are by definition unable to obey commands, or to utter recognizable sounds. The fifth and final outcome category was Death. This scale has now been widely adopted as the usual way to record the outcome of severe head injury.

More recently Bond has shown that it is possible to separate "good recovery" and "moderate disability" each into two categories, thus making a sevenpoint scale, without losing much of the precision of definition of the five-point scale (Bond and Brooks 1976). For the purposes of attaining a prognosis, however, the use of even the five-point scale imposes tremendous statistical burdens on the data base. It has become widespread practice, therefore, to collapse the five-point scale into two categories, either death versus survival, or death and dependence versus independent recovery. Probably the best compromise would be a three-point outcome scale where "good recovery" and "moderate disability" are linked, as are "severe disability" and "vegetative state".

A crucial factor is the time after injury at which the outcome declaration is made. Most deaths occur within the first month after injury, therefore if the outcome categories are to be simply stated as death versus survival, this declaration can be made early. If dependence versus independence is important, then a longer period must elapse. Jennett and his colleagues (1979) have shown that while two-thirds of a series of severely head injured patients reached their final outcome status (as declared at two years) by three months from the injury, 95 percent attained this final status by six months. For this reason the Glasgow group and their coworkers have declared outcomes at six months from the time of injury. Miller and his colleagues (1981) found a smaller change in outcome status between three and six months and defended the use of three-month outcome declaration.

It is not to be denied that further improvements in the performance of surviving head injured patients can be seen between one and two years after injury and even later. Seldom, however, do these improvements in performance attain sufficient significance to move the patient from one major outcome category to another.

## F. Generation of a Data Base

Once systematic collection of input and outcome data in head injured patients has been started, the next major question is how big should be the data base. Teasdale *et al.* (1979) have indicated that when data is being collected simultaneously using the same terminology in two different centres it is only when the two patient populations reach 300 each that the mean values and distribution of the important prognostic variables become the same. In practice, however, most centres have made a declaration of their mortality rates and disability levels in series of patients ranging between 100 and 300 cases.

### G. Development and Testing of a Prognostic Algorithm

Once an adequate data base has been assembled it is possible to link mathematically the input data with the actual outcome of the patients. There are various statistical techniques to carry out this exercise, each of which has its own advantages and disadvantages. The two most popular methods are the Bayesian approach, which compares the distribution of input factors among patients with different given outcomes, assumes independence of the input factors, but is relatively unaffected by missing data items and is in practice an extremely robust method (Jennett *et al.* 1979). Another is the linear logistic regression technique (Stablein *et al.* 1980). This method permits interdependence of prognostic factors, something that is present in real life, but is adversely affected by missing data. In practice, both of these techniques produce similar performance. By their use it is possible, once the prognostic algorithm has been calculated, to take any subsequent individual patient and insert his input data into an equation the solution of which will produce a figure that represents this individual patient's chance of attaining a particular outcome state, usually the percentage chance of dying from the injury.

Once this has been carried out, the next stage is to take a small series of new patients from the same centre and fit their input data into the prognostic algorithm and see whether outcome in the group of new patients is predicted accurately from the system based on data obtained from previous patients (Narayan *et al.* 1981).

## Individual Prognostic Factors in Head-Injured Patients

### A. Preinjury Factors

There is a continuous relationship between age and mortality from head injury, with older patients more likely to die, and younger patients to survive (Table 3). When account is taken of the mode of death from the injury the influence of age appears to be an increased liability of older patients in prolonged coma to die from the medical complications of that state. If only those patients who die from intracranial complications of injury are considered, the relationship between age and mortality is less

236        J. D. Miller:

Table 3. *Age and Mortality in Moderate (GCS 9–12) and Severe (GCS 8 or less) Head Injury*

| Age (years) | Moderate (n = 188) | | Severe (n = 93) | |
|---|---|---|---|---|
| | Number | Mortality (%) | Number | Mortality (%) |
| 0–20 | 51 | 0 (0%) | 35 | 12 (34%) |
| 20–40 | 52 | 0 (0%) | 24 | 9 (38%) |
| 40–60 | 43 | 1 (2%) | 18 | 9 (50%) |
| 60–90 | 24 | 5 (21%) | 16 | 12 (75%) |
| Total | 170 | 6 (7%) | 93 | 42 (45%) |

Miller, J. D., Jones, P. A. (1985).

evident. There is also a somewhat complicated interrelationship between advancing age and the liability of a comatose head injury patient to harbor an intracranial hematoma; this factor is also associated with a higher mortality (Becker *et al.* 1977).

The sex of the head injured patient is important, not only because there are so many more males then females (four times as many in most series) but because males seem more likely to sustain head injuries associated with greater violence and, therefore, more severe degrees of diffuse axonal injury (Braakman *et al.* 1980).

The psychosocial status of the head injured patient is important in survivors with minor and moderate degrees of disability, as the evidence suggests that those patients in higher social classes are more likely to attain the outcome categories of "good recovery" or "moderate disability" than head injured patients from lower psychosocial class. Whether this difference in outcome capability is purely environmental remains to be determined (Rimel *et al.* 1981, 1982).

The previous state of health of the head injured patient is extremely important. Obviously, the presence of preexisting medical disorders such as diabetes mellitus, chronic emphysema, arterial hypertension, all prejudice the safe recovery of a severely head injured patient in the Intensive Care Unit. The importance of previous brain damage is even greater. Patients who have made an apparently good recovery from a previous head injury, stroke or hydrocephalus, may be devastated by what is apparently a relatively minor head injury. Such patients may have been operating at the limits of their capacity and the further neuronal loss produced by the head injury sufficient to tip the patient into a state of incapacity (Becker *et al.* 1982).

Finally, preexisting physical factors related to the dimensions and volume of the intracranial CSF space and the configuration of the skull, dura, tentorium and other intracranial structures may all play a part in determining the response of that individual patient to a particular type of injury. Most obvious is the capacity of the patient with a large CSF space to tolerate the presence of a sizeable intracranial hematoma before betraying any signs of neurological deterioration. This may not, however, always operate to the patient's advantage because diagnosis of an intracranial hematoma is delayed. The effect of these factors on prognosis is, therefore, not consistent.

## B. Injury-Related Factors

### 1. Type of Injury

The cause of the brain injury is extremely important in terms of prognosis. A person who has become comatose as the result of brain compression due to a hematoma is statistically more likely to die than a patient without a hematoma but may recover provided that surgical decompression is effected sufficiently soon (Mendelow *et al.* 1979, Seelig *et al.* 1981). A person rendered comatose to the same degree as the result of a high speed acceleration/deceleration injury, such as a motor cycle accident, is much more likely to remain disabled, even if he survives. With respect to depressed skull fractures, penetrating or missile wounds, the prognosis for these wounds is also related to the development of infection and the site of injury (Miller and Jennett 1968). Patients with unilateral frontal lobe injuries may make a satisfactory recovery, whereas the prognosis for transventricular missile wounds is extremely poor. Injuries that result in destruction of the right (nondominant) parietal cortex seem to result in particularly severe disabilities.

### 2. Level of Consciousness

This is probably the single most important determinant of prognosis in blunt and missile head injury. There is a strong relationship between increasing mortality and decreasing levels on the coma scale (Table 4). Of the three elements of the Glasgow coma scale the most important for prognosis is the motor scale. On the motor scale the most critical difference is unfortunately the one that is hardest to define at the bedside, namely the difference between normal and abnormal flexion (between 4 and 3 on the six-point motor scale) (Table 5.). The prognostic value of the eye-opening scale is clear only during the first days after the onset of coma (Jennett and Teasdale 1977). During the second week there is a tendency towards

Table 4. *Level of Consciousness on Glasgow Coma Scale on Admission vs. Mortality in Two Series of Cases of Severe Head Injury (defined as GCS 8 or less on admission)*

| GCS score sum | Med. College Va. | | Univ. of Edinburgh | |
|---|---|---|---|---|
| | Number | Mortality (%) | Number | Mortality (%) |
| 8 | 68 | 9 (13%) | 7 | 0 (0%) |
| 5–7 | 109 | 32 (29%) | 47 | 14 (30%) |
| 3–4 | 48 | 35 (73%) | 39 | 28 (72%) |
| Total | 225 | 76 (34%) | 93 | 42 (45%) |

N. B.: While the mortality rate at the same levels of coma are the same in the two series, the overall mortality is quite different. This is a good illustration of the importance of differences in "patient mix".

Table 5. *Motor Score on Glasgow Coma Scale vs. Mortality in Two Series of Cases of Severe Head Injury*

| Motor score on GCS | Med. College Va. | | Univ. of Edinburgh | |
|---|---|---|---|---|
| | Number | Mortality (%) | Number | Mortality (%) |
| Localize/normal flex | 157 | 33 (21%) | 24 | 5 (21%) |
| Abnormal flexor | 17 | 7 (41%) | 29 | 9 (31%) |
| Extensor | 34 | 23 (68%) | 9 | 3 (33%) |
| Nil | 17 | 13 (76%) | 31 | 25 (81%) |
| Total | 225 | 76 (34%) | 93 | 42 (45%) |

spontaneous eye-opening, even in patients who show no other signs of regaining consciousness and still are unable to obey commands or to utter any formed verbal response. Most patients in a permanent vegetative state have spontaneous eye-opening and may even have sleep/wake cycles.

## 3. Signs of Brain Stem Dysfunction

When combined with the features of the Glasgow coma scale, information as to whether there is normal or abnormal function in the brain stem is of powerful prognostic value. Even on its own the information that a

Table 6. *Oculocephalic Response\* and Pupillary Light Response vs. Mortality in Patients with Severe Head Injury*

| Oculocephalic response | Number | Mortality (%) |
|---|---|---|
| Present | 114 | 20% |
| Impaired/absent | 83 | 54% |
| Total | 197 | 34% |

| Pupil light response | Number | Mortality (%) |
|---|---|---|
| Present | 173 | 21% |
| Bilateral absent | 53 | 75% |
| Total | 226 | 34% |

\* OCR not obtained in all cases.

patient has absent oculocephalic reflexes or bilateral failure of the pupillary responses to light is associated with tripling of the mortality from a head injury (Table 6).

Where abnormalities are unilateral, there may be difficulty in distinguishing signs of brain stem dysfunction from isolated cranial nerve dysfunction. Traumatic third nerve palsy is not uncommon following head injuries which are of otherwise minor significance and does not always signal tentorial herniation. Similarly, loss of function of the optic nerve on one side may be a local consequence of a fracture extending to the apex of the orbit and be dissociated from the degree of associated brain damage. For that reason isolated cranial nerve palsies are not of great prognostic value unless associated with the syndrome complex of tentorial herniation.

Marshall has recently drawn attention to the value of oval fixed pupils as a sign of impending brain death. While this is true, this clinical sign is of limited value since the majority of patients who are clinically diagnosed as having suffered brain death do not have this particular sign. This raises an important point in prognosis. While certain clusters of abnormal neurological signs can have a powerful association with a particular outcome, their rate of occurrence may be so infrequent that their value is limited.

The most important of the many brain stem reflexes that can be tested are the pupil light reflex, the corneal reflex, the oculocephalic and oculovestibular reflexes, and gag and cough reflexes. In the United Kingdom it is not permissible to make a diagnosis of absence of brain stem reflex activity unless oculovestibular reflexes have been tested using iced water irrigated into the ears. (Conference of Medical Royal Colleges and their Faculties 1976, 1979.)

## C. Secondary Systemic Insults to the Injured Brain

The concurrence of hypoxemia or arterial hypotension with severe head injury is associated with doubling or mortality and poorer quality recovery (Price and Murray 1972). These insults are relatively common. Hypoxemia was recorded in 30 percent of a series of 220 comatose head-injured patients reported by Miller and his colleagues in Virginia (1978) and arterial hypotension was present on admission in 15 percent of the same population. In a subsequent series of 93 severely injured patients seen in Edinburgh the proportion of hypotension on admission was 16 percent (Miller and Jones 1985).

## D. Intracranial Hematoma

One of the major concerns of the surgeon who is managing a patient with a head injury is that an intracranial hematoma may develop in the extradural or subdural space or in the substance of the brain. The presence of a sizeable intracranial hematoma in a comatose patient more than doubles the mortality. In comatose patients with intracranial hematomas there is a higher incidence of clinical signs held to have an adverse prognostic significance, such as extension or abnormal flexion on the motor scale or the presence of impaired brain stem function. Patients who are comatose and have intracranial hematomas also tend to be older than comatose patients without intracranial hematomas. There is, therefore, an interaction between presence of a hematoma, age, neurological status and outcome (Becker et al. 1977, 1982). The incidence of elevated intracranial pressure is also higher, both in patients who are harbouring a hematoma and after the hematoma has been surgically decompressed (Miller et al. 1977, 1981). The complexity of these interactions related to prognosis should be recognized by those who look after head injured patients.

## E. Injury-Related Factors—Special Investigations

### 1. Intracranial Pressure

Elevations of intracranial pressure above 20 mm Hg (normal range 0–10 mm Hg) are quite common in head-injured patients. Miller and his colleagues (1981) found such elevations of pressure in just over half of a series of over 200 comatose head-injured patients. There was a clear relationship between the highest levels of ICP that were attained during the period of intensive care of such patients and the mortality. No patients survived in whom ICP had risen above 60 mm Hg for more than five minutes (Table 7). Because of this, most neurosurgeons believe that the continuous monitoring of intracranial pressure is of importance in the management of the more severely head-injury patient and that elevations of

Table 7. *Highest Level of Intracranial Pressure vs. Mortality*

| ICP level (mm Hg) | Med. Coll. Va. | |
| --- | --- | --- |
| | Number | Mortality (%) |
| 0–20 | 95 | 18 (19%) |
| 20–40 | 67 | 19 (28%) |
| 40–60 | 21 | 13 (62%) |
| 60–80 | 18 | 18 (100%) |
| Total | 201 | 68 (34%) |

ICP should be treated. It is fair to point out, however, that the benefits to the patient of recording and treating elevated ICP have not been conclusively shown. In a series of cases recently reported from Australia, ICP monitoring was not practiced at all, yet the overall outcome for the series compared favorably with other reported series in which ICP monitoring had been used routinely (Stuart *et al.* 1983).

## 2. CT Scan

Apart from its obvious value in the early stage after head injury in the diagnosis of extracerebral or intracerebral hematomas requiring surgical decompression, CT scanning also provides prognostic information. The presence of bilateral subfrontal contusions is an indicator that the patient is likely to have a period of posttraumatic confusion and behavioural disturbance (Sweet *et al.* 1978). Strategically related contusions may correspond with clinical signs of focal neurological deficit such as dysphasia or visual field disturbance. CT scanning carried out at a later stage, two weeks or three months, after injury may be an aid towards the differentiation between those patients who have a recoverable neurological deficit and those in whom the deficit is permanent (Clifton *et al.* 1980). Patients with fixed neurological deficits often show changes suggestive of infarction on the late CT scan. The incidence of severe disability is higher in patients who demonstrate enlargement of the ventricles at three months and the incidence of ataxia and dysarthria is higher in patients in whom the CSF spaces in the posterior fossa are enlarged (van Dongen and Braakman 1980).

### 3. Measurements of Regional Cerebral Blood Flow

At the present time these measurements are technically quite difficult to make, the equipment is expensive and they have, therefore, only been carried out in a limited number of centers. Resting flow levels that are abnormally high or abnormally low both carry an adverse prognostic significance (Obrist *et al.* 1979). Normalization of cerebral blood flow during the first days after injury is an encouraging sign. Loss of responsiveness of cerebral vessels to changes in arterial pressure in areas of cortical brain damage is not uncommon after head injury, but complete loss of cerebrovascular response to changes in carbon dioxide tension is seen only in the most severely injured patients and carries a very bad prognosis (Overgaard and Tweed 1974).

Simpler measurements of cerebral circulatory transit time are of limited prognostic value. While group differences can be seen, individual variations in circulation time measurements even in normal subjects make it difficult to assess the significance of a measurement in an injured patient.

### 4. Measurement of Evoked Cortical Potentials

With appropriate instrumentation, it is possible to obtain records in comatose head injured patients of the visual, somatosensory and auditory evoked potentials, including information on the early waves that are held to reflect the passage of the electrical impulse from the auditory apparatus throught the cell stations in the brain stem. Greenberg (1977) and Narayan (1981) and their colleagues have shown that this information, when coupled with clinical data, produces a high accuracy of prediction of outcome in two categories, and at an acceptably high confidence level in individual head injured patients. The drawback is that the measurements are time consuming and arguments about the threshold levels of differing degrees of abnormality are still taking place. Sources of artefact are many and this is a measurement that should at the present time be left to the expert.

### 5. Recording of Respiratory Pattern

In patients who are breathing spontaneously after a head injury, a record of the pattern of respiration may yield information that can be correlated with the patient's clinical status and outcome. Bedside observation of respiratory pattern is virtually useless and a chart-written record must be obtained. Extensive studies of respiratory pattern in brain injured patients were carried out by North and Jennett (1974). They concluded that it was not possible to localise the area of brain damage by a particular form of respiratory abnormality, but that the more severe and centrally located the damage, the more likely it was that the patient would have an abnormal respiratory pattern.

## 6. Measurements of Substances in CSF and Blood

A wide variety of substances have been assayed in samples of blood and CSF drawn in head injured patients and attempts made to correlate the laboratory findings with outcome. Examples include CSF lactate, blood levels of brain specific antigen, CSF levels of cyclic AMP and blood levels of brain specific creatine phosphokinase. While it is possible with all of these measurements to differentiate between groups of head injured patients with injuries of differing prognostic significance ranging from minor to major and severe, the scatter of values is virtually always so great that it is seldom possible when presented with a single measurement in an individual patient to state with confidence that this particular substance level will be associated with a particular outcome.

## Current Status of Outcome Prediction

### A. Predicting the Chances of Death or Survival

In patients with severe head injury (scoring less than 8 on the Glasgow coma scale, including no eye opening whatsoever for at least six hours after injury) it is possible to make a 95 percent confident individual prediction of the outcome, expressed in the two categories of Death versus Survival, in at least two thirds of the patients within a matter of hours from the time of injury or admission to hospital. The factors that are significant in predicting a poor outcome include advancing age, presence of an intracranial hematoma, low score on the motor part of the coma scale, presence of brain stem dysfunction, presence of systemic insult. This predictive exercise has been repeated in several different series of cases, using differing statistical techniques and broadly the same information has emerged.

In the United Kingdom the diagnosis of brain death following intra-cranial hemorrhage or head injury is made entirely on observations recorded at the bedside. The clinician must, therefore, record a constellation of clinical signs which exclude the possibility of any spontaneous recovery from the injury. The criteria include the observations that the cause of the coma is known, the patient is not hypothermic and not under the influence of sedative or relaxant drugs. There must be no response to pain applied above the neck and no signs of brain stem reflex activity including the pupillary light reflexes, corneal reflexes, oculovestibular reflexes, tested with iced water in both ears, and the gag and cough reflexes. There must be no spontaneous respiration despite a period of apnoeic oxygenation sufficient to elevate the arterial $PCO_2$ to levels that would, under normal circumstances, provide a strong stimulus to spontaneous respiration. These tests are carried out by two doctors and on two separate occasions. After the second tests the patient can legally be declared dead. This is a crucial example of the use of clinical information related to prognosis because the prognosis must always be correct. As a matter of deliberate policy in the U.K. it has been decided not to rely upon technological studies such as EEG or perfusion brain scan. These studies may erroneously indicate no brain activity for purely technical reasons and cannot, therefore, fulfil the rigorous criterion of never producing a false negative result.

With information that is now available concerning the influence of various preinjury and clinical factors upon outcome it is now possible to examine the reported results of head injury treatment much more realistically and critically—provided, of course, that the authors include the necessary information in their publication! All the indications are, however, that this is being done. It is possible therefore to adjust reported data so as to ensure compatibility and comparability with other series and thereby to determine whether there has been a difference in outcome, or whether the results really are the same.

One intriguing possibility for prognostic information is to apply the prognostic algorithm derived from a "standard" series of head injury patients to a series of head injured patients treated by a newer mode of therapy. The actual outcome of the treated patients can be compared with the predicted outcome obtained from previous data from "untreated" patients. It can then be seen whether there is a significant improvement in outcome in the "treated" group. The advantage of this method is that it takes account of differences in patient population and in the distribution of the most important prognostic factors and it may well be the most rigorous test yet of the efficacy of treatment.

It is unfortunately that to date the application of this method to a large series of head injured patients has failed to demonstrate the efficacy of any currently used treatment modality, including artificial ventilation, intracranial pressure monitoring or steroid therapy. One is left at this stage, therefore, with the nagging doubt that while it is probably true that these treatments have not greatly improved outcome, this method of assessing treatment may be incapable of demonstrating a small effect on outcome when one does truly exist (Jennett *et al.* 1980, Cooper *et al.* 1979, Braakman *et al.* 1983).

## B. Forecasting Morbidity

Early detection of those head injured patients likely to remain disabled after injury is of great importance to the rehabilitationist. It would be an attractive proposition if patients liable to suffer disability could be identified at a very early stage and appropriate rehabilitation measures begun. The problem is that at that early stage many severely head injured patients die, and none of the prognostic factors which so reliably predict death after injury are of much value in predicting disability in survivors (Bricolo *et al.* 1980). There is some suggestion that certain findings on CT and moderate intracranial hypertension may identify patients likely to suffer prolonged disability (Miller *et al.* 1981, Miller 1983).

## Conclusions

The enormous amount of activity that has been devoted in the last few years to the prediction of outcome of severely head injured patients has had many useful spin-offs. The need to use tight, precise terminology and objective descriptions has been of value to all concerned in the management of head-injured patients. The identification of those factors which are of the greatest significance in determining death after head injury has directed the attention of the treating physician to the factors that should be given the highest priority for treatment. Early detection of intracranial hematoma has emerged as a most important factor. The area is still developing and it is to be hoped that a more critical approach to therapy and a selective approach to rehabilitation therapy may result. It is also to be hoped that the lessons learned from the care of the head-injured patient may be more widely applied across the field of neurosurgery.

## References

1. Becker, D. P., Miller, J. D., Greenberg, R. P., 1982: Prognosis after head injury. In: Neurological Surgery, Vol. 4, 2nd Edition, pp. 2137–2174. Philadelphia: Saunders.
2. Becker, D. P., Miller, J. D., Ward, J. D., Greenberg, R. P., Young, H. F., Sakalas, R., 1977: The outcome from severe head injury with early diagnosis and intensive management. J. Neurosurg. *47*, 491–502.
3. Bond, M. R., Brooks, D. N., 1976: Understanding the process of recovery as a basis for the investigation of rehabilitation for the brain injured. Scand. J. Rehab. Med. *8*, 127–133.
4. Braakman, R., Gelpke, G. J., Habbema, J. D. F., Maas, A. I. R., Minderhoud, J., 1980: Systematic selection of prognostic features in patients with severe head injury. Neurosurgery *6*, 362–370.
5. Braakman, R., Schouten, H. J. A., Blaauw-van Dishoeck, M., Minderhoud, J. M., 1983: Megadose steroids in severe head injury: results of a prospective double-blind clinical trial. J. Neurosurg. *58*, 326–330.

6. Bricolo, A., Turazzi, S., Feinotto, G., 1980: Prolonged post-traumatic unconsciousness. Therapeutic assets and liabilities. J. Neurosurg. *52*, 625–634.

7. Clifton, G. L., Grossman, R. G., Makela, M. E., Miner, M. E., Handel, S., Sadhu, V., 1980: Neurological course and correlated computerized tomography findings after severe closed head injury. J. Neurosurg. *52*, 611–624.

8. Conference of Medical Colleges and their Faculties (U.K.), Diagnosis of Brain Death. Lancet *2*, 1069–1070, 1976. Brit. Med. J. *1*, 322, 1979.

9. Cooper, P. R., Moody, S., Clark, W. K., Kirkpatrick, J., Maravilla, K., Gould, A. L., Drane, W., 1979: Dexamethasone and severe head injury. A prospective double-blind study. J. Neurosurg. *51*, 307–316.

10. Greenberg, R. P., Becker, D. P., Miller, J. D., Mayer, D. J., 1977: Evaluation of brain function in severe human head trauma with multi-modality evoked potentials: Part II. Localization of brain dysfunction and correlation with post-traumatic neurological conditions. J. Neurosurg. *47*, 163–177.

11. Jennett, B., Bond, M. R., 1975: Assessment of outcome after severe brain damage. Lancet *1*, 480–484.

12. Jennett, B., Plum, F., 1972: Persistent vegetative state after brain damage. Lancet *1*, 734–737.

13. Jennett, B., Teasdale, G., 1977: Aspects of coma after severe head injury. Lancet *1*, 878–881.

14. Jennett, B., Teasdale, G., Braakman, R., et al., 1976: Predicting outcome in individual patients after severe head injury. Lancet *i*, 1031–1034.

15. Jennett, B., Teasdale, G., Braakman, R., Minderhoud, J., Heiden, J., Kurze, T., 1979: Prognosis of patients with severe head injury. Neurosurgery *4*, 283–289.

16. Jennett, B., Teasdale, G., Fry, J., Braakman, R., Minderhoud, J., Heiden, J., Kurze, T., 1980: Treatment for severe head injury. J. Neurol. Neurosurg. Psychiat. *43*, 289–295.

17. Mendelow, A. D., Karmi, M. Z., Paul, K. S., Fuller, G. A. G., Gillingham, F. J., 1979: Extradural haematoma: effect of delayed treatment. Brit. Med. J. *1*, 1240–1242.

18. Miller, J. D., 1983: Neurosurgery—triumphs and tragedies. J. Roy. Coll. Surg. Ed. *28*, 1–7.

19. Miller, J. D., Becker, D. P., Sullivan, H. G., Adams, W. E., Rosner, M. J., 1977: Significance of intracranial hypertension in severe head injury. J. Neurosurg. *47*, 503–516.

20. Miller, J. D., Butterworth, J. F., Gudeman, S. K., Faulkner, J. E., Choi, S. C., Selhorst, J. B., Harbison, J. W., Lutz, H., Young, H. F., Becker, D. P., 1981: Further experience in the management of severe head injury. J. Neurosurg. *54*, 289–299.

21. Miller, J. D., Jennett, W. B., 1968: Complications of depressed skull fracture. Lancet *2*, 991–995.

21 a. Miller J. D., Jones P. A., 1985: The work of a regional head injury service. Lancet *1*, 1141–1144.

22. Miller, J. D., Sweet, R. C., Narayan, R., Becker, D. P., 1978: Early insults to the injured brain. J. Amer. Med. Ass. *240*, 439–442.

23. Narayan, R. K., Greenberg, R. P., Miller, J. D., Enas, G. G., Choi, S. C., Kishore, P. R. S., Selhorst, J. B., Lutz, H. L., Becker, D. P., 1981: Improved confidence of outcome prediction in severe head injury. J. Neurosurg. *54*, 751−762.
24. North, J. B., Jennett, S., 1974: Abnormal breathing patterns associated with acute brain damage. Arch. Neurol. *31*, 338−344.
25. Obrist, W. D., Gennarelli, T. A., Segawa, H., Dolinskas, C. A., Langfitt, T. W., 1979: Relation of cerebral blood flow to neurological status and outcome in head-injured patients. J. Neurosurg. *51* (3), 292−300.
26. Overgaard, J., Tweed, W. A., 1974: Cerebral circulation after head injury: cerebral blood flow and its regulation after closed head injury with emphasis on clinical correlations. J. Neurosurg. *41*, 531−541.
27. Price, D. J. E., Murray, A., 1972: The influence of hypoxia and hypotension on recovery from head injury. Injury *3* (4), 218−224.
28. Rimel, R. W., Giordani, B., Barth, J. T., Jane, J. A., 1982: Moderate Head Injury: Completing the clinical spectrum of brain trauma. Neurosurgery *II* (3), 344−351.
29. Rimel, R. W., Giordani, B., Barth, J. T., Boll, T. J., Jane, J. A., 1981: Disability caused by minor head injury. Neurosurgery *9* (3), 221−228.
30. Seelig, J. M., Becker, D. P., Miller, J. D., Greenberg, R. P., Ward, J. D., Choi, S. C., 1981: Traumatic acute subdural hematoma. Major mortality reduction in comatose patients treated within four hours. New Engl. J. Med. *304*, 1511−1518.
31. Stablein, D. M., Miller, J. D., Choi, S. C., Becker, D. P., 1980: Statistical methods for determining prognosis in severe head injury. Neurosurgery *6*, 243−248.
32. Stuart, G. G., Merry, G. S., Smith, J. D., Yelland, J. N., 1983: Severe head injury managed without intracranial pressure monitoring. J. Neurosurg. *59*, 601−605.
33. Sweet, R. C., Miller, J. D., Lipper, M., *et al.,* 1978: The significance of bilateral abnormalities on the CT scan in patients with severe head injury. Neurosurgery *3*, 16−24.
34. Teasdale, G., Jennett, B., 1974: Assessment of coma and impaired consciousness. A practical scale. Lancet *2*, 81−84.
35. Teasdale, G., Knill-Jones, R., van der Sande, J., 1978: Observer variability in assessing impaired consciousness and coma. J. Neurol. Neurosurg. Psychiat. *41*, 603−610.
36. Teasdale, G., Parker, L., Murray, G., *et al.,* 1979 b: On comparing series of head injured patients. Acta Neurochir. (Wien) (Suppl.) *28*, 205−208.
37. Van Dongen, K. J., Braakman, R., 1980: Late computed tomography in survivors of severe head injury. Neurosurgery *7*, 14−22.

## Epilogue

The chapters which constitute the first volume of this series have been selected to explore in depth the present concepts of the pathophysiology, diagnosis, and management of traumatic intracranial hemorrhage. The authors have been selected on the basis of their respective areas of expertise and the information included in each chapter is based on many years of concentrated experience. It is hoped by the editors of this volume that the sections devoted to "How to do it" will be of assistance to those individuals who are called on only occasionally to deal with intracranial hemorrhage of traumatic origin.

A word of caution may be appropriate in this summarizing statement. During the past few years several reports have appeared concerning the nonsurgical treatment of both subdural and epidural hematomas. This mode of management carries considerable risk and should be utilized only under exceptional and well-controlled circumstances. The risk of surgical evacuation of a surface hematoma is far less than the hazards of simple observation, and the potential for permanent neural damage is minimized by surgical intervention.

The chapter concerning intracranial pressure monitoring was included because this has become such a routine, and helpful, method of monitoring severe craniocerebral trauma. Again, one finds in current literature reports which appear to deny the value of this tool but the consensus favors ICP monitoring. In general, it is recommended in any patient whose Glasgow Coma Score is 5 or less and in other patients whose score is 6 or 7 if other risk factors, *e.g.*, skull fracture or CT evidence of cerebral contusion or swelling, are present. The increased risk for intracranial hematoma in those patients with impaired consciousness and/or skull fracture has been clearly documented.

Finally, the chapter concerning outcome predictions has provided evidence that based on careful observation and recording of large numbers of traumatized patients, certain prognostic criteria may be derived. These clearly have value in dealing with head injured patients when limited medical resources are available as well as providing reasonable expectations to families and dependents in individual cases.

The volume may be deficient in neglecting the various types of traumatic hematomas occurring in the neonatal and infancy periods. This deficiency is not the result of attaching less importance to these lesions than to hematomas occurring at older ages; indeed, it may be argued that the brain damage which may result from birth trauma or injury during infancy has a more prolonged and devastating effect on the person's ability to learn and then become productive. The deficiency is attributable only to limitations of the volume length so that it will address the majority of related problems.

The editors express gratitude to the individual authors for their efforts and any shortcomings of the volume may be attributed entirely to the organizing and editorial staff. At the same time it is hoped that this and subsequent volumes in this series will serve to enhance the quality of care in the field of craniocerebral trauma which accounts for worldwide devastation of millions of persons annually.

Robert L. McLaurin, M.D.
Cincinnati, Ohio, U.S.A.

# Subject Index

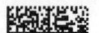